# Autoimmune Blistering Diseases: Part I – Pathogenesis and Clinical Features

*Guest Editor*

DÉDÉE F. MURRELL, MA, BMBCh, FAAD, MD, FACD

# DERMATOLOGIC CLINICS

www.derm.theclinics.com

*Consulting Editor*
BRUCE H. THIERS, MD

July 2011 • Volume 29 • Number 3

SAUNDERS an imprint of ELSEVIER, Inc.

**W.B. SAUNDERS COMPANY**
*A Division of Elsevier Inc.*

1600 John F. Kennedy Boulevard • Suite 1800 • Philadelphia, PA 19103-2899

http://www.theclinics.com

**DERMATOLOGIC CLINICS Volume 29, Number 3**
**July 2011 ISSN 0733-8635, ISBN-13: 978-1-4557-1033-1**

Editor: Stephanie Donley
Developmental Editor: Teia Stone

*Dermatologic Clinics* (ISSN 0733-8635) is published quarterly by Elsevier Inc., 360 Park Avenue South, New York, NY 10010-1710. Months of publication are January, April, July, and October. Business and editorial offices: 1600 John F. Kennedy Blvd., Suite 1800, Philadelphia, PA 19103-2899. Customer service office: 11830 Westline Drive, St. Louis, MO 63146. Periodicals postage paid at New York, NY, and additional mailing offices. Subscription prices are USD 317.00 per year for US individuals, USD 474.00 per year for US institutions, USD 371.00 per year for Canadian individuals, USD 568.00 per year for Canadian institutions, USD 434.00 per year for international individuals, USD 568.00 per year for international institutions, USD 148.00 per year for US students/residents, and USD 214.00 per year for Canadian and international students/residents. International air speed delivery is included in all *Clinics* subscription prices. All prices are subject to change without notice. **POSTMASTER:** Send address changes to *Dermatologic Clinics*, Elsevier Health Sciences Division, Subscription Customer Service, 3251 Riverport Lane, Maryland Heights, MO 63043. **Customer Service: 1-800-654-2452 (U.S. and Canada); 314-447-8871 (outside U.S. and Canada). Fax: 314-447-8029. E-mail: journalscustomerservice-usa@elsevier.com (for print support); journalsonlinesupport-usa@elsevier.com (for online support).**

*Reprints.* For copies of 100 or more, of articles in this publication, please contact the Commercial Reprints Department, Elsevier Inc., 360 Park Avenue South, New York, New York 10010-1710. Tel.: (212) 633-3813; Fax: (212) 462-1935; Email: reprints@elsevier.com.

The *Dermatologic Clinics* is covered in *MEDLINE/PubMed (Index Medicus)*, *Current Contents/Clinical Medicine, Excerpta Medica, Chemical Abstracts,* and *ISI/BIOMED*.

Printed in the United States of America.

# Contributors

## CONSULTING EDITOR

**BRUCE H. THIERS, MD**
Professor and Chairman, Department
of Dermatology and Dermatologic Surgery,
Medical University of South Carolina,
Charleston, South Carolina

## GUEST EDITOR

**DÉDÉE F. MURRELL, MA, BMBCh,
FAAD, MD, FACD**
Professor and Head, Department of
Dermatology, St George Hospital, University
of New South Wales, Kogarah, Sydney,
New South Wales, Australia

## AUTHORS

**MARISA ANDRÉ, MD**
Clínica Universitária de Dermatologia, Hospital
de Santa Maria, Centro Hospitalar Lisboa
Norte, Lisbon, Portugal

**VALERIA AOKI, MD**
Assistant Professor of Dermatology,
Department of Dermatology, University of São
Paulo Medical School, São Paulo, Brazil

**LUCA BORRADORI, MD**
Department of Dermatology, Inselspital,
University Hospital of Bern, Bern, Switzerland

**ADELA RAMBI G. CARDONES, MD**
Assistant Professor, Department of
Dermatology, Duke University, Durham,
North Carolina

**FRÉDÉRIC CAUX, MD, PhD**
Department of Dermatology and Reference
Center on Autoimmune Bullous Diseases,
Bobigny, France

**SHIEN-NING CHEE, MBBS**
Department of Dermatology, St George
Hospital, Sydney, New South Wales, Australia

**DONNA A. CULTON, MD, PhD**
Assistant Professor, Department of
Dermatology, University of North Carolina at
Chapel Hill, Chapel Hill, North Carolina

**ROCCO DELLA TORRE, MD**
Department of Dermatology, Inselspital,
University Hospital of Bern, Bern,
Switzerland

**LUIS A. DIAZ, MD**
Professor and Chair, Department of
Dermatology, University of North Carolina at
Chapel Hill, Chapel Hill, North Carolina

**JOHN W. FREW, MBBS, M. Clin Epi**
Resident Medical Officer, Department of
Dermatology, St George Hospital, Kogarah;
Faculty of Medicine, University of New South
Wales, Sydney, New South Wales, Australia

**VIBHA K. GUPTA, BS**
Division of Dermatology and Cutaneous
Sciences, Center for Investigative
Dermatology, Michigan State University,
East Lansing, Michigan

**RUSSELL P. HALL III, MD**
J Lamar Callaway Professor and Chair,
Department of Dermatology, Duke University,
Durham, North Carolina

**HELMUT HINTNER, MD**
Professor of Dermatology, Head of the
Department of Dermatology, Paracelsus
Medical University Salzburg, Salzburg,
Austria

**LIZBETH R.A. INTONG, MD, DPDS**
Dermatology Fellow, Department of
Dermatology, St George Hospital; Associate
Lecturer, Faculty of Medicine, University of
New South Wales, Kogarah, Sydney, New
South Wales, Australia

**KIRK A. JAMES, BS**
Student Research Fellow, Department of
Dermatology, University of North Carolina at
Chapel Hill, Chapel Hill, North Carolina

**SAROLTA KÁRPÁTI, MD, PhD, DrSc**
Professor, Department of Dermatology,
Venereology and Dermato-Oncology,
Semmelweis University; Hungarian Academy
of Sciences, Molecular Research Group,
Budapest, Hungary

**THEODORE E. KELBEL, BS**
Division of Dermatology and Cutaneous
Sciences, Center for Investigative
Dermatology, Michigan State University,
East Lansing, Michigan

**A. SHADI KOUROSH, MD**
Department of Dermatology, University
of Texas Southwestern Medical Center in
Dallas, Dallas, Texas

**RALF J. LUDWIG, MD**
Department of Dermatology, University of
Lübeck, Lübeck, Germany

**KATHERINE C. MELONAKOS, BS**
Division of Dermatology and Cutaneous
Sciences, Center for Investigative
Dermatology, Michigan State University,
East Lansing, Michigan

**EMILY M. MINTZ, MD**
Dermatology Resident, Department of
Dermatology, Columbia University,
New York, New York

**MARYIA MITEVA, MD**
Department of Dermatology and Cutaneous
Surgery, University of Miami, Miller School
of Medicine, Miami, Florida

**KIMBERLY D. MOREL, MD, FAAD, FAAP**
Associate Professor of Clinical Dermatology
and Clinical Pediatrics, Department of
Dermatology, Columbia University,
New York, New York

**ANDREW MULLARD, MS**
Biomedical Research and Informatics
Center, Michigan State University,
East Lansing, Michigan

**DÉDÉE F. MURRELL, MA, BMBCh,
FAAD, MD, FACD**
Professor and Head, Department of
Dermatology, St George Hospital, University
of New South Wales, Kogarah, Sydney,
New South Wales, Australia

**DANIELA NGUYEN, MS**
Department of Dermatology, Weill Medical
College of Cornell University, New York,
New York

**WATARU NISHIE, MD, PhD**
Department of Dermatology, Hokkaido
University Graduate School of Medicine,
Kita-ku, Sapporo, Japan

**GABRIELA POHLA-GUBO, PhD**
Head, Laboratory for Immunology,
Allergology and Molecular Diagnostics,
Department of Dermatology, Paracelsus
Medical University Salzburg, Salzburg,
Austria

**PHILIP L. REED, MSc, PhD**
Director, Biomedical Research and
Informatics Center, Michigan State
University, East Lansing, Michigan

**ENNO SCHMIDT, MD, PhD**
Department of Dermatology; Comprehensive
Center for Inflammation Medicine, University
of Lübeck, Lübeck, Germany

**DESHAN F. SEBARATNAM, MBBS (Hons)**
Intern, Royal Prince Alfred Hospital; Research
Student, Faculty of Medicine, Department of
Dermatology, St George Hospital, Kogarah,
Sydney, New South Wales, Australia

**KRISTINA SEIFFERT-SINHA, MD**
Research Assistant Professor, Division of
Dermatology and Cutaneous Sciences,
Center for Investigative Dermatology,
Michigan State University, East Lansing,
Michigan; Department of Dermatology,
State University of New York at Buffalo
and Roswell Park Cancer Center,
Buffalo, New York

**HIROSHI SHIMIZU, MD, PhD**
Department of Dermatology, Hokkaido
University Graduate School of Medicine,
Kita-ku, Sapporo, Japan

**ANIMESH A. SINHA, MD, PhD**
Ralph and Rita Behling Professor and
Chair of Dermatology, Department of
Dermatology, State University of
New York at Buffalo and Roswell
Park Cancer Institute, Buffalo,
New York

**JOAQUIM XAVIER SOUSA Jr, MD**
Post-Doctoral Fellow, Department of
Dermatology, University of São Paulo
Medical School, São Paulo, Brazil

**ANTONELLA TOSTI, MD**
Department of Dermatology and Cutaneous
Surgery, Miller School of Medicine, University
of Miami, Miami, Florida

**HIDEYUKI UJIIE, MD, PhD**
Department of Dermatology, Hokkaido
University Graduate School of Medicine,
Kita-ku, Sapporo, Japan

**VANESSA A. VENNING, BMBCh, DM, FRCP**
Consultant Dermatologist and Honorary
Senior Lecturer, Department of Dermatology,
Churchill Hospital, Oxford, United Kingdom

**SUPRIYA S. VENUGOPAL, MBBS,
MMed (USYD)**
Dermatology Registrar, Department of
Dermatology, Westmead Hospital, Westmead;
PhD Student, Department of Dermatology,
St George Hospital, University of New South
Wales, Kogarah, Sydney, New South Wales,
Australia

**YAN XIE, MS**
Senior Statistician, Center for Statistical
Training and Consulting, Michigan State
University, East Lansing, Michigan

**KIM B. YANCEY, MD**
Department of Dermatology, University of
Texas Southwestern Medical Center in Dallas,
Dallas, Texas

**DETLEF ZILLIKENS, MD**
Department of Dermatology, University of
Lübeck, Lübeck, Germany

# Contents

> DIF and IIF evaluates in vivo bound and circulating autoantibodies and are the preferred methods for diagnosing AIBDs. In pemphigus diseases and dermatitis herpetiformis, the titer of circulating autoantibodies reflects the disease activity. In patients with a classical clinical picture, the DIF confirms the diagnosis. Furthermore, this technique is essential in subtypes of AIBDs with atypical clinical manifestations (eg, no blisters or erosions) or clinically similar presenting manifestations, such as bullous pemphigoid, MMP, or EBA. A direct or indirect SSST is often crucial for the differential diagnosis between subtypes of these diseases, leading to proper treatment for severely affected patients.

> Autoimmune bullous diseases are associated with autoimmunity against structural components that maintain cell-cell and cell-matrix adhesion in the skin and mucous membranes. They include those where the skin blisters at the basement membrane zone and those where the skin blisters within the epidermis (pemphigus vulgaris, pemphigus foliaceus, and other subtypes of pemphigus). The variants of pemphigus are determined according to the level of intraepidermal split formation. There are 5 main variants of pemphigus: pemphigus vulgaris, pemphigus foliaceus, pemphigus erythematosus, drug-induced pemphigus, and paraneoplastic pemphigus. This review focuses only on pemphigus vulgaris.

> Pemphigus vulgaris (PV) is an autoimmune blistering disorder with a complex etiology involving an interplay of genetic as well as environmental factors, most of which remain unknown. Despite the identification of several human leukocyte antigen (HLA) alleles as risk factors for disease, no other non-HLA genes have clearly been implicated in disease susceptibility. Newer candidate gene and whole-genome approaches are needed to illuminate the full palate of genetic risk elements in PV. Based on this information, genetic-based tools can be expected to provide a scientific rationale for future clinical decision-making by physicians and facilitate an era of personalized medicine.

> The authors developed an anonymous, Web-based survey instrument available globally, and collected data from 171 pemphigus vulgaris (PV) patients to assemble

morbidity. It has usually a chronic course with spontaneous exacerbations. The cutaneous manifestations of BP can be extremely protean. While diagnosis of BP in the bullous stage is straightforward, in the non-bullous stage or in atypical variants of BP signs and symptoms are frequently non-specific with eg, only itchy excoriated, eczematous, papular and/or urticarial lesions that may persist for several weeks or months. Diagnosis of BP critically relies on immunopathologic examinations including direct immunofluorescence microscopy and detection of serum autoantibodies by indirect immunofluorescence microscopy or BP180-ELISA.

## Pathogenesis of Bullous Pemphigoid

Hideyuki Ujiie, Wataru Nishie, and Hiroshi Shimizu

Bullous pemphigoid, the most common autoimmune blistering disease, is induced by autoantibodies against type XVII collagen. Passive transfer of IgG or IgE antibodies against type XVII collagen into animals has revealed not only the pathogenicity of these antibodies but also the subsequent immune responses, including complement activation, mast cell degranulation, and infiltration of neutrophils and/or eosinophils. In vitro studies on ectodomain shedding of type XVII collagen have also provided basic knowledge on the development of bullous pemphigoid. The pathogenic role of autoreactive CD4+ T lymphocytes in the development of the pathogenic autoantibodies to type XVII collagen should also be noted.

## Pemphigoid Gestationis: Pathogenesis and Clinical Features

Lizbeth R.A. Intong and Dédée F. Murrell

Pemphigoid gestationis is a rare, autoimmune bullous disease of pregnancy that involves autoantibodies directed against type XVII collagen in the basement membrane zone. This article discusses the immunopathogenesis, diagnostic methods, and clinical features of this fascinating disease.

## Linear IgA Disease: Clinical Presentation, Diagnosis, and Pathogenesis

Vanessa A. Venning

Linear IgA disease is one of the rarer subepidermal blistering diseases. Linear IgA disease is a chronic, acquired, autoimmune blistering disease that is characterized by subepidermal blistering and linear deposition of IgA basement membrane antibodies. The disease affects both children and adults and, although there are some differences in their clinical presentations, there is considerable overlap with shared immunopathology and immunogenetics.

## Clinical Features, Diagnosis, and Pathogenesis of Chronic Bullous Disease of Childhood

Emily M. Mintz and Kimberly D. Morel

Chronic bullous disease of childhood (CBDC) is the most common acquired autoimmune blistering disorder of childhood and is characterized by linear IgA staining of the basement membrane zone on direct immunofluorescence. This autoimmune attack on structural proteins, usually proteolytic fragments of collagen XVII, renders the dermal-epidermal junction prone to blistering. Diagnosis is confirmed by characteristic histology and direct immunofluorescence. Prognosis is generally favorable, with spontaneous remission usually occurring by puberty; however, cases with severe morbidity and cases persisting into adulthood have been reported. This article discusses the clinical features, diagnosis, and pathogenesis of CBDC in more detail.

Dermatitis herpetiformis (DH) is characterized by chronic, itching papules, seropapules, small vesicles and, exceptionally, large blisters. The distribution of these polymorphic symptoms around the elbow, knee, buttock, and back is suggestive of the diagnosis. DH is further confirmed by the accumulation of granulocytes at the papillary dermis, resulting in a subepidermal split formation and by the presence of a unique, granular IgA precipitate in the uppermost dermis. Prognosis is predominantly determined by other autoimmune pathologies, malabsorption, or very rarely by lymphomas. Some of these diseases can be prevented by an early-onset, strict gluten-free diet, which is therefore the suggested treatment option.

Dermatitis herpetiformis (DH) is an autoimmune blistering skin disease in which antigen presentation in the gastrointestinal mucosa results in cutaneous IgA deposition and distinct, neutrophil-driven cutaneous lesions. Our findings suggest that the qualitatively different immune response to gluten in the intestinal mucosa of patients with DH results in minimal clinical symptoms, allowing the continued ingestion of gluten and the eventual development of DH. Our model may provide a new way to understand the pathogenesis of other skin diseases associated with gastrointestinal inflammation such as pyoderma gangrenosum or erythema nodosum, or explain association of seronegative inflammatory arthritis with inflammatory bowel disease.

Mucous membrane pemphigoid (MMP) is the clinical phenotype of a group of autoimmune blistering diseases characterized by autoantibodies directed against different structural proteins in epidermal basement membranes. The clinical course and prognosis of MMP are affected by the specific autoantigen targeted, the titer and bioactivity profile of corresponding autoantibodies, and the specific mucosal sites of disease activity. Irreversible scarring and loss of function must be prevented by early diagnosis and appropriate interventions.

Epidermolysis bullosa acquisita (EBA) is a rare autoimmune subepidermal blistering disease characterized by immune deposits on anchoring fibrils of cutaneous and mucosal basement membrane zones. It is due to circulating antibodies directed to type VII collagen. Clinical manifestations include a classical form with skin fragility, blisters and scars on trauma-prone surfaces, an inflammatory form, and a cicatricial pemphigoid–like form. Specialized tests available in only certain laboratories are necessary to confirm a diagnosis of EBA, such as immunoelectron microscopy, immunoblotting, or ELISA using recombinant proteins. A frequent association between EBA and Crohn disease has been observed.

## Pathogenesis of Epidermolysis Bullosa Acquisita

Ralf J. Ludwig and Detlef Zillikens

Epidermolysis bullosa acquisita (EBA) is an autoimmune blistering skin disease characterized by autoantibodies to type VII collagen. Clinically, a noninflammatory and an inflammatory variant of EBA can be distinguished. Despite major achievements in the understanding of EBA, current therapeutic options are far from optimal. However, with an emerging and more detailed understanding of the events ultimately leading to blister formation in EBA, novel therapeutic options may become available for patients with EBA. Therefore, this article reviews the current understanding of the pathogenesis of EBA and may indicate possible avenues towards a more targeted therapy for EBA and possibly other antibody-mediated autoimmune diseases.

## Hair Loss in Autoimmune Cutaneous Bullous Disorders

Maryia Miteva, Dédée F. Murrell, and Antonella Tosti

The expression of the basement membrane zone (BMZ) components in the anagen hair follicles of the human scalp is similar to that of interfollicular epidermis. Expression of the BMZ components varies according to the different follicular portions. Blistering of the scalp, involving lamina lucida and below, usually leads to scarring alopecia secondary to the inflammatory process in the interfollicular epidermis and in the upper portion of the hair follicle. This article discusses the presence of alopecia in the most common acquired forms of bullous disorders.

## Nail Involvement in Autoimmune Bullous Disorders

Antonella Tosti, Marisa André, and Dédée F. Murrell

Autoimmune bullous disorders frequently cause nail abnormalities, particularly paronychia and onychomadesis. In pemphigus vulgaris (PV) nail abnormalities can even precede skin findings. Nail lesions often relapse just before generalized disease exacerbation or recurrence. Severe nail changes are often associated with extensive and severe disease. Fingernails are more commonly affected. A report in the literature associates hemorrhagic nail abnormalities with poor prognosis in patients with PV. Nail scarring and pterygium are a rare complication of bullous pemphigoid. Nail loss has been occasionally reported in epidermolysis bullosa acquisita.

## Objective Scoring Systems for Disease Activity in Autoimmune Bullous Disease

Deshan F. Sebaratnam and Dédée F. Murrell

Objectively evaluating disease activity in autoimmune bullous disease (AIBD) is important in terms of the clinical assessment of patients and as an outcome measure for clinical trials. Measures need to be general enough to capture the issues specific to each of the bullous dermatoses but specific enough to capture any changes to disease status for a patient. Different tools have been put forward over the last 15 years, but presently the Autoimmune Bullous Skin Disorder Intensity Score and Pemphigus Disease Area Index seem to be the most promising tools to assess disease activity in AIBD.

## Pemphigus and Quality of Life

Shien-Ning Chee and Dédée F. Murrell

Measuring the impact of disease on quality of life (QOL) is important for evaluating effectiveness of care and capturing aspects of health that may not correlate with clinical severity. Few QOL studies have been conducted on pemphigus, and a disease-specific QOL questionnaire for this condition has not been developed. The 5 previous studies of the effect of pemphigus on QOL used generic health or skin-specific measures. These measures have limitations, and results from these studies have sometimes been conflicting. The development of a disease-specific measure for pemphigus would allow for better monitoring of patients' QOL and improve management.

# Dermatologic Clinics

**THE CLINICS ARE NOW AVAILABLE ONLINE!**

Access your subscription at:
**www.theclinics.com**

# Preface

# Autoimmune Blistering Diseases: Part I – Pathogenesis and Clinical Features

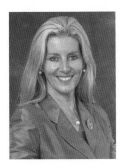

Dédée F. Murrell, MA, BMBCh, FAAD, MD, FACD
*Guest Editor*

When invited to edit a special issue of *Dermatologic Clinics* on Autoimmune Blistering Diseases by Bruce Thiers, I was delighted and honored to accept.

There have been very few textbooks devoted to autoimmune blistering diseases (AIBD), with some focusing on the pathology and others on management.

Unlike a textbook, where the articles may be over a year or two out of date by the time the book is published, these articles have been written in the last 6 months and by respected leaders in the particular aspects of AIBD. The issue has been organized such that a leading AIBD clinician has written about the clinical aspects of that form of AIBD followed by a leading investigator writing about the pathogenesis of the subtype of AIBD. Unlike a textbook, these articles can be found on Medline and PubMed and are accessible online. The individual issues of the journal may be purchased for much less cost than either a textbook or the articles individually.

There was so much to cover about AIBD that it was decided to cover clinical features, diagnostic testing, and pathogenesis in the first issue. This issue starts with an article explaining the key diagnostic immunofluorescence testing needed for AIBD from the leading European group, led by Gabriela Pohla-Gubo and Helmut Hinter in Salzburg, Austria. After this there are articles on pemphigus vulgaris, covering clinical features by

our group, and genetic risk factors and epidemiology by Animesh Sinha's group. Following this are articles on pemphigus foliaceus (PF) with the clinical features covered by the master in the field, Luis Diaz, and a separate article on pathogenesis of endemic PF, fogo selvagem, by Luis' Brazilian collaborator, Valeria Aoki. Paraneoplastic pemphigus is covered for clinical features but so little is known about its pathogenesis at present that this gap will hopefully be filled in coming years.

Bullous pemphigoid clinical features are covered by Luca Borradori and his team, pathogenesis by Hiroshi Shimizu and his laboratory, and pemphigoid gestationes clinical features by our group, drawn mainly from the work of Martin Black's team. Linear IgA disease is covered from clinical features, diagnosis, and pathogenesis by Vanessa Venning and the team at Oxford, which stemmed from Fenella Wojanarowska's work on the subject over many years. Kimberly Morel and her pediatric dermatology team have covered chronic bullous disease of childhood. On dermatitis herpetiformis we have experts, Sarolta Kárpáti, writing about the clinical features, and Russell Hall, writing about the pathogenesis, both of whom have devoted years to the understanding of this condition.

Kim Yancey's group has written about mucous membrane pemphigoid, a disease in which his group made seminal discoveries. For epidermolysis bullosa acquisita, experts Frédéric Caux in France and Detlef Zillikens and his group in

Dermatol Clin 29 (2011) xv–xvi
doi:10.1016/j.det.2011.03.021

Germany have written on the clinical features and pathogenesis. Last, hair and nails expert, Antonella Tosti, has contributed her overall knowledge of how AIBD affect the hair and nails, an area relatively neglected in AIBD.

Last, in transition to the second issue, which will cover diagnosis and management of AIBD in detail, we introduce articles on important outcome measures in the assessment of AIBD, quality of life, and physical extent assessment tools that are in use and have been developed by the collaboration of an international team of blistering disease experts, many of whom are contributing articles to the second issue.

The contributors deserve many thanks for their time and effort in writing these articles at relatively short notice and in a succinct manner with excellent color photographs and figures.

Hopefully these two issues will be educational not only for dermatologists but for all clinicians who interact with patients with AIBD, as well as scientists, family members, and the patients themselves. Understanding what is known so far about a disease leads to improved clinical practice, better research, and improved compliance with therapy.

Dédée F. Murrell, MA, BMBCh, FAAD, MD, FACD
Department of Dermatology
St George Hospital
University of New South Wales
Gray Street
Kogarah, Sydney, NSW 2217, Australia

E-mail address:
d.murrell@unsw.edu.au

# Direct and Indirect Immunofluorescence for the Diagnosis of Bullous Autoimmune Diseases

Gabriela Pohla-Gubo, PhD[a],*, Helmut Hintner, MD[b]

## KEYWORDS

- Immunofluorescence • Bullous diseases
- Differential diagnosis

Acquired autoimmune bullous diseases (AIBDs) are characterized by a pathogenic immune response against structural proteins of keratinocytes or of the dermoepidermal basement membrane zone (BMZ). Autoantibodies, both tissue-bound and circulating, account for the pathogenicity of this group of diseases known to be rare and also severe. The laboratory diagnosis includes histologic, immunohistochemical, and sometimes ultrastructural assessment. Immunofluorescence microscopy is a technique to rapidly show the reaction of an antigen (structural protein) and the pathogenic autoantibody in a patient suspected to have an AIBD.[1] Direct immunofluorescence (DIF) is the method to show the deposition of immunoreactants (in vivo bound autoantibodies) in skin or mucous membranes. Indirect immunofluorescence (IIF) quantitates the respective circulating autoantibodies in the serum of the patient. Thus, immunofluorescence is the key instrument for diagnosing the three major groups of AIBDs: (1) pemphigus diseases, (2) BMZ diseases, including pemphigoid diseases such as bullous pemphigoid, mucous membrane pemphigoid (MMP), and epidermolysis bullosa acquisita (EBA) and (3) dermatitis herpetiformis, or Duhring disease. This article describes the method, practical application for the differential diagnosis of AIBDs, method to discern between subtypes within groups of those disorders (salt-split skin test [SSST]), and importance of the method to diagnose AIBDs representing with an atypical clinical picture.

## MATERIALS AND METHODS
### Biopsy and Blood Sample

If an AIBD is suspected, the biopsy for DIF should be taken when the routine lesional biopsy is taken within the edge of an active blister for routine pathology sent in formalin. A 4- to 6-mm punch or excision biopsy of patient skin or mucous membrane should be taken from an area of perilesional or clinically normal appearing skin or mucous membrane. For cosmetic reasons, the authors prefer to take the immunofluorescence biopsy from the (non–sun exposed) inner aspect of the upper arm if the blistering is widespread. If the immunofluorescence laboratory is nearby, such as within the same institution or hospital, the biopsy simply can be placed in a plastic tube (without any liquid) and transferred immediately to a freezer at $-20°C$. Alternatively, if the biopsy is to be sent to an immunofluorescence laboratory elsewhere, it can be placed in a small transport tube containing Michel's medium.[2,3] Samples

[a] Laboratory for Immunology, Allergology & Molecular Diagnostics, Department of Dermatology, Paracelsus Medical University Salzburg, Muellner Hauptstrasse 48, 5020 Salzburg, Austria
[b] Department of Dermatology, Paracelsus Medical University Salzburg, Muellner Hauptstrasse 48, 5020 Salzburg, Austria
* Corresponding author.
E-mail address: g.pohla-gubo@salk.at

Dermatol Clin 29 (2011) 365–372
doi:10.1016/j.det.2011.03.001
0733-8635/11/$ – see front matter © 2011 Elsevier Inc. All rights reserved.

can be stored in this medium for up to 28 days at room temperature or in the fridge (specimen should not be frozen in Michel's medium) and sent worldwide to any specialized laboratory that performs diagnostic immunofluorescence.[4]

A 2- to 5-mL sample of whole blood (without any additives) is centrifuged and the serum is used for IIF to discover circulating autoantibodies in AIBDs. The authors recommend always taking a biopsy and a blood sample from each patient.

### Direct Immunofluorescence

For the DIF test, three to six cryocut sections (4- to 6-$\mu$ thick) from the patient's skin or mucous membrane are placed on each of five microscope glass slides, air-dried for 10 minutes, and rinsed in phosphate buffered saline (PBS). For routine DIF, each slide is then covered with an appropriate dilution of one of the antisera against IgG, IgA, IgM, complement factor C3, and fibrinogen. The antibodies are conjugated to a fluorescent dye, most commonly fluorescein-iso-thio-cyanate (FITC). Incubation in a moist chamber (30 minutes, room temperature) is followed by two washings of 15 minutes each with PBS. The sections are then mounted with a drop of buffered glycerin or a special embedding medium containing anti-bleaching reagent (eg, EUROIMMUN Order no. ZF 1200–0130). For FITC conjugated antibodies, the results are read with a fluorescence ultraviolet microscope at 450 to 490 nm.

### Indirect Immunofluorescence

Different commercially available animal tissues, such as the frequently used monkey or guinea pig esophagus, serve as antigenic substrates. For special purposes, such as for the SSST, normal human skin (NHS) is used as a substrate. The source for the NHS samples is excess cutaneous material from the Dermatosurgery Unit of the authors' Department of Dermatology, provided that the respective patient has given informed consent for use, but other places use donated abdominopexy skin. In the first step, circulating autoantibodies bind to their respective antigens (mostly keratinocyte or BMZ structural proteins) in the tissue. For this purpose the substrate is covered with a series of dilutions of patient serum in PBS (mostly starting with 1:10), incubated in a moist chamber for 30 minutes at room temperature, and rinsed then twice for 15 minutes in PBS. In the next step the tissue sample is incubated for 30 minutes with a second antibody directed against various immunoglobulin classes of the autoantibody that has bound in vitro in the first step. Typically these second antibodies are raised in mice (usually mouse anti-human IgG1), swine, or rat and are conjugated to a fluorescent dye like FITC. Again the slides are washed twice, mounted, and viewed under the microscope.

### SSST

Salt-split skin is the substrate of choice for the differential diagnosis between subtypes of AIBDs with autoantibodies directed against proteins of the dermoepidermal BMZ (for example bullous pemphigoid vs epidermolysis bullosa acquisita). Ray Gammon at the University of North Carolina, Chapel Hill first described using incubation in 1M sodium chloride (NaCl) to separate the skin between the epidermis and dermis in the lamina lucida (**Fig. 1**).[5] This technique can be performed on the patient's skin (direct SSST) and on separated NHS using patient serum (indirect SSST).[5,6]

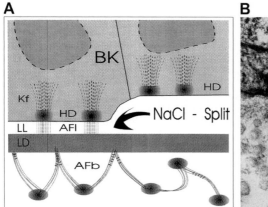
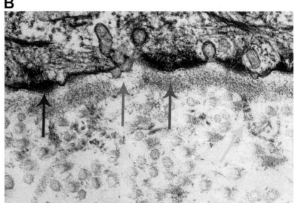

**Fig. 1.** Salt-split skin test (SSST). On incubation of a skin sample with 1M NaCl, an artificial blister is produced within the lamina lucida. (*A*) Localization of the split. (*B*) Electron micrograph of the BMZ of the skin (*blue arrows*: hemidesmosomes; *red arrows*: lamina lucida; *green arrows*: lamina densa; *yellow arrows*: anchoring fibrils).

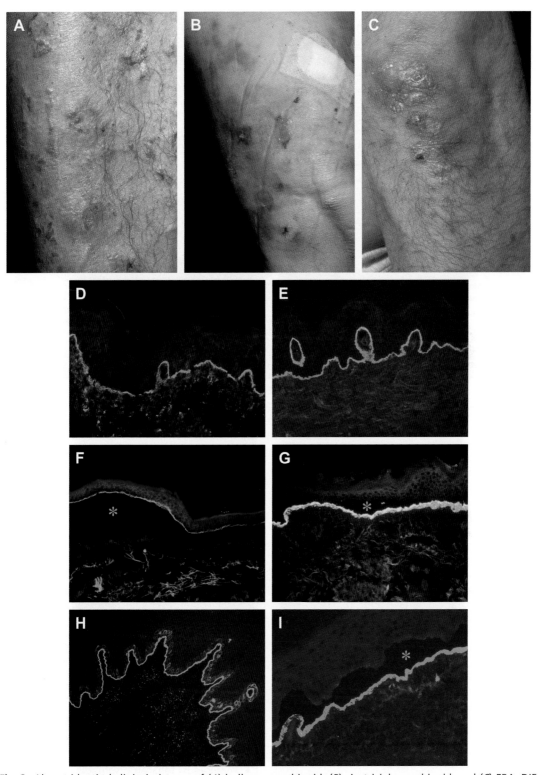

**Fig. 2.** Almost identical clinical pictures of (*A*) bullous pemphigoid, (*B*) cicatricial pemphigoid, and (*C*) EBA. DIF showing linear, band-like deposition of IgG within the BMZ of (*D*) bullous pemphigoid and (*E*) EBA. Direct SSST of (*F*) bullous pemphigoid with IgG at blister roof and (*G*) EBA at blister floor (blister indicated with *asterisk*). Circulating anti-BMZ autoantibodies on monkey esophagus as seen in bullous pemphigoid and sometimes in EBA (*H*) and indirect SSST on NHS in EBA (*I*). Circulating autoantibodies localize to the floor of the artificial blister.

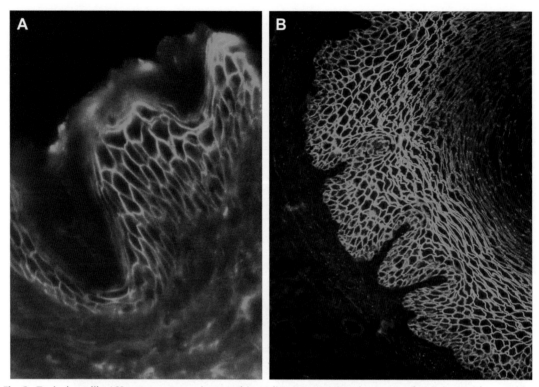

**Fig. 3.** Typical net-like ICS pattern as seen in pemphigus diseases. IIF using the serum of a patient with pemphigus foliaceus on NHS, anti-IgG (*A*), and on monkey esophagus, anti-IgG (*B*).

### Direct SSST

Usually a biopsy that has already been investigated with routine DIF is prepared for the direct SSST. If two biopsies (normal and perilesional) were obtained, the authors prefer the one from normal-appearing skin. If only a perilesional biopsy from the patient is available, the authors also use this one. When the biopsy is prepared for the SSST, the sample is lost for a reinvestigation using routine DIF because it is placed overnight in 1M NaCl. This technique produces an artificial blister within the lamina lucida (see **Fig. 1**). The DIF is then repeated on cryostat sections of the salt-split sample, as described earlier. The distribution of in vivo bound autoantibodies can then be seen on either the epidermal or the dermal side of the artificial blister (ie, on the blister roof or blister floor; **Fig. 2**F, G). This method allows one to distinguish, for example, between bullous pemphigoid (epidermal staining) and the BP-variant of EBA (dermal staining), which clinically may look identical (see **Fig. 2**A–C).

### Indirect SSST

For indirect SSST, NHS is incubated for 1 night in 1M NaCl. An IIF with the serum of the patient is then performed on cryostat sections of that substrate as described. The test, which is more sensitive than routine IIF, shows circulating autoantibodies binding to either the epidermal or the dermal or both sides of the artificial blister. This technique again allows, for example, differentiation between bullous pemphigoid and EBA (see **Fig. 2**H).

## PATTERNS OF STAINING
### Pemphigus Diseases

Pemphigus diseases are characterized by intraepithelial blister formation from acantholysis as the result of autoantibody reactivity directed against (desmosomal) intercellular adhesion proteins of keratinocytes such as desmoglein 1 or 3. On a biopsy, a typical net-like (chicken

---

**Box 1**
**Pemphigus diseases (with ICS pattern)**

- Pemphigus vulgaris
- Pemphigus vegetans
- Pemphigus foliaceus, sporadic or endemic (fogo selvagem)
- Pemphigus erythematosus
- Paraneoplastic pemphigus
- Drug-induced pemphigus

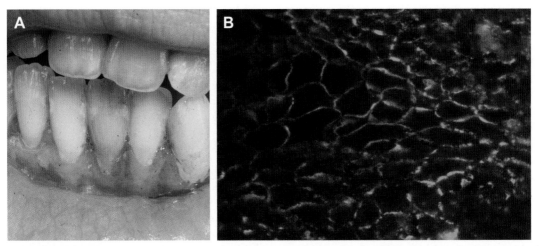

**Fig. 4.** (*A*) Atypical clinical picture of a pemphigus vegetans presenting as desquamative gingivitis. (*B*) DIF of oral mucosa with an ICS pattern with anti-IgG.

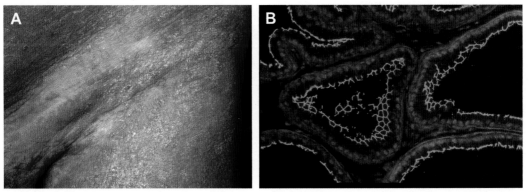

**Fig. 5.** (*A*) Paraneoplastic pemphigus manifesting as lichenoid dermatitis. (*B*) IIF showing ICS pattern on rat urinary bladder epithelium.

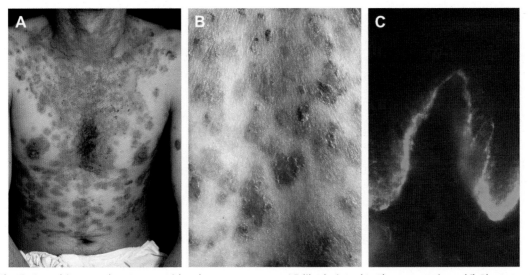

**Fig. 6.** Pemphigus erythematosus with subacute cutaneous LE-like lesions (*A*, *B*); note erosions. (*C*) Photograph focused on the lupus band in DIF, anti-IgG.

> **Box 2**
> **BMZ diseases (with linear deposits of immunoglobulins and complement components in the BMZ)**
>
> - Bullous pemphigoid
> - MMP, cicatricial pemphigoid
> - Pemphigoid gestationis
> - Linear IgA disease
> - Chronic bullous disease of childhood
> - Lichen planus pemphigoides
> - Epidermolysis bullosa acquisita
> - Bullous systemic lupus erythematosus

wire–like) intercellular substance pattern (ICS) (**Fig. 3**A) is seen in the DIF with anti-IgG and anti-C3, and rarely also with anti-IgA (in IgA pemphigus) (**Box 1**). IIF on monkey esophagus shows circulating IgG autoantibodies in the serum of the patients (see **Fig. 3**B). The amount of autoantibodies is reflected in the ICS titer, and correlates with the disease activity in pemphigus diseases. Patient follow-up is performed through monitoring the ICS titer with IIF. To detect technical pitfalls in the immunofluorescence technique (eg, decrease in brightness because of the time span of the microscope lamp), the authors study the actual serum together with a former sample on one slide containing two cuts of the substrate to see an increase or decrease of the titer. In addition to DIF and IIF, enzyme-linked immunosorbent assays (ELISA) or immunoblot techniques are used to specify the autoantibodies against different antigens, such as desmoglein 3 and 1.

The method of immunofluorescence is particularly important in patients presenting with atypical clinical manifestations of the pemphigus diseases, such as a desquamative gingivitis (**Fig. 4**A), in which the corresponding DIF of the oral mucosa (or even NHS) shows the ICS pattern (see **Fig. 4**B). Further examples are the paraneoplastic pemphigus (obligatorily associated with a malignant disease), which may manifest as lichenoid dermatitis (**Fig. 5**A). This diagnosis is confirmed with IIF using rat urinary bladder as substrate (see **Fig. 5**B). Also in this category is pemphigus erythematosus (Senear-Usher syndrome), which clinically may present with symptoms of subacute cutaneous lupus erythematosus (**Fig. 6**A, B). In the DIF a lupus band can be seen (see **Fig. 6**C), and occasionally antinuclear antibodies are found with IIF.

### Basement membrane zone diseases

A subepidermal blister formation is seen in all pemphigoid diseases and EBA, which immunohistochemically present with a linear band of immunoglobulin or complement component C3 in the BMZ. In most of the pemphigoid disorders, the blisters result from an autoantibody reaction directed mainly against type 17 collagen (180-kD bullous pemphigoid antigen) of the dermoepidermal BMZ (**Box 2**). In EBA, the autoantibodies are directed and localize to the anchoring fibrils (type 7 collagen in and below the lamina densa), resulting in a comparably thicker BMZ band (see **Fig. 2**D, E). Because variants of the pemphigoid diseases and the EBA, with its bullous pemphigoid, MMP, and classic subtype, may present

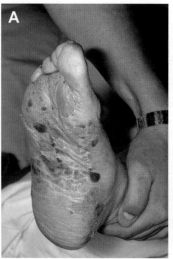 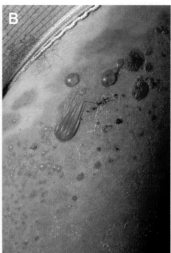 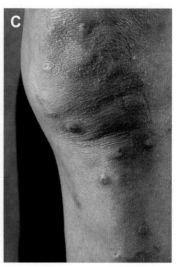

**Fig. 7.** Subtypes of bullous pemphigoid. (*A*) Dyshidrosiform bullous pemphigoid. (*B*) Vesicular (drug-induced) bullous pemphigoid. (*C*) Nodular bullous pemphigoid. DIF finally led to the right diagnosis.

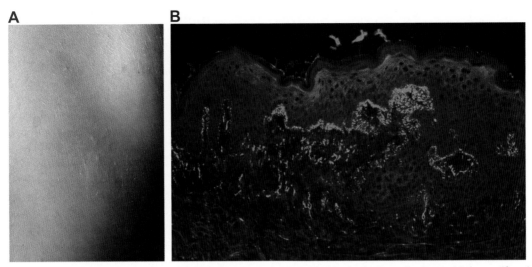

**Fig. 8.** (*A*) Very unspectacular clinical presentation (mainly strong itching) of a juvenile dermatitis herpetiformis. (*B*) Granular deposits of IgA along the dermoepidermal junction and in the papillary dermis.

with a very similar clinical picture (see **Fig. 2**A, B, C), the SSST is important for distinguishing them (see **Fig. 2**F, G).

DIF, IIF, and direct and indirect SSST are also important to diagnose special manifestations of BMZ-AIBDs that either lack characteristic signs of the bullous autoimmune disease (eg, blisters, erosions) or mimic completely different dermatoses. Examples are variants of bullous pemphigoid, such as the dyshidrosiform, vesicular (drug-induced), or nodular bullous pemphigoid (**Fig. 7**).

Most patients with a BMZ disease also present with circulating IgG–anti-BMZ autoantibodies (see **Fig. 2**H), and an indirect SSST can help distinguish the disorders (see **Fig. 2**I). In contrast to the pemphigus diseases, no correlation exists between the autoantibody titer and the disease activity.

### Dermatitis herpetiformis (Duhring disease)
Dermatitis herpetiformis (**Fig. 8**A) is a chronic, pruritic, papulovesicular dermatosis and a cutaneous manifestation of celiac disease (gluten-sensitive enteropathy). It is characterized by IgA autoantibodies directed against epidermal transglutaminase and tissue transglutaminase located on dermal microfibrils. In the nonlesional skin, DIF shows regular granular IgA and C3 deposits along the dermoepidermal junction, and especially in the tips of the papillary dermis (see **Fig. 8**B). For circulating IgA autoantibodies against tissue transglutaminase, ELISA-based assays are the preferred tests, but IIF may also be used to show IgA autoantibodies directed against the

endomysium and found on substrates containing smooth muscle, such as monkey esophagus.

### SUMMARY

DIF and IIF evaluates in vivo bound and circulating autoantibodies and are the preferred methods for diagnosing AIBDs. In pemphigus diseases and dermatitis herpetiformis, the titer of circulating autoantibodies reflects the disease activity. In patients with a classical clinical picture, the DIF confirms the diagnosis. Furthermore, this technique is essential in subtypes of AIBDs with atypical clinical manifestations (eg, no blisters or erosions) or clinically similar presenting manifestations, such as bullous pemphigoid, MMP, or EBA. A direct or indirect SSST is often crucial for the differential diagnosis between subtypes of these diseases, leading to proper treatment for severely affected patients.

### REFERENCES

1. Hintner H, Stingl G, Schuler G, et al. Immunofluorescence mapping of antigenic determinants within the dermal-epidermal junction in mechanobullous diseases. J Invest Dermatol 1981;76:113–8.
2. Michel B, Milner Y, David K. Preservation of tissue-fixed immunoglobulins in skin biopsies of patients with lupus erythematosus and bullous diseases. J Invest Dermatol 1973;59:449.
3. Vaughan Jones SA, Bhogal BS, Black MM. The use of Michel's transport media for immunofluorescence and immunoelectron microscopy in autoimmune bullous diseases. J Cutan Pathol 1995;22:365–70.

4. Pohla-Gubo G, Cepeda-Valdes R, Hintner H. Immu-nofluorescence mapping for the diagnosis of epider-molysis bullosa. Dermatol Clin 2010;28:201–10.

5. Gammon WR, Kowalewski C, Chorzelski TP, et al. Direct immunofluorescence studies of sodium chloride-separated skin in the differential diagnosis of bullous pemphigoid and epidermolysis bullosa acquisita. J Am Acad Dermatol 1990;22:664–70.

6. Pohla-Gubo G, Becher E, Romani N, et al. 'Salt-split' test on normal, non-sun-exposed skin of patients with autoimmune subepidermal bullous diseases. Dermatology 1994;189(Suppl 1):123.

# Diagnosis and Clinical Features of Pemphigus Vulgaris

Supriya S. Venugopal, MBBS, MMed[a,b],
Dédée F. Murrell, MA, BMBCh, FAAD, MD, FACD[b,*]

## KEYWORDS

- Pemphigus vulgaris • Desmoglein 3 • Diagnosis

## CLINICAL PRESENTATION OF PEMPHIGUS VULGARIS

Autoimmune bullous diseases are associated with autoimmunity against structural components that maintain cell-cell and cell-matrix adhesion in the skin and mucous membranes.[1] They include those where the skin blisters at the basement membrane zone (bullous pemphigoid, herpes gestationis, mucous membrane pemphigoid, linear immunoglobulin (Ig)A dermatosis, epidermolysis bullosa acquisita, bullous lupus, and dermatitis herpetiformis) and those where the skin blisters within the epidermis (pemphigus vulgaris [PV], pemphigus foliaceus [PF], and other subtypes of pemphigus).

Because of the considerable overlap in the clinical presentation of these conditions, diagnosis of autoimmune bullous skin conditions can be challenging. Detection of tissue-bound and circulating serum autoantibodies and characterization of their molecular specificity is an important modality for diagnosis. In the past decade, there have been several advances in diagnostic modalities for autoimmune bullous skin conditions.

Pemphigus, a word derived from the Greek word "pemphix" meaning bubble or blister, is a life-threatening autoimmune blistering disease characterized by intraepithelial blister formation.[2–4] Damage to intercellular adhesion structures, desmogleins, are the target of circulating autoantibodies resulting in the hallmark of this condition, acantholysis.[5,6] Acantholysis may result in the development of the Tzanck phenomenon, which is the rounding of single epidermal cells caused by the loss of cell-cell attachment.

## EPIDEMIOLOGY

The incidence of pemphigus is approximately 1 in 100,000 people. Pemphigus vulgaris is the most common variant of pemphigus with an incidence of 0.1 to 0.5 per 100,000 population and higher among Jewish patients.[7] In India, Malaysia, China, and the Middle East, pemphigus vulgaris accounts for 70% of all pemphigus cases and may be the most common autoimmune blistering disease.[8–10]

Various environmental and pharmacologic etiological factors have been reported in pemphigus. These factors include medications, pesticides, malignancy, ultraviolet radiation, and stress.[11–18]

Foods containing an allium, phenol, thiol, or urushiol group have also been reported to trigger pemphigus.[19,20]

### Pathogenesis

PV is an autoimmune condition that is more likely to develop in patients with HLA types after certain triggers. PV is associated with several autoantibodies. The main autoantibodies target the desmosomal protein, desmoglein 3 (dsg3), a 130-kDa glycoprotein cadherin.[5] Later, there is secondary

Financial Disclosure/Conflict of Interest Statement: The authors of this article have no financial disclosures or conflict of interest to express.
a Department of Dermatology, Westmead Hospital, Westmead, Sydney, NSW, Australia
b Department of Dermatology, St George Hospital, University of New South Wales, Ground floor, James Laws House, Gray Street, Kogarah, Sydney, New South Wales 2217, Australia
* Corresponding author.
E-mail address: d.murrell@unsw.edu.au

Dermatol Clin 29 (2011) 373–380
doi:10.1016/j.det.2011.03.004
0733-8635/11/$ – see front matter © 2011 Elsevier Inc. All rights reserved.

derm.theclinics.com

development of antibodies to another desmo-somal cadherin, desmogleins 1, which is a 160-kDa glycoprotein dsg1 antigen, when the skin is involved.[21] Further potential target antigens in PV are acetylcholine receptors on keratinocytes.[22–24] Pincelli's group has shown that apoptosis pathways are triggered early in PV and are followed by desmosomal endocytosis.[25,26] In addition, David Rubenstein's group has shown that the signaling molecule p38 is rapidly phosphorylated when PV IgG is added to human keratinocytes and that inhibiting p38 blocks dsg3 endocytosis, keratin retraction, and actin reorganization. P38 is phosphorylated in the skin of neonatal mice tested with either PV or PF IgG. P38 inhibitors block blistering in both the PV and PF passive transfer mouse models. Similarly, p38 is phosphorylated in the skin of human patients with PV and PF.[27,28]

PV is strongly associated with the HLA serotypes HLA-DR4 and HLA-DR6.[29] 48% of healthy relatives of patients with PV had low levels of autoantibody and the inheritance of autoantibody positivity was linked to the DR4 and DR6 haplotype. Although population studies report differing prevalences of alleles in various ethnic groups, greater than 95% of patients with PV possess one or both of these haplotypes.[30] In 2006, Lee and colleagues[30] concluded that in the non-Jewish population, 8 alleles were positively associated and 1 allele was negatively associated with PV. The 2 candidate alleles most likely to contribute to disease susceptibility in the Non-Jewish population included DRB1*0402 and DQB1*0503. DRB1*0402 was determined to be the sole allele likely to confer susceptibility to PV in Ashkenazi Jewish patients.

## CLINICAL FEATURES
### Clinical Presentation

The variants of pemphigus are determined according to the level of intraepidermal split formation. There are 5 main variants of pemphigus: pemphigus vulgaris, pemphigus foliaceus, pemphigus erythematosus, drug-induced pemphigus, and paraneoplastic pemphigus. This review focuses only on PV.

Patients suffering from PV present with oral erosions and then subsequently develop cutaneous involvement.[31,32] Mucosal erosions usually precede the cutaneous manifestations of the disease and often result in a protracted course of misdiagnosis with conditions, such as aphthous ulceration. In some cases, oral ulceration may be the only manifestation of the disease. The mucosal surfaces that may be involved include the oropharynx, esophagus, conjunctiva, nasal, larynx, urethra, vulva, and cervix.[33–38]

Cutaneous involvement may be localized or generalized. Skin lesions have a predilection for the trunk, groins, axillae, scalp, face, and pressure points (**Figs. 1–4**).[39] Flaccid blisters develop on these sites and may coalesce; these blisters eventually rupture and result in painful erosions. PV usually presents in adults and can affect anywhere in the body but predominantly affects the buccal and labial mucosa (**Fig. 5**). This condition is characterized by Nikolsky's sign; the direct Nikolsky is when the application of slight pressure on a blister results in extension of the blistering to adjacent skin and the indirect Nikolsky is when rubbing on clinically normal skin causes shearing. These signs are not always 100% reliable for the diagnosis of PV, but they are suggestive if present.[40]

Other more rare clinical manifestations include nail dystrophy, paronychia, subungual hematomas, and neonatal pemphigus vulgaris.[41,42]

## DIFFERENTIAL DIAGNOSIS

Patients are often treated for multiple other blistering conditions before the diagnosis of pemphigus vulgaris is made with diagnostic investigations, in particular a skin or mucosal biopsy for DIF.

The differentials for mucosal lesions include stomatitis secondary to herpes simplex virus;

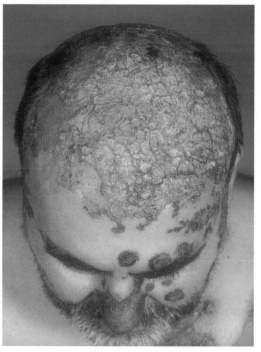

**Fig. 1.** Patient with pemphigus vulgaris presenting with crusted erosions on his scalp and face.

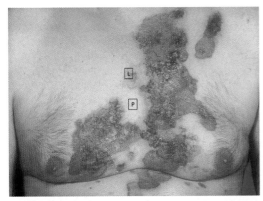

Fig. 2. Crusted, superficial erosions on the chest and abdomen of the same patient with pemphigus vulgaris. Boxed *L* indicates an appropriate site for a lesional biopsy for routine histology and boxed *P* indicates a site that is good for the perilesional biopsy for direct immunofluorescence.

aphthous ulcers; lichen planus; paraneoplastic pemphigus; or autoimmune disease, such as lupus erythematosus or dermatitis herpetiformis. Differentials for cutaneous involvement include other autoimmune blistering skin conditions, such as pemphigus foliaceus, pemphigus vegetans, IgA pemphigus, paraneoplastic pemphigus,

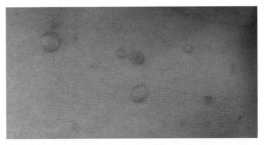

Fig. 4. Some tense and flaccid, well-circumscribed bullae and superficial erosions on the abdomen of a young woman with pemphigus vulgaris.

bullous pemphigoid, linear IgA disease, erythema multiforme, Grover disease, and Hailey-Hailey disease.

There are a variety of blistering conditions that must be taken into consideration when suspecting that patients have pemphigus vulgaris. The etiology of blistering diseases may be broadly divided into autoimmune, infective, or inflammatory.

## DIAGNOSIS

The diagnosis of PV can be made using 4 major criteria:

1. Clinical findings
2. Light microscopic findings
3. Direct immunofluorescence findings
4. Indirect immunofluorescence findings.[4,43]

The clinical findings assisting in the diagnosis of PV, a potentially life-threatening autoimmune vesiculobullous disorder, include nonscarring, fragile vesicles, and bullae involving the mucosae with varying cutaneous involvement.

The biopsies should be carefully performed on lesional and perilesional skin. The most recent, untreated lesion is the most preferable site for

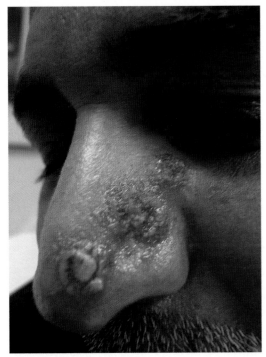

Fig. 3. Vegetative erosions on the nose of a patient with pemphigus vulgaris.

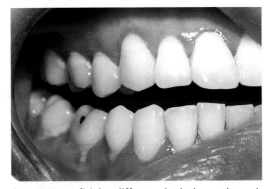

Fig. 5. Superficial, diffuse gingival erosions in a patient with pemphigus vulgaris. (*Courtesy of Dr Schifter, Skin and Cancer Foundation, Westmead, Sydney.*)

biopsy. At the edge of a blister (lesional) is the best site for hematoxylin and eosin (H+E) analysis to discern the presence and level of blistering or acantholysis (see **Fig. 2**). The type, density, and level of inflammatory infiltrate in conjunction with the direct immunofluorescence findings assist in making the diagnosis of pemphigus vulgaris. Lesional biopsies for H+E can be transported in formalin.

Perilesional biopsies taken within 2 cm of active blistering (see **Fig. 2**) should be taken for DIF analysis and transported in normal saline if they can get to the laboratory straight away for the best results[44] or Michel's medium otherwise. These characteristically show netlike, intercellular staining with IgG, C3, IgM, or IgA (discussed in the next section).

Patients with isolated mucosal disease should have lesional and perilesional mucosal biopsies performed for H+E and DIF to confirm the diagnosis of pemphigus vulgaris in conjunction with biopsies of cutaneous lesions, if clinically warranted.

## HISTOPATHOLOGY

PV is usually characterized by suprabasalar loss of adhesion leaving a single layer of basal keratinocytes attached to the dermoepidermal basement membrane (tombstone pattern). This characteristic is distinguished from PF, which is associated with a more superficial split formation in the subcorneal layer. Histologic findings in PV lesions on hematoxylin and eosin demonstrate suprabasalar acantholysis and infiltration with predominantly neutrophils and eosinophils (**Fig. 6**). The early findings of pemphigus may be subtle and include suprabasalar acantholysis associated with a mild, superficial mixed inflammatory infiltrate, including some eosinophils. These changes can also be present in more developed lesions (see **Fig. 6**).

On direct immunofluorescence, IgG or C3 binding to the intercellular cement substance in the mid-lower or entire epidermis of perilesional skin or mucosa is characteristic (**Fig. 7**).[45–48]

Desmoglein 3[5] and desmoglein 1[21] are the targets for autoantibodies in PV and PF, respectively. Tissue-bound IgG, C3, IgM, or IgA in a characteristic netlike intercellular distribution pattern within the epidermis is demonstrated on direct immunofluorescence microscopy (see **Fig. 7**). Anti-dsg1 and anti-dsg3 antibodies predominantly belong to the IgG4 subclass.[49–52] Anti-IgA and IgE subclass antibodies have also been detected. Patients with predominantly mucosal involvement have antibodies only against dsg3; however, a significant proportion of mucosal-dominant disease will also have dsg1 autoantibodies.[53,54] The phenotypic presentation of pemphigus vulgaris with respect to mucosal and generalized cutaneous involvement has been attributed to the presence of desmoglein 3 and desmoglein 1 autoantibodies, respectively.[55–62]

Indirect immunofluorescence microscopy reveals the presence of serum autoantibodies against desmosomal antigens. Pemphigus sera show a characteristic netlike intercellular staining of IgG with human skin as a substrate. Other substrates, such as monkey esophagus, guinea pig esophagus or rat bladder epithelium, may be used in the diagnosis of paraneoplastic pemphigus.[63]

Enzyme-linked immunosorbent assay (ELISA) has provided higher sensitivity and specificity in making the diagnosis of pemphigus subtypes.[64] ELISA results can be used to determine pemphigus vulgaris disease activity and be used for longitudinal monitoring of treatment response. Antibodies can be detected in patients without clinical signs of pemphigus and can be found in patients with staphylococcal scalded skin,[65] penicillin adverse drug reactions,[66] toxic epidermolysis

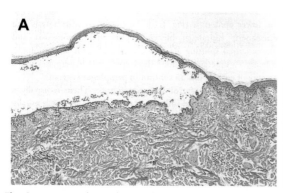
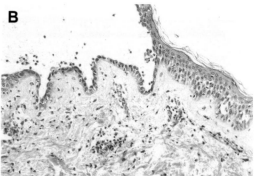

**Fig. 6.** Hematoxylin and eosin findings of an acute lesion of pemphigus vulgaris showing suprabasal acantholysis (*A, B*) (*From* Weedon D, Strutton G, Rubin AI. The vesiculobullous reaction pattern. In: Weedon D, ed. Weedon's Skin Pathology, 3rd edition. Philadelphia: Churchill-Livingston; 2010; with permission.)

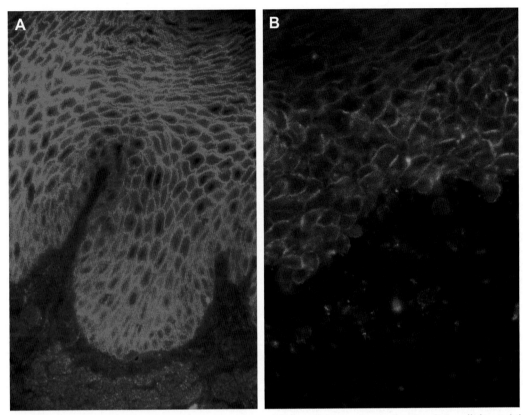

**Fig. 7.** Direct immunofluorescence results in a patient with pemphigus vulgaris showing intercellular staining with IgG (*A*) and C3 (*B*). (*Courtesy of* Professor Kossard, Skin and Cancer Foundation, Darlinghurst, Sydney.)

necrosis,[67] and burns.[68] In addition, patients with blood group O who have antibodies to blood groups A and B may give low false positives on indirect immunofluorescence testing,[69] which is avoided by preabsorbing their sera with these blood group antigens.

In active PV, immunoblot analysis with recombinant dsg3 demonstrated that anti-dsg3 of the IgG4, IgA, and IgE subtypes predominate; however, chronic remittent PV is characterized by IgG1 and IgG4 autoantibodies.[50,53]

## DISEASE ACTIVITY CATEGORIZATION

The Consensus Statement on Disease Endpoints and Therapeutic Response for Pemphigus[70] divides pemphigus disease activity into the following categories:

- Early endpoints
  Baseline
  Control of disease activity
  End of consolidation phase
- Late endpoints
  Complete remission off therapy
  Complete remission on therapy

Minimal therapy
Minimal adjuvant therapy
Partial remission off therapy
Partial remission on minimal therapy
- Relapse/flare
- Treatment failure.

Early endpoints provide a useful clinical indicator for clinicians regarding the commencement of differing treatment regimes. The *baseline* is classified as the day that the treating practitioner initiates treatment. *Control of disease activity* is defined as the time at which there is cessation of new lesions in conjunction with the healing of preexisting lesions. In the majority of cases the expected time period in this stage is weeks. The *end of the consolidation phase* is the time period in which no new lesions have developed over a minimum period of 2 weeks. This phase is also characterized by the healing of most lesions, and most medical practitioners would consider the weaning of steroids.

Late endpoints of disease activity may be reached with or without therapy. *Complete remission off therapy* is characterized by the absence of new lesions over a 2-month period after cessation of therapy. *Minimal therapy* constitutes treatment with less than or equal to 10 mg/day of prednisone or the equivalent or the use of minimal adjuvant therapy for a duration of at least 2 months. *Minimal adjuvant therapy* comprises of half the dose required to be defined as treatment failure. *Partial remission off therapy* is classified as development of lesions after cessation of treatment that heal within 1 week without treatment. Patients must be off systemic therapy for 2 months to be classified in this category. Patients may suffer a partial remission on minimal therapy when they develop new lesions that heal within 1 week while receiving minimal therapy. Topical steroids also constitute minimal therapy.

A *relapse/flare* is defined by the development of 3 or more new lesions that persist without healing for greater than 1 week or by the extension of preexisting established lesions. Treatment failure results when there is no change in disease activity despite treatment on therapeutic doses of systemic steroids and other agents whose doses and durations were agreed by international consensus.[70]

## ACKNOWLEDGMENTS

This article was supported in part by the University of NSW Postgraduate Awards for Dr Venugopal's PhD studies with Dedee Murrell.

## REFERENCES

1. Mihai S, Sitaru C. Immunopathology and molecular diagnosis of autoimmune bullous diseases. J Cell Mol Med 2007;11(3):462–81.
2. Lever WF. Pemphigus. Medicine 1953;32:1–123.
3. Huilgol SC, Black MM. Management of the immunobullous disorders. II. Pemphigus. Clin Exp Dermatol 1995;20:283–93.
4. Hertl M. Humoral and cellular autoimmunity in autoimmune bullous skin disorders. Int Arch Allergy Immunol 2000;122:91–100.
5. Amagai M, Klaus-Kovtun V, Stanley JR. Auto-Ab against a novel epithelial cadherin in pemphigus vulgaris, a disease of cell adhesion. Cell 1991;67:869–77.
6. Bedane C, Prost C, Thomine E, et al. Binding of autoantibodies is not restricted to desmosomes in pemphigus vulgaris: comparison of 14 cases of pemphigus vulgaris and 10 cases of pemphigus foliaceus studied by western immunoblot and immunoelectron microscopy. Arch Dermatol Res 1996;288:343–52.
7. Ahmed AR, Yunis EJ, Khatri K. Major histocompatibility complex haplotype studies in Ashkenazi Jewish patients with pemphigus vulgaris. Proc Natl Acad Sci U S A 1991;87:7658–62.
8. Wilson C, Wojnarowska F, Mehra NK, et al. Pemphigus in Oxford, UK, and New Delhi, India: a comparative study of disease characteristics and HLA antigens. Dermatology 1994;189(Suppl 1):108–10.
9. Adam BA. Bullous diseases in Malaysia: epidemiology and natural history. Int J Dermatol 1992;31:42–5.
10. Chams-Davatchi C, Valikhani M, Daneshpazhooh M, et al. Pemphigus: analysis of 1209 cases. Int J Dermatol 2005;44:470–6.
11. Mashiah J, Brenner S. Medical pearl: First step in managing pemphigus–addressing the etiology. J Am Acad Dermatol 2005;53(4):706–7.
12. Brenner S, Mashiah J, Tamir E, et al. Pemphigus: an acronym for a disease with multiple etiologies. Skinmed 2003;2:163–7.
13. Brenner S, Bialy-Golan A, Ruocco V. Drug-induced pemphigus. Clin Dermatol 1998;163:393–7.
14. Goldberg I, Kashman Y, Brenner S. The induction of pemphigus by phenol drugs. Int J Dermatol 1999;38:888–92.
15. Brenner S, Wolf R, Ruocco V. Contact pemphigus: a subgroup of induced pemphigus. Int J Dermatol 1994;33:843–5.
16. Brenner S, Bar-Nathan EA. Pemphigus vulgaris triggered by emotional stress. J Am Acad Dermatol 1984;11:524–5.
17. Brenner S, Tur E, Shapiro J, et al. Pemphigus vulgaris: environmental factors. Occupational, behavioral, medical, and qualitative food frequency questionnaire. Int J Dermatol 2001;40:562–9.
18. Jacobs SE. Pemphigus erythematosus and ultraviolet light. A case report. Arch Dermatol 1965;91:139–41.
19. Brenner S, Ruocco V, Wolf R, et al. Pemphigus and dietary factors. In vitro acantholysis by allyl compounds of the genus Allium. Dermatology 1995;190:197–202.
20. Tur E, Brenner S. Diet and pemphigus. In pursuit of exogenous factors in pemphigus and fogo selvagem. Arch Dermatol 1998;134:1406–10.
21. Emery DJ, Diaz LA, Fairley LA, et al. Detection and characterization of pemphigus foliaceus autoantibodies that react with the desmoglein-1 ectodomain. J Invest Dermatol 1995;104:323–8.
22. Grando SA. Autoimmunity to keratinocyte acetylcholine receptors in pemphigus. Dermatology 2000;201(4):290–5.
23. Sison-Fonacier L, Bystryn JC. Heterogeneity of pemphigus vulgaris antigens. Arch Dermatol 1987;123:1507–10.
24. Vu TN, Lee TX, Ndoye A, et al. The pathophysiological significance of nondesmoglein targets of pemphigus autoimmunity. Development of antibodies against keratinocyte cholinergic receptors in patients with pemphigus vulgaris and pemphigus foliaceus. Arch Dermatol 1998;134(8):971–80.

25. Grando SA, Bystyrn JC, Chernyvavsky AI, et al. Apoptolysis: novel mechanism of skin blistering in pemphigus vulgaris linking the apoptotoc pathways to basal cell shrinkage and suprabasal acantholysis. Exp Dermatol 2009;18(9):764–70.

26. Berkowitz P, Hu P, Warren S, et al. p38MAPK inhibition prevents disease in pemphigus vulgaris mice. Proc Natl Acad Sci U S A 2006;103:12855–60.

27. Berkowitz P, Chua M, Liu Z, et al. Autoantibodies in the autoimmune disease pemphigus foliaceus induce blistering via p38 mitogen-activated protein kinase-dependent signaling in the skin. Am J Pathol 2008;173:1628–36.

28. Szafer F, Brautbar C, Tzfoni E, et al. Detection of disease-specific restriction fragment length polymorphisms in pemphigus vulgaris linked to the DQw1 and DQw3 alleles of the HLA-D region. Proc Natl Acad Sci U S A 1987;84:6542.

29. Todd JA, Acha-Orbea H, Bell JI, et al. A molecular basis for MHC class II–associated autoimmunity. Science 1988;240:1003.

30. Lee E, Lendas KA, Chow S, et al. Disease relevant HLA class II alleles isolated by genotypic, haplotypic, and sequence analysis in North American Caucasians with pemphigus vulgaris. Hum Immunol 2006;67(1-2):125–39.

31. Meurer M, Millns JL, Rogers RS III, et al. Oral pemphigus vulgaris. A report of ten cases. Arch Dermatol 1977;113:1520–4.

32. Sirois DA, Fatahzadeh M, Roth R, et al. Diagnostic patterns and delays in pemphigus vulgaris: experience with 99 patients. Arch Dermatol 2000;136:1569–70.

33. Hodak E, Kremer I, David M, et al. Conjunctival involvement in pemphigus vulgaris: a clinical, histopathological and immunofluorescence study. Br J Dermatol 1990;123:615–20.

34. Hale EK, Bystryn JC. Laryngeal and nasal involvement in pemphigus vulgaris. J Am Acad Dermatol 2001;44:609–11.

35. Lurie R, Trattner A, David M, et al. Esophageal involvement in pemphigus vulgaris: report of two cases and review of the literature. Dermatologica 1990;181:233–6.

36. Trattner A, Lurie R, Leiser A, et al. Esophageal involvement in pemphigus vulgaris: a clinical, histologic, and immunopathologic study. J Am Acad Dermatol 1991;24:223–6.

37. Marren P, Wojnarowska F, Venning V, et al. Vulvar involvement in autoimmune bullous diseases. J Reprod Med 1993;38:101–7.

38. Sagher F, Bercovici B, Romem R. Nikolsky sign on cervix uteri in pemphigus. Br J Dermatol 1974;90:407–11.

39. Korman N. Pemphigus. J Am Acad Dermatol 1988; 18:1219–38.

40. Uzun S, Durdu M. The specificity and sensitivity of Nikolsky sign in the diagnosis of pemphigus. J Am Acad Dermatol 2006;54:411–5.

41. Berker DD, Dalziel K, Dawber RP, et al. Pemphigus associated with nail dystrophy. Br J Dermatol 1993;129:461–4.

42. Kolivras A, Gheeraert P, Andre J. Nail destruction in pemphigus vulgaris. Dermatology 2003;206: 351–2.

43. Mutasim DF. Autoimmune bullous diseases: diagnosis and management. Dermatol Nurs 1999;11:15–21.

44. Vodegel RM, de Jong MC, Meijer HJ, et al. Enhanced diagnostic immunofluorescence using biopsies transported in saline. BMC Dermatol 2004;4:10.

45. Ahmed AR, Graham J, Jordan RE, et al. Pemphigus: current concepts. Ann Intern Med 1980;92:396–405.

46. Lever WF. Pemphigus and pemphigoid. J Am Acad Dermatol 1979;1:2–31.

47. Scully C. A review of mucocutaneous disorders affecting the mouth and lips. Ann Acad Med Singapore 1999;28:704–7.

48. Scott JE, Ahmed AR. The blistering diseases. Med Clin North Am 1998;82:1239–83.

49. Ding X, Diaz LA, Fairley JA, et al. The anti-desmoglein 1 autoantibodies in pemphigus vulgaris sera are pathogenic. J Invest Dermatol 1999;112:739–43.

50. Kricheli D, David M, Frusic-Zlotkin M, et al. The distribution of pemphigus vulgaris-IgG subclasses and their reactivity with desmoglein 3 and 1 in pemphigus patients and their first-degree relatives. Br J Dermatol 2000;143:337–42.

51. Ayatollahi M, Joubeh S, Mortazavi H, et al. IgG4 as the predominant autoantibody in sera from patients with active state of pemphigus vulgaris. J Eur Acad Dermatol Venereol 2004;18:241–2.

52. David M, Katzenelson V, Mimouni D, et al. The distribution of pemphigus vulgaris-IgG subclasses in patients with active disease. J Eur Acad Dermatol Venereol 2006;20:232.

53. Spaeth S, Riechers R, Borradori L, et al. IgG, IgA and IgE autoantibodies against the ectodomain of desmoglein 3 in active pemphigus vulgaris. Br J Dermatol 2001;144:1183–8.

54. Mentink LF, de Jong MCJM, Kloosterhuis GJ, et al. Coexistence of IgA antibodies to desmogleins 1 and 3 in pemphigus vulgaris, pemphigus foliaceus and paraneoplastic pemphigus. Br J Dermatol 2007;156:635–41.

55. Amagai M, Tsunoda K, Zillikens D, et al. The clinical phenotype of pemphigus is defined by the anti-desmoglein autoantibody profile. J Am Acad Dermatol 1999;40:167–70.

56. Jamora MJJ, Jiao D, Bystryn JC. Antibodies to desmoglein 1 and 3, and the clinical phenotype of pemphigus vulgaris. J Am Acad Dermatol 2003;48:976–7.

57. Miyagawa S, Amagai M, Iida T, et al. Late development of antidesmoglein 1 antibodies in pemphigus vulgaris: correlation with disease progression. Br J Dermatol 1999;141:1084–7.

58. Amagai M. Towards a better understanding of pemphigus autoimmunity. Br J Dermatol 2000;143: 237–8.

59. Harman KE, Gratian MJ, Bhogal BS, et al. A study of desmoglein 1 autoantibodies in pemphigus vulgaris: racial differences in frequency and the association with a more severe phenotype. Br J Dermatol 2000;143:343–8.

60. Ding X, Aoki V, Mascaro JM Jr, et al. Mucosal and mucocutaneous (generalized) pemphigus vulgaris show distinct autoantibody profiles. J Invest Dermatol 1997;109:592–6.

61. Harman KE, Seed PT, Gratian MJ, et al. The severity of cutaneous and oral pemphigus is related to desmoglein 1 and 3 antibody levels. Br J Dermatol 2001;144:775–80.

62. Olszewska M, Gerlicz Z, Blaszczyk M. Cutaneous pemphigus vulgaris. J Eur Acad Dermatol Venereol 2007;21:698–9.

63. Jiao D, Bystryn JC. Sensitivity of indirect immunofluorescence, substrate specificity and immunoblotting in the diagnosis of pemphigus. J Am Acad Dermatol 1997;37:211–6.

64. Ishii K, Amagai M, Hall RP, et al. Characterization of autoantibodies in pemphigus using antigen-specific enzyme linked immunosorbent assays with baculovirus expressed recombinant desmogleins. J Immunol 1997;159:2010–7.

65. Anzai H, Stanley JR, Amagai M. Production of low titers of anti-desmoglein 1 IgG autoantibodies in some patients with staphylococcal scalded skin syndrome. J Invest Dermatol 2006;126:2139–41.

66. Fellner MJ, Mark AS. Penicillin- and ampicillin-induced pemphigus vulgaris. Int J Dermatol 1980; 19:392–3.

67. Ahmed A, Workman A. Anti-intercellular substance antibody: presence in serum of 14 patients without pemphigus. Arch Dermatol 1983;119:17–21.

68. Thivolet J, Beyvin A. Recherche par immunofluorescence d'anticorps seriques vis-vis des constituants de l'epiderme chez les brutes. Experientia 1968; 24:945–6.

69. Lee FJ, Silvestrini R, Fulcher DA. False positive intercellular cement substance antibodies due to group A/B red cell antibodies: frequency and approach. Pathology 2010;42(6):574–6.

70. Murrell DF, Amagai M, Barnadas MA, et al. Consensus statement on definitions of disease endpoints and therapeutic response for pemphigus. J Am Acad Dermatol 2008;58(6):1043–6.

# The Genetics of Pemphigus

Animesh A. Sinha, MD, PhD

**KEYWORDS**

- Genetics • Pemphigus • Autoimmunity
- Blistering disorders

Pemphigus is 1 of 4 major groups of autoimmune blistering diseases (AIBD) characterized by autoantibodies against intercellular junctions in the skin. Pemphigus vulgaris (PV) is representative of the pemphigus group. It is a prototypical organ-specific human autoimmune disease that presents clinically with flaccid blister formation on the skin and mucous membranes. Histologically, there is an intraepidermal split resulting from acantholysis of suprabasilar keratinocytes.[1] Autoantibodies against desmoglein 3 (Dsg3) in humans have been primarily implicated in lesional disorders,[2] and can passively transfer the disease in mice.[3] More than 50% of patients with PV also have circulating autoantibodies against desmoglein 1 (Dsg1), and their presence may be required for the development of nonmucosal lesions.[4] More recently, nondesmoglein targets are also being uncovered in PV.[5,6] Nevertheless, the etiopathogenesis of PV, particularly the role of genetic factors in the generation of autoantibodies that are relevant to disease development and clinical presentation, remains poorly understood.

Numerous studies provide support for the importance of genetic factors in PV.[7–12] As for many autoimmune conditions, several lines of evidence make a compelling argument for a complex, polygenic basis for disease involving multiple, but an unknown number of genetic loci, as well as nongenetic factors. Genetic and nongenetic/environmental elements are believed to contribute to the dysregulation of normal immune tolerance that ultimately leads to the development of autoimmunity in the skin. At present, the full complement of susceptibility loci remain unidentified, and it is not possible to identify individuals at risk.

This article reviews the evidence for the genetic basis of disease from studies on (1) population analyses, (2) autoimmune comorbidity, and (3) familial aggregation. It reviews the data implicating specific (1) human leukocyte antigen (HLA) and (2) non-HLA genes in the development of PV. It also outlines current and emerging strategies intended to identify disease susceptibility loci including (1) candidate gene and (2) whole-genome approaches. The role of genetics in terms of biologic and clinical relevance to our understanding and management of disease is also discussed.

## GENETIC BASIS OF DISEASE: WHAT IS THE EVIDENCE?
### Population Studies

The overall prevalence and incidence of PV is low, but it varies significantly in various ethnic populations. As discussed by Gupta and colleagues elsewhere in this issue, the incidence of PV to is reported to range between 0.076 per 100,000 person years and 5 per 100,000 person years.[13–17] This wide range of incidence across worldwide geographic locations supports the hypothesis that genetic factors linked to specific racial and ethnic populations affect disease incidence. However, population-associated environmental factors such as those related to microbial variance and social-psychological and economic variables cannot be ruled out and are likely to be intertwined with relevant genetic factors. In general, PV incidence seems lower in more northern locations. A north-south gradient has previously been observed in type 1 diabetes mellitus and multiple sclerosis and has been suggested to be related

Conflict of interest: none to report.

Department of Dermatology, State University of New York at Buffalo and Roswell Park Cancer Institute, MRC 234, Buffalo, NY 14263, USA

E-mail address: asinha@msu.edu

Dermatol Clin 29 (2011) 381–391

doi:10.1016/j.det.2011.03.020

to the relative dominance of Th1-type versus Th2-type pathogens in particular geographic locations. It remains to be determined how specific genetic and environmental factors influence the development of PV across the globe.

Similarly, the literature and our own studies indicate a female predominance in PV, as is often reported in autoimmune conditions. The female/male ratio ranges from 1.1:1 to 2.25:1 (see the article by Gupta and colleagues elsewhere in this issue). This female bias can be interpreted as evidence for the role of genetics in disease. Nongenetic mechanisms may be involved, likely in concert with heritable elements, in influencing the expression of PV in women rather than men.

For several autoimmune conditions, twin and adoption studies have been able to provide strong evidence for genetic susceptibility. The comparison of concordance rates among monozygotic versus dizygotic individuals allows a focus on the relative contribution of genetic risk to disease. However, because large-scale population-based assessments are required and the prevalence of PV is low, twin and/or adoption studies are not available.

### Autoimmune Comorbidity

It has long been observed that patients with 1 autoimmune condition have an increased likelihood to develop 1 or more other autoimmune diseases.[18,19] Work from others, as well as our group, indicates that this is the case in PV. In a survey of 171 patients with PV, we found that nearly 21% of patients report having a comorbid autoimmune condition (please refer to Fig. 1 in the article by Gupta and colleagues elsewhere in this issue). Thyroid disease was by far the most common PV-associated condition, occurring in nearly half of those reporting a concomitant autoimmune disorder. Autoimmunity affecting the thyroid has been similarly linked with several autoimmune diseases.[20] This may be, at least in part, because of the higher incidence of thyroid disease compared with other autoimmune conditions. Nevertheless, these data suggest that PV and autoimmune thyroid disease may share at least some pathogenetic factors. Recently, a common-cause theory for the development of autoimmunity based on shared disease genes and polymorphisms has emerged. Data from our laboratory on overlapping gene expression changes within several autoimmune skin diseases, such as alopecia areata, psoriasis, and vitiligo, and with other nonskin autoimmune conditions, lend experimental support to this hypothesis.[21,22] The subset of PV-associated susceptibility loci that are disease specific and those that are related to an overall autoimmune diathesis remain to be determined.

### Familial Aggregation

Additional support for the genetic basis of disease comes from the increased incidence of autoimmunity in blood relatives of autoimmune patients.[18,19,23] In our survey of 171 patients with PV, we found that 48% reported having 1 or more relatives with autoimmune disease (please refer to Fig. 2 in the article by Gupta and colleagues elsewhere in this issue). Type 1 diabetes was reported most commonly, followed by autoimmune thyroid disease. PV itself was reported less commonly, occurring in the relatives of 2.9% of patients. Although familial cases of PV have been cited in the literature,[24–27] they are rare.

Multiple PV cases within families are most likely to occur in first-degree relatives. There is a significantly higher incidence of all autoimmune diseases in first-degree relatives of patients with PV compared with second-degree and third-degree relatives (**Fig. 1**). These findings, in which autoimmunity correlates more strongly with an increased genetic commonality (first>second>third degree), strongly support the genetic basis of PV. However, the influence of environmental factors cannot be ruled out.

## HLA AND PV

Most of the literature on the genetic susceptibility to PV has centered on the investigation of major histocompatibility complex (MHC) genes. The MHC in humans is termed the HLA and spans approximately 4000 kb on chromosome 6p21. HLA associations are a hallmark of autoimmunity and have been established for a large number of conditions.[7,8,28]

### HLA Class II

A plethora of HLA typing studies have been performed in PV in numerous worldwide populations. Early studies based on serologic reagents showed associations between PV and the HLA class II specificities DR4 and DR6.[29] Further molecular sequencing by the author and others highlighted 2 HLA class II subtypes, now known as DRB1*0402 and DQB1*0503[7,8,28,30]; more than 95% of patients with PV carry 1 of these risk factors. The subsequent ubiquitous availability of DNA sequencing and genotyping techniques implicated numerous other DRB1 and DQB1 allelic variants in various studies, leading to confusion regarding which alleles truly confer disease risk. A variety of confounding factors, particularly the strong linkage disequilibrium within the HLA region

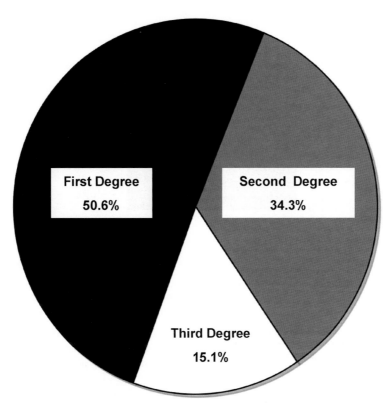

**Fig. 1.** Family history of autoimmune disease in patients with PV. There is a significant increase in the prevalence of autoimmune disease in relatives of patients (48%) versus controls. Of these, first-degree relatives are most commonly affected.

(especially between DR and DQ), has made it difficult to precisely designate HLA risk alleles. The full list of HLA and PV associations is not reviewed here, but can be referenced in several other articles[9–12,31–33] and public databases.

In an effort to pinpoint the relevant susceptibility alleles among overrepresented sequences, our group applied a stepwise reductionist analysis based on 3 factors: (1) determination of the degree of linkage disequilibrium between purportedly associated alleles, (2) haplotype frequencies comparisons, and (3) primary sequence comparisons of disease-associated versus non–disease-associated alleles to identify crucial differences in amino acid residues in putative peptide binding pockets.[9] This analysis provided extended support that the disease-relevant HLA associations in patients with PV map to DRB1*0402 and DQB1*0503 alone, at least in non-Asian patients. The association between HLA-DRB1*0402 and DQB1*0503 is particularly strong in the Ashkenazi Jewish population. The high prevalence of DRB1*0402 among the general Ashkenazi population may account for an increased prevalence of PV in this group.[34] Analysis of the sequence and structure of these PV susceptibility alleles

reveals key HLA peptide binding site pockets and residues that distinguish these molecules from non–disease-associated sequences[9,35] (**Fig. 2**). These data highlight the exquisite specificity of the immune response and suggest mechanisms by which autoimmune reactions are initiated. HLA II associations in PV are consistent with the prevailing model of disease development in which the activation of class II restricted, desmoglein-specific CD4 T effector cells drives autoreactive B cell activity and autoantibody production (**Fig. 3**).[36]

### HLA Class Ia

Although HLA II associations with PV are well documented, additional disease associations have been reported with several classic HLA class I (Ia) molecules, including HLA-A3,[37] A10,[38] A26, and HLA-B15,[39] B35,[40] B38,[41] B44,[40] and B60.[37] The significance of these findings to disease susceptibility remains unclear. These associations may simply be based on linkage disequilibrium to the true disease linked alleles at HLA II, or contribute to risk along disease-associated extended haplotypes.[41,42]

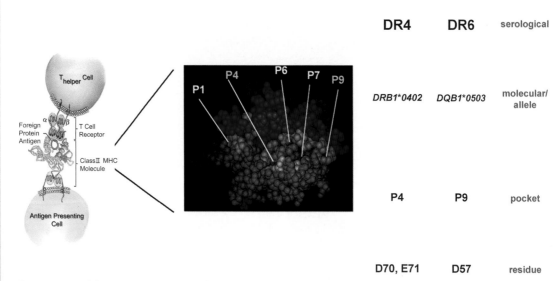

**Fig. 2.** Susceptibility to PV is most strongly associated within the HLA II peptide DRB1*0402 and DQB1*0503. These risk alleles vary from nonrisk alleles at precise pockets and specific residues within the HLAII peptide binding pocket.

## HLA Class Ib

To date, there has been limited work regarding nonclassic HLA class Ib alleles (HLA- E, F, and G) and PV. Gazit and colleagues[43] reported an increased frequency of a 14-bp deletion variant at HLA-G in patients with PV. In addition, this group found 4 informative SNP (single nucleotide polymorphisms) markers that mapped to HLA-G in a cohort of 26 Jewish patients.[12] Corroborative studies are required to define the role of HLA-G in disease susceptibility.

Recently, our group found an association between HLA-E and PV. The HLA-E genetic region is located between the classical class 1a loci at HLA-C and HLA-A on the telomeric (distal) end of the short arm of chromosome 6p21. HLA-E is a highly conserved molecule with only 4 reported-nonsynonymous alleles: HLA-E*0101, HLA-E*0102, HLA-E*0103, and HLA-E*0104. In genotyping

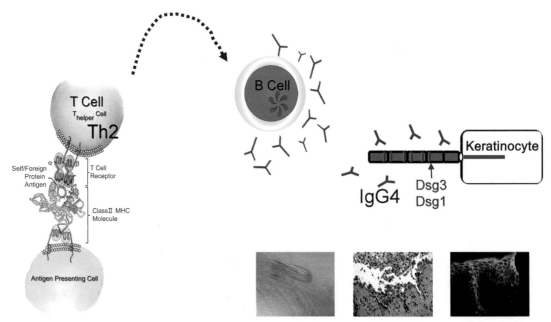

**Fig. 3.** HLA and autoimmune initiation. HLA risk alleles are believed to activate Th2 type T cells that promote the activation of autoreactive B cells and the generation of autoantibodies to Dsg3, Dsg1 (primarily the IgG4 subtype), and perhaps other autoantigenic targets.

studies of 52 patients with PV and 51 healthy controls, the HLA-E*0103 allele was significantly increased in the patient population.[44] HLA-E*0103 confers increased risk for Behcet disease and childhood onset of type I diabetes. HLA-E polymorphisms have also been linked to experimental autoimmune encephalomyelitis, multiple sclerosis, and celiac disease.[45–49] The functional role of HLA-E in PV disease development remains unclear. However, recent functional work in model systems[50,51] indicates that HLA-E may be a key modulator in self/nonself discrimination and contributes to the development of autoimmunity. An intriguing possibility is that HLA-E (and/or classical HLA 1a) restricted responses are relevant to the activation and/or functional activity of CD8 T cells with a suppressor phenotype that are capable of down-regulating CD4 activity in vitro that our group has recently identified in the blood of remittent patients with PV.[52] A schematic overview of the HLA region and key loci and alleles with disease relevance to PV is illustrated in **Fig. 4**.

## NON-HLA GENES

Although there are many data on the importance of HLA genes, susceptibility to PV is clearly polygenic. Currently, there are no non-HLA genes that have been definitively linked to disease. To date, only a handful of studies have been performed on a limited number of genes in PV. Polymorphisms

in autoantigens have been identified in or near other autoimmune conditions, including type I diabetes (insulin gene[53]) and myasthenia gravis (acetylcholine receptor α subunit gene[54]). This background prompted the investigation of the desmoglein 3 gene in PV. Examining 5 SNPs, Capon and colleagues[55] observed a significant association between PV and the DSG3*TCCTC haplotype in 2 case-controlled datasets of British and northern Indian patients with PV. Another small study of 12 patients found an association with a VH3 polymorphism of the immunoglobulin heavy chain constant region gene.[56] However, French patients with PV were not associated with allotypic markers of immunoglobulin κ.[57] There have been conflicting reports regarding transporter associated with antigen processing (TAP) genes and PV.[58]

More recently, our group investigated the genetic association between protein tyrosine phosphatase N22 (PTPN22) and PV. Alterations in the protein PTPN22 gene have been shown to affect the threshold required for T lymphocyte activation. The PTPN22 1858T polymorphism leads to uninhibited T cell receptor cascade propagation and has been positively associated with several human autoimmune diseases including rheumatoid arthritis,[59,60] type 1 diabetes,[61] and systemic lupus erythematosus.[62] Although blister formation in PV is ultimately caused by autoantibody attack on keratinocytes, it is clear that T cell activation is a necessary step in the generation of autoreactive

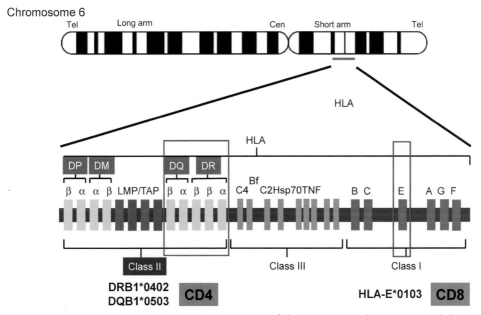

**Fig. 4.** HLA and PV. The HLA region is located on the short arm of chromosome 6 in humans. Several class II, class I, and nonclassic class Ib associations have been reported in PV. The strongest associations are with DRB1*0402, DQB1*0503. Recent work suggests an association with HLA-E*0103.

B cells, providing a rationale to explore the link between PTPN22 and PV. However, in a study of 102 patients with PV and 102 healthy controls, we were unable to find an association between the PTPN22 1858T polymorphism and disease.[63] Thus, the search for non-HLA risk genes in PV continues.

## STRATEGIES FOR THE IDENTIFICATION OF DISEASE SUSCEPTIBILITY GENES

The status of PV as a genetically complex trait has posed several hurdles for genetic analysis. Although the evidence for HLA-associated risk is strong, an unknown number of non-HLA genetic loci, along with nongenetic factors, are yet to be identified. Adding to the difficulty of defining genetic elements at play in PV is the rare nature of the disease. Large numbers of cases and controls are required for statistically robust studies. Even in studies involving hundreds, if not thousands, of subjects, the search for consensus disease susceptibility loci in complex traits has proved to be of low yield. Two basic approaches remain applicable: candidate gene and genome-wide investigation. In the past 2 to 3 decades, genetic markers used in these studies have progressed from fragment length polymorphisms, to variable number tandem repeats, to the more recent ubiquitous use of SNPs that now offer tremendous coverage of large parts of the genome. Newer study designs and emerging technologies offer the possibility of increased success in future studies.

### Candidate Gene Search

In this strategy, a focused, hypothesis-driven approach is applied to directly assess 1 or more of the usual suspects that are considered to be potential disease risk candidates. For autoimmune conditions, this includes genes for known or possible autoimmune targets (autoantigens), cytokines, lymphocyte structure or function related proteins, and general immune response molecules. As noted earlier, a few such candidates have been studied in PV. However, these studies have generally been hampered by small study sample sizes and a lack of validation studies in alternate populations, and no clear associations have been uncovered.

Despite the technical and statistical barriers, an increasing number of genetic associations are being implicated in human autoimmune conditions. With more robust methods, the list of candidates will probably expand significantly in the coming years. The common gene hypothesis for autoimmune diseases provides a rationale for targeting associations first defined in other conditions for future study in PV.

Another promising strategy involves leveraging functional information to inform genetic analysis (Fig. 5). Specifically, gene expression profiles can provide an enriched set of candidate genes. This strategy is based on the hypothesis that among the genes that are transcriptionally dysregulated in diseased tissues, at least a subset owe their altered gene expression to genetic variance. Previous studies have shown that mRNA levels are heritable traits useful for genetic analysis.[64,65] Each gene differentially expressed between diseased and healthy individuals represents a candidate for genetic investigation. This focus can be extended to a targeted pathway analysis to include a larger set of genes relating to a unifying cellular process (eg, interferon pathway, apoptosis) that is found to be central to disease. Our group has used this reverse genetics approach to highlight potential disease susceptibility loci with functional impact in cutaneous lupus[66] and alopecia areata.[67] Moreover, we identified transcriptional hot spots in both conditions where differentially expressed genes are concentrated with statistically increased frequency. These hot spots may represent particularly high-yield destinations for genetic investigation. Recently completed gene expression profiles in PV blood by our group will allow us to apply similar strategies to facilitate the search for risk-associated genetic markers in this disease.

### Genome-wide Investigation

In contrast with the candidate gene approach, genome-wide investigation is not hypothesis driven. The search for susceptibility loci is undertaken without a priori knowledge of disease risk factors. This shotgun strategy is particularly appealing if there is a paucity of existing genetic information. In recent years, the genome-wide association studies (GWAS) have become the go-to approach in complex diseases. However, after much scientific and financial investment, the results of GWAS have been collectively disappointing. For most chronic diseases, GWAS have not offered any better prediction of risk than simple family history.[68] It has been argued that the focus should be shifted from common sequence variants detected by most SNPs to the search for rare variants with potentially stronger effects.[69] Newer strategies such as whole-genome sequencing and exon sequencing may give better access to rare and novel variants, including insertions, deletions, and single nucleotide changes.[70]

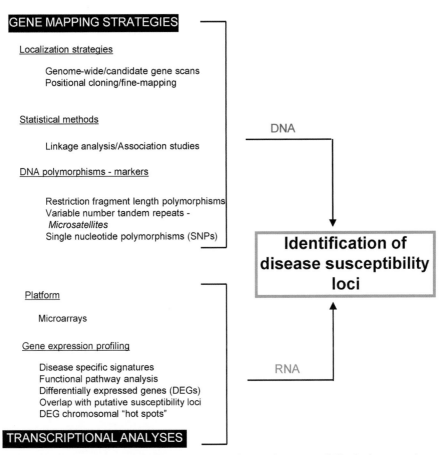

**Fig. 5.** Differentially expressed genes (DEGs) overlapping with putative susceptibility loci. Integrating genetic and DEG transcriptional hot spots can help to pinpoint disease risk genes.

The advancement of genetic studies in PV is critically dependent on the development of large-scale disease registries with correlated biorepositories. To this end, the International Pemphigus and Pemphigoid Foundation has recently launched a blistering disorders registry as a first step toward this goal. A well-archived DNA/RNA sample collection through national and international cooperation is required to support the application of modern genetic technologies to this rare disease. It is likely that a combination of candidate gene and whole-genome approaches with newly considered study designs, including those involving integrated transcriptional and chromosomal profiling, will be needed to unravel the complex interplay of genes and environment that drive the development of disease.

## CLINICAL RELEVANCE

Ultimately, future investigations can be expected to illuminate more clearly defined links between specific genetic markers, alterations in biologic pathways, and clinical expression (**Fig. 6**). The goal here is to better understand the precise biologic and clinical consequences of carrying specific sets of disease-risk and disease-modifying genes. Based on these enhanced insights, genetic information will increasingly affect clinical care at several levels to usher in a new era of personalized medicine (**Fig. 7**).

First, once disease-predisposing genes are identified, genetic tests can be developed to identify individuals at risk. Although screening could begin with a limited set of genes, the more complete the set of disease susceptibility loci, the more accurate the screening process. Although more than 95% of patients with PV type as HLA-DRB1*0402 and/or HLA-DQB1*0503, most individuals carrying these alleles are not at risk for PV. Thus, a larger set of risk alleles, particularly those with high disease specificity, need to be identified to be of practical value.

Second, future genetic data may allow the prediction of clinical course. Autoimmune diseases are notoriously variable in terms of extent and

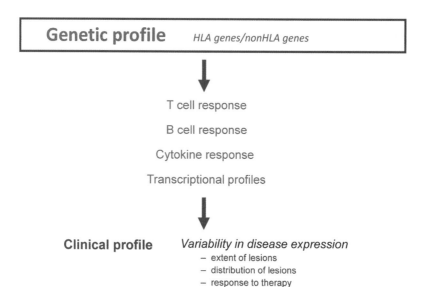

**Fig. 6.** Linking genetic, biologic, and clinical profiles to gain insights into disease. Emerging data will help to define the genetic elements that direct the dysregulation of specific biologic pathways and determine disease phenotypes.

expression. At present, it is not possible to identify the subset of patients that will have mild versus extensive disease, or those that will have mucosal dominant versus mucocutaneous disease. If refined genetic markers can be linked to defined clinical profiles that stratify patients based on disease variables such as severity and distribution of lesions, appropriately matched management protocols can be instituted early in the most vulnerable patients. Key phenotype-associated gene markers with predictive clinical value can be expected to accelerate the development of next-generation prognostic tools.

Third, at present there are no consensus guidelines for therapy in PV. Moreover, the subset of patients that will be responders versus nonresponders to any given drug cannot be identified. Thus, many therapies are given to patients with PV on a trial-and-error basis, leading to significant inefficiencies and delays in effective management. Genetic markers linked to therapeutic response represent a holy grail of clinical management. Moreover, mechanistic knowledge of how genes affect specific functional pathways will undoubtedly uncover new targets for therapeutic intervention. Genetic-based tools are likely to provide a scientific rationale behind future clinical decision making by physicians and facilitate the implementation of individually tailored therapy.

- Identify individuals at risk  *develop new genetic screening tests*

- Predict course of disease  *early intervention*

- Predict response to therapy  *tailored therapy*

- Understand disease mechanisms  *new therapeutic targets*

New era of ***personalized*** medicine

**Fig. 7.** Clinical relevance of genetic information. Knowledge of disease susceptibility genes can potentially affect patient management at several levels.

# REFERENCES

1. Becker BA, Gaspari AA. Pemphigus vulgaris and vegetans. Dermatol Clin 1993;11:429–52.
2. Amagai M, Tsunoda K, Zillikens D, et al. The clinical phenotype of pemphigus is defined by the anti-desmoglein autoantibody profile. J Am Acad Dermatol 1999;40:167–70.
3. Anhalt GJ, Labib RS, Voorhees JJ, et al. Induction of pemphigus in neonatal mice by passive transfer of IgG from patients with the disease. N Engl J Med 1982;306:1189–96.
4. Mahoney MG, Wang Z, Rothenberger K, et al. Explanations for the clinical and microscopic localization of lesions in pemphigus foliaceus and vulgaris. J Clin Invest 1999;103:461–8.
5. Kalantari-Dehaghi M, Molina DM, Farhadieh M, et al. New targets of pemphigus vulgaris antibodies identified by protein array technology. Exp Dermatol 2011;20:154–6.
6. Patel M, Furstenberg G, Hazelton J, et al. Development of protein microarrays to investigate autoantibody profiles in pemphigus vulgaris. J Invest Dermatol 2010;130:S19 [abstract: 549].
7. Sinha AA, Brautbar C, Szafer F, et al. A newly characterized HLA DQ beta allele associated with pemphigus vulgaris. Science 1988;239:1026–9.
8. Sinha AA, Lopez MT, McDevitt HO. Autoimmune diseases: the failure of self tolerance. Science 1990;248:1380–8.
9. Lee E, Lendas KA, Chow S, et al. Disease relevant HLA class II alleles isolated by genotypic, haplotypic, and sequence analysis in North American Caucasians with pemphigus vulgaris. Hum Immunol 2006;67:125–39.
10. Tron F, Gilbert D, Joly P, et al. Immunogenetics of pemphigus: an update. Autoimmunity 2006;39:531–9.
11. Tron F, Gilbert D, Mouquet H, et al. Genetic factors in pemphigus. J Autoimmun 2005;24:319–28.
12. Gazit E, Loewenthal R. The immunogenetics of pemphigus vulgaris. Autoimmun Rev 2005;4:16–20.
13. Salmanpour R, Shahkar H, Namazi MR, et al. Epidemiology of pemphigus in south-western Iran: a 10-year retrospective study (1991–2000). Int J Dermatol 2006;45:103–5.
14. Asilian A, Yoosefi A, Faghini G. Pemphigus vulgaris in Iran: epidemiology and clinical profile. Skinmed 2006;5:69–71.
15. Langan SM, Smeeth L, Hubbard R, et al. Bullous pemphigoid and pemphigus vulgaris–incidence and mortality in the UK: population based cohort study. BMJ 2008;337:a180.
16. Bystryn JC, Rudolph JL. Pemphigus. Lancet 2005;366:61–73.
17. Nanda A, Dvorak R, Al-Saeed K, et al. Spectrum of autoimmune bullous diseases in Kuwait. Int J Dermatol 2004;43:876–81.
18. Humbert P, Dupond JL, Vuitton D, et al. Dermatological autoimmune diseases and the multiple autoimmune syndromes. Acta Derm Venereol Suppl (Stockh) 1989;148:1–8.
19. Mohan MP, Ramesh TC. Multiple autoimmune syndrome. Indian J Dermatol Venereol Leprol 2003;69:298–9.
20. Weetman AP. Diseases associated with thyroid autoimmunity: explanations for the expanding spectrum. Clin Endocrinol (Oxf) 2011;74(4):411–8.
21. Coda AB, Qafalijaj Hysa V, Seiffert-Sinha K, et al. Peripheral blood gene expression in alopecia areata reveals molecular pathways distinguishing heritability, disease and severity. Genes Immun 2010;11:531–41.
22. Subramanya RD, Coda AB, Sinha AA. Transcriptional profiling in alopecia areata defines immune and cell cycle control related genes within disease-specific signatures. Genomics 2010;96:146–53.
23. Bordel-Gomez MT, Sanchez-Estella J, Yuste-Chaves M, et al. Familial pemphigus vulgaris: immunogenetic study of HLA class II antigens. Actas Dermosifiliogr 2006;97:509–13 [in Spanish].
24. Laskaris G, Sklavounou A, Stavrou A, et al. Familial pemphigus vulgaris with oral manifestations affecting two Greek families. J Oral Pathol Med 1989;18:49–53.
25. Katzenelson V, David M, Zamir R, et al. Familial pemphigus vulgaris. Dermatologica 1990;181:48–50.
26. Feinstein A, Yorav S, Movshovitz M, et al. Pemphigus in families. Int J Dermatol 1991;30:347–51.
27. Stavropoulos PG, Zarafonitis G, Petridis A, et al. Pemphigus vulgaris in two sisters. Acta Derm Venereol 2001;81:149.
28. Todd JA, Acha-Orbea H, Bell JI, et al. A molecular basis for MHC class II–associated autoimmunity. Science 1988;240:1003–9.
29. Szafer F, Brautbar C, Tzfoni E, et al. Detection of disease-specific restriction fragment length polymorphisms in pemphigus vulgaris linked to the DQw1 and DQw3 alleles of the HLA-D region. Proc Natl Acad Sci U S A 1987;84:6542–5.
30. Scharf SJ, Friedmann A, Brautbar C, et al. HLA class II allelic variation and susceptibility to pemphigus vulgaris. Proc Natl Acad Sci U S A 1988;85:3504–8.
31. Shams S, Amirzargar AA, Yousefi M, et al. HLA class II (DRB, DQA1 and DQB1) allele and haplotype frequencies in the patients with pemphigus vulgaris. J Clin Immunol 2009;29:175–9.
32. Brick C, Belgnaoui FZ, Atouf O, et al. Pemphigus and HLA in Morocco. Transfus Clin Biol 2007;14:402–6.
33. Saenz-Cantele AM, Fernandez-Mestre M, Montagnani S, et al. HLA-DRB1*0402 haplotypes without DQB1*0302 in Venezuelan patients with pemphigus vulgaris. Tissue Antigens 2007;69:318–25.

34. Slomov E, Loewenthal R, Goldberg I, et al. Pemphigus vulgaris in Jewish patients is associated with HLA-A region genes: mapping by microsatellite markers. Hum Immunol 2003;64:771–9.

35. Tong JC, Tan TW, Sinha AA, et al. Prediction of desmoglein-3 peptides reveals multiple shared T-cell epitopes in HLA DR4- and DR6-associated pemphigus vulgaris. BMC Bioinformatics 2006; 7(Suppl 5):S7.

36. Takahashi H, Amagai M, Nishikawa T, et al. Novel system evaluating in vivo pathogenicity of desmoglein 3-reactive T cell clones using murine pemphigus vulgaris. J Immunol 2008;181:1526–35.

37. Geng L, Wang Y, Zhai N, et al. Association between pemphigus vulgaris and human leukocyte antigen in Han nation of northeast China. Chin Med Sci J 2005; 20:166–70.

38. Hashimoto K, Miki Y, Nakata S, et al. HLA-A10 in pemphigus among Japanese. Arch Dermatol 1977; 113:1518–9.

39. Miyagawa S, Niizeki H, Yamashina Y, et al. Genotyping for HLA-A, B and C alleles in Japanese patients with pemphigus: prevalence of Asian alleles of the HLA-B15 family. Br J Dermatol 2002;146:52–8.

40. Birol A AR, Tutkak H, Gürgey E. HLA-class 1 and class 2 antigens in Turkish patients with pemphigus. Int J Dermatol 2002;41:79–83.

41. Ahmed AR, Yunis EJ, Khatri K, et al. Major histocompatibility complex haplotype studies in Ashkenazi Jewish patients with pemphigus vulgaris. Proc Natl Acad Sci U S A 1990;87:7658–62.

42. Ahmed AR, Wagner R, Khatri K, et al. Major histocompatibility complex haplotypes and class II genes in non-Jewish patients with pemphigus vulgaris. Proc Natl Acad Sci U S A 1991;88: 5056–60.

43. Gazit E, Slomov Y, Goldberg I, et al. HLA-G is associated with pemphigus vulgaris in Jewish patients. Hum Immunol 2004;65:39–46.

44. Bhanusali D, Sachdev A, Rahmanian A, et al. HLA-E*0103 is associated with susceptibility to pemphigus vulgaris. J Invest Dermatol 2008;128:86 [abstract: 139].

45. Jabri B, de Serre NP, Cellier C, et al. Selective expansion of intraepithelial lymphocytes expressing the HLA-E-specific natural killer receptor CD94 in celiac disease. Gastroenterology 2000; 188:867–79.

46. Hu DIK, Lu L, Sanchirico ME, et al. Analysis of regulatory CD8 T cells in Qa-1-deficient mice. Nat Immunol 2004;5:516–23.

47. Tennakoon DK, Mehta RS, Ortega SB, et al. Therapeutic induction of regulatory, cytotoxic CD8+ T cells in multiple sclerosis. J Immunol 2006;176: 7119–29.

48. Hodgkinson AD, Millward BA, Demaine AG. The HLA-E locus is associated with age at onset and susceptibility to type 1 diabetes mellitus. Hum Immunol 2000;61:290–5.

49. Park KS, Park JS, Nam JH, et al. HLA-E*0101 and HLA-G*010101 reduce the risk of Behcet's disease. Tissue Antigens 2007;69:139–44.

50. Sullivan LC, Clements CS, Rossjohn J, et al. The major histocompatibility complex class Ib molecule HLA-E at the interface between innate and adaptive immunity. Tissue Antigens 2008;72: 415–24.

51. Jiang H. CL: Qa-1/HLA-E-restricted regulatory CD8+ T cells and self-nonself discrimination: an essay on peripheral T-cell regulation. Hum Immunol 2008;69:721–7.

52. Lee E, Chow S, Dionsio R, et al. Identification of two distinct CD8+ T cell populations associated with remittent disease in pemphigus vulgaris. J Invest Dermatol 2006;126:13 [abstract: 76].

53. Vafiadis P, Bennett ST, Todd JA, et al. Insulin expression in human thymus is modulated by INS VNTR alleles at the IDDM2 locus. Nat Genet 1997;15: 289–92.

54. Garchon HJ, Djabiri F, Viard JP, et al. Involvement of human muscle acetylcholine receptor alpha-subunit gene (CHRNA) in susceptibility to myasthenia gravis. Proc Natl Acad Sci U S A 1994; 91:4668–72.

55. Capon F, Bharkhada J, Cochrane NE, et al. Evidence of an association between desmoglein 3 haplotypes and pemphigus vulgaris. Br J Dermatol 2006;154:67–71.

56. Gibson WT, Walter MA, Ahmed AR, et al. The immunoglobulin heavy chain and disease association: application to pemphigus vulgaris. Hum Genet 1994;94:675–83.

57. Zitouni M, Martel P, Ben Ayed M, et al. Pemphigus is not associated with allotypic markers of immunoglobulin kappa. Genes Immun 2002;3:50–2.

58. Niizeki H, Kumagai S, Kanagawa S, et al. Exclusion of the TAP1 and TAP2 genes within the HLA class II region as candidate susceptibility genes to pemphigus in the Japanese population. J Dermatol Sci 2004;36:122–4.

59. Michou L, Lasbleiz S, Rat AC, et al. Linkage proof for PTPN22, a rheumatoid arthritis susceptibility gene and a human autoimmunity gene. Proc Natl Acad Sci U S A 2007;104:1649–54.

60. Farago B, Talian GC, Komlosi K, et al. Protein tyrosine phosphatase gene C1858T allele confers risk for rheumatoid arthritis in Hungarian subjects. Rheumatol Int 2008;29:793–6.

61. Howson JM, Dunger DB, Nutland S, et al. A type 1 diabetes subgroup with a female bias is characterised by failure in tolerance to thyroid peroxidase at an early age and a strong association with the cytotoxic T-lymphocyte-associated antigen-4 gene. Diabetologia 2007;50:741–6.

62. Balada E, Villarreal-Tolchinsky J, Ordi-Ros J, et al. Multiplex family-based study in systemic lupus erythematosus: association between the R620W polymorphism of PTPN22 and the FcgammaRIIa (CD32A) R131 allele. Tissue Antigens 2006;68:432–8.

63. Sachdev A, Bhanusali D, Zamora MB, et al. PTPN22 1858T is not a risk factor for North American pemphigus vulgaris. Experimental Dermatology 2011, in press.

64. Cheung VG, Conlin LK, Weber TM, et al. Natural variation in human gene expression assessed in lymphoblastoid cells. Nat Genet 2003;33:422–5.

65. Brem RB, Yvert G, Clinton R, et al. Genetic dissection of transcriptional regulation in budding yeast. Science 2002;296:752–5.

66. Sinha AA, Baumgarten J, Pan H, et al. Gene expression profiling in cutaneous lupus erythematosus [abstract]. J Invest Dermatol 2002; 119:266.

67. Coda A, Sinha AA. Linking alopecia areata to atopy: evaluation of transcriptionally regulated genes in patient subsets suggests a shared basis for genetic susceptibility. J Invest Dermatol 2010;130:S92 [abstract: 549].

68. Couzin-Frankel J. Major heart disease genes prove elusive. Science 2010;328:1220–1.

69. McClellan J, King MC. Genetic heterogeneity in human disease. Cell 2010;141:210–7.

70. Nielsen R. Genomics: in search of rare human variants. Nature 2010;467:1050–1.

# A Globally Available Internet-Based Patient Survey of Pemphigus Vulgaris: Epidemiology and Disease Characteristics

Vibha K. Gupta, BS[a], Theodore E. Kelbel, BS[a],
Daniela Nguyen, MS[b], Katherine C. Melonakos, BS[a],
Dédée F. Murrell, MA, BMBCh, FAAD, MD, FACD[c],
Yan Xie, MS[d], Andrew Mullard, MS[e],
Philip L. Reed, MSc, PhD[e], Kristina Seiffert-Sinha, MD[a,f],
Animesh A. Sinha, MD, PhD[a,f,*]

**KEYWORDS**

- Pemphigus vulgaris • Epidemiology • Online survey
- Autoimmune disease comorbidity and family history
- Trigger factors

Pemphigus vulgaris (PV) is a prototypic organ-specific autoimmune disease characterized by the presence of circulating autoantibodies against desmoglein (Dsg) 3, and in some cases Dsg1, causing blister formation in the skin and mucous membranes. Previous studies have reported the incidence of PV to range from 0.076 per 100,000 person-years to 5 per 100,000 person-years.[1–5]

While PV is rare, for those affected the disease presents a lifetime physical, emotional, and monetary burden. There is no cure, and only palliative treatment, mostly based on general immunosuppression, is available at this time.

As with all autoimmune diseases, the etiology of PV is multifactorial, with complex interactions of genetic and environmental factors contributing

The authors V.K.G. and T.E.K. contributed equally to this article.
The authors have no conflict of interest to disclose.
[a] Division of Dermatology and Cutaneous Sciences, Center for Investigative Dermatology, Michigan State University, 4179 Biomedical and Physical Sciences Building, East Lansing, MI 48824, USA
[b] Department of Dermatology, Weill Medical College of Cornell University, 1300 York Avenue, New York, NY 10021, USA
[c] Department of Dermatology, St George Hospital, University of New South Wales, Gray Street, Kogarah, Sydney, NSW 2217, Australia
[d] Center for Statistical Training and Consulting, 152 Giltner Hall, Michigan State University, East Lansing, MI 48824, USA
[e] Biomedical Research & Informatics Core, Department of Epidemiology, 100 Conrad Hall, Michigan State University, East Lansing, MI 48824, USA
[f] Department of Dermatology, State University of New York at Buffalo and Roswell Park Cancer Center, Buffalo, NY 14263, USA
* Corresponding author. Department of Dermatology, State University of New York at Buffalo and Roswell Park Cancer Center, MRC 234, Buffalo, NY 14263.
E-mail address: asinha@msu.edu

Dermatol Clin 29 (2011) 393–404
doi:10.1016/j.det.2011.03.016

to disease development and exacerbation.[6] Although there is a strong link to the HLA DR4 and DR6 associated alleles, specifically DRB*0402 and DQB1*0503,[7,8] the vast majority of individuals carrying these PV associated alleles do not develop PV. There are limited data regarding additional genetic or environmental factors relevant to the initial expression of disease and the subsequent disease course in the current literature, and to date there are no published national or international registries for autoimmune bullous skin diseases with large databases of clinical information.

Comprehensive demographic and epidemiologic data collection can potentially help to elucidate questions of disease etiology. To date, studies regarding the epidemiology of PV have focused on narrowly defined demographic populations,[1,9–14] and the data collected have typically been restricted to a limited set of disease characteristics. To bridge this gap, and to overcome limitations in patient recruitment due to the rarity of PV, the authors developed an anonymous, Web-based survey instrument available globally. It has been reported that 80% of American adults have used the Internet to search for health-related information; as such, the Internet is an increasingly useful tool to conduct research.[15] In fact, anonymous Web-based questionnaire techniques are increasingly being used to assess patient attitudes toward medical care[16,17] and to collect disease-relevant medical history data in an expedient and efficient manner.[18,19] In this study, self reported demographic and epidemiologic data pertaining to a wide range of clinical parameters was collected, including disease onset, phase, and morphology, comorbid disease, family history of autoimmunity, and possible trigger factors in PV.

Two hundred and fifty-one patients affected by a variety of autoimmune blistering conditions took part in the online survey, of which 171 reported a diagnosis of PV. The study supports the viability and usefulness of an online mechanism for the investigation of a rare disease. The authors have successfully collected a comprehensive set of disease-relevant data that provide insights into disease expression and disease association.

This newly developed survey tool for blistering skin disorders facilitates patient participation across broad demographic areas, and has the potential to be used to follow patients longitudinally in order to track disease development over time.

## MATERIALS AND METHODS
### Online Study Tool

To collect epidemiologic data from a diverse group of people affected by pemphigus and pemphigoid, the authors devised a comprehensive, anonymous, online survey available globally to all individuals with Internet access and English language proficiency. The Longitudinal Study Engine (LSE) hosted at the Biomedical Research & Informatics Core at Michigan State University was used.[20] The LSE supports a fully anonymous data collection protocol and can track multiple logins as separate entries for a given patient identification number, hence providing the possibility of longitudinal data analysis.

### Patient Recruitment

The study was approved by Michigan State University's Institutional Review Board (IRB, X06-943, status exempt). Patients were recruited to participate in the online questionnaire primarily by the International Pemphigus and Pemphigoid Foundation (IPPF) research Web site link to the study, and subsequent patient promotion through Internet support group forums and message boards. Other methods included a link on the homepage of the Division of Dermatology and Cutaneous Sciences, Michigan State University, and direct contact with patients who had previously expressed interest to be contacted when new research projects became available.

### Data Acquisition

After logging into the survey, patients were prompted to create a username, accept a consent form, and review a short instructional page on how to use the survey. Depending on the question, answer choices included yes-or-no options, drop-down boxes, or open text fields. The entire survey requires approximately 15 to 20 minutes to complete. LSE is housed on 2 Dell PowerEdge 2850 (Dell Inc, Round Rock, TX, USA) servers hosted in the Michigan State University HealthTeam Data Center. The data center is physically and logically controlled to meet National Institute of Standards and Technology definitions of HIPAA (Health Insurance Portability and Accountability Act of 1996) security.

### Data Analysis

Participants were first grouped by diagnosis (PV, pemphigus foliaceus, pemphigus vegetans, pemphigus erythematosus, IgA pemphigus, bullous pemphigoid, herpes gestationis, cicatricial pemphigoid, ocular pemphigoid) and descriptive statistics for the largest cohort, PV, are reported as frequencies and percentages. In a subsequent analysis within the PV population the authors compared North American and non–North American populations. To investigate whether the distribution of categorical variables differs between populations, chi-square or Fisher's exact test values and unadjusted odds ratios (OR) with 95% confidence intervals were calculated. All analyses were performed using SAS software, Version 9.1 (SAS Institute Inc, Cary, NC, USA). Because of the online nature of the survey, entries that failed to answer any questions and entries that only provided demographic information were removed. In addition, uninterpretable data were excluded from analysis.

## RESULTS

### Study Population

A total of 251 pemphigus and pemphigoid patients were enrolled over a time interval of 8 months. The majority of patients reported a diagnosis of PV (n = 171), followed by cicatricial pemphigoid (n = 33), bullous pemphigoid (n = 28), pemphigus foliaceous (n = 25), ocular pemphigoid (n = 13), pemphigus vegetans (n = 2), IgA pemphigus (n = 1), paraneoplastic pemphigus (n = 1) and pemphigus erythematosus (n = 1). A majority of PV patients originated from North America (United States, n = 125; Canada, n = 11; Mexico, n = 1) while the remainder originated from Great Britain (n = 13), Israel (n = 7), the Netherlands (n = 4), India (n = 3), Australia (n = 2), Belgium (n = 1), Germany (n = 1), Greece (n = 1), Pakistan (n = 1), and Trinidad (n = 1). In this report the analysis is focused on the PV population.

Eighty percent of PV respondents to the survey reside in North America (United States, Canada, Mexico). Differences in genetic background, specifically HLA haplotypes in various ethnic groups, have been described in PV.[8] Because genetic as well as environmental factors can potentially vary across geographic regions,[21] the authors undertook an initial strategy to compare disease characteristics of North American PV (NAPV) patients with non–North American PV (non-NAPV) subjects. However, as few significant differences were detected in regards of demography (racial breakdown, see later discussion) and disease characteristics (history and development of lesion morphology, see later discussion), both populations were merged for most analyses.

### Demography

The demographic breakdown of the PV populations participating in this study is shown in **Table 1**. Of the 171 PV patients, 52 were male and 117 female, with a male to female ratio of 1:2.25. The mean age was 51.8 years, ranging from 25 to 80 years. Most patients identified themselves as Caucasian (n = 142, 83.0%), followed by

**Table 1**
**PV population demographics**

|  | PV (n = 171) | |
| --- | --- | --- |
| Age in years, mean (range) | 51.8 (25–80) | |
| Male/Female ratio | 1:2.25 | |
|  | n | % |
| Sex | | |
| Male | 52 | 30.8 |
| Female | 117 | 69.2 |
| Race | | |
| White/Caucasian | 142 | 83.0 |
| Asian | 12 | 7.0 |
| Black/African American | 4 | 2.3 |
| American Indian/Alaskan Native | 1 | 0.6 |
| Native Hawaiian/Pacific Islander | 1 | 0.6 |
| Hispanic/Latino | 6 | 3.5 |
| Other | 5 | 2.9 |
| Jewish Descent | | |
| Jewish | 74 | 43.3 |
| Ashkenazi Jewish[a] | 58 | 73.8 |

PV demographic information is presented as raw number of respondents and percent of respondents (n = 171).
[a] Ashkenazi Jewish descent is presented as raw number of patients and percent of Jewish participants within the Jewish subgroup (n = 74).

Asian (n = 12, 7.0%), Hispanic (n = 6, 3.5%) and Black (n = 4, 2.3%). However, in the NAPV population, significantly more patients identified themselves as Caucasian than in the non-NAPV population (OR 13.14, 95% confidence limit [CL] 5.48–31.52, P<.001). Congruent with the fact that PV and the PV-associated HLA haplotype DRB1*0402 are highly prevalent in Ashkenazi Jewish populations,[22] nearly one-half of the 171 patients in the study reported being Jewish (n = 74, 43.3%); of these 74, 58 (73.8%) reported Ashkenazi descent (see **Table 1**).

### Disease Characteristics

To assess disease characteristics several defined clinical variables were evaluated: the age of onset of disease, the current phase of disease (active vs remittent), the morphology of lesions (mucosal-only vs mucocutaneous vs cutaneous-only), and lesion distribution. Because differences were found between NAPV and non-NAPV patients in terms of lesion morphology, data for both groups are listed in **Table 2**.

**Table 2**
**Disease characteristics**

| | ALL PV (n = 171) | | NAPV (n = 137) | | non-NAPV (n = 34) | | | | |
|---|---|---|---|---|---|---|---|---|---|
| Age of onset in years, mean (range) | 45.2 (17–74) | | 45.2 (17–74) | | 45.4 (23–61) | | | | |
| | n | % | n | % | n | % | OR | CL | P value |
| Disease Phase | | | | | | | | | |
| Active | 83 | 48.53 | 67 | 48.91 | 16 | 47.06 | 1.16 | 0.54–2.47 | .70 |
| Remittent | 83 | 48.53 | 65 | 47.44 | 18 | 52.94 | | | |
| No response | 5 | 2.94 | 5 | 3.65 | 0 | 0 | | | |
| History of Lesion Morphology[a] | | | | | | | | | |
| Cutaneous only | 19 | 11.59 | 12 | 9.16 | 7 | 21.21 | 0.37 | 0.13–1.03 | .0495 |
| Mucosal only | 37 | 22.56 | 28 | 21.37 | 9 | 27.27 | 0.71 | 0.30–1.70 | .44 |
| Mucocutaneous | 108 | 65.85 | 91 | 69.47 | 17 | 51.52 | 1.98 | 0.93–4.23 | .08 |
| Development of Lesion Morphology[b] | | | | | | | | | |
| Mucosal before cutaneous | 71 | 65.74 | 64 | 70.33 | 7 | 41.18 | 0.26 | 0.10–0.86 | .02 |
| Cutaneous before mucosal | 19 | 17.59 | 13 | 14.29 | 6 | 35.29 | 0.26 | 0.10–0.86 | .02 |
| No response | 18 | 16.67 | 14 | 15.38 | 4 | 23.53 | 3.27 | 1.03–10.39 | .04 |

Differences between the NAPV and non-NAPV population are represented as odds ratio (OR), 95% confidence limit (CL), and P value. Disease characteristics are presented as raw number of patients and percent of respondents (n = 171), or out of each subgroup (NAPV, n = 137; non-NAPV, n = 34), or percent of patients who responded to the respective questions.
    [a] History of lesion morphology (all PV n = 164; NAPV, n = 131; non-NAPV, n = 33).
    [b] Development of lesion morphology (all PV n = 108; NAPV, n = 77; non-NAPV, n = 13).

The average age of onset for disease in the combined (NAPV and non-NAPV) PV population was 45.2 years (range 17–74 years). The diagnosis of PV was confirmed by biopsy in nearly all participants (n = 168, 98%). In a considerable number of patients, however, the initial biopsy did not reveal the diagnosis of PV (n = 24, 14.0%). Of those who were initially misdiagnosed, the length of time that patients experienced symptoms before being correctly diagnosed ranged from 1 to 24 months (mean, 8 months).

Half of all PV survey respondents were in an active phase of disease (continuous presence of nontransient lesions), whereas the other half was in remission (no lesions or transient lesions only; transient defined as lasting less than a week) (see **Table 2**).[23]

65.85% of patients reported a history of mucocutaneous lesions (n = 108), followed by a history of mucosal-only (22.56%, n = 37) and a history of cutaneous-only (11.59%, n = 19) lesions (see **Table 2**). Of note, the history of cutaneous-only disease morphology (ie, never had mucosal lesions) was significantly less frequent in the NAPV population (OR 0.37; 95% CL 0.13–1.03;

P = .0495). Among participants who had experienced both mucosal and cutaneous lesions, a greater number manifested with mucous membrane lesions before the development of cutaneous lesions in both populations (65.7%, n = 71) than cutaneous before mucous membrane lesions (17.6%, n = 19), However, the percentage of NAPV patients who presented with mucosal lesions before cutaneous lesions was significantly higher than those in the non-NAPV group. Conversely, the non-NAPV population had a significantly higher percentage of patients who developed cutaneous lesions before mucosal lesions than that reported by the NAPV population (see **Table 2**).

Both mucosal and cutaneous lesion sites in patients were widely distributed over all areas of the body. Patients with mucosal disease (in both the mucosal-only and mucocutaneous disease manifestation) reported predominantly oral lesions (97.24%, n = 141), followed by involvement of the nasal passages, and less commonly anogenital or conjunctival lesions. Subjects with cutaneous disease (in both the cutaneous-only and mucocutaneous disease manifestation) reported lesions mainly on the scalp and face (n = 106, 83.46%;

n = 61, 48.06%, respectively), less on the torso (chest n = 95, 74.80%; back n = 89, 70.08%; abdomen n = 72, 56.67%), followed by the extremities (arms n = 66, 51.97%; legs n = 53, 41.73%; hands n = 32, 25.20%; feet n = 19, 14.96%).

The difference between the NAPV and non-NAPV populations regarding mucosal lesion distribution was calculated in patients experiencing mucosal-only or mucocutaneous lesions. Cutaneous lesion distribution was calculated in patients experiencing cutaneous-only or mucocutaneous lesions. To address whether patients with distinct morphologic profiles exhibit different lesion distribution patterns, this analysis was repeated for each of the 3 morphologic groups described above: mucosal-only, mucocutaneous, and cutaneous-only. The authors find that regardless of the subgroup analyzed, the general distribution patterns remained the same, and there were only negligible differences between the NAPV and non-NAPV populations (data not shown).

## Comorbidity

Because several comorbidities have been reported with various autoimmune diseases,[24,25] it was next assessed whether other autoimmune diseases and cancers were prevalent among patients in the study population. Thirty-five of all 171 PV patients (20.5%) reported an additional autoimmune diagnosis. Nearly half (n = 16) of these were affected by autoimmune thyroid disease (**Fig. 1**). A history of cancer was reported

in 19 of the 171 PV patients (11%). Twelve of these 19 patients reported a history of skin cancer of an unspecified type. A limited number of patients listed cervical- (n = 2), prostate- (n = 2), breast- (n = 1), stomach/colon- (n = 1), or thyroid cancer (n = 1), and thymoma (n = 1). No patients reported a history of lymphoma or leukemia.

## Genetics/Family History

Autoimmune diseases tend to run in families, and patients with a particular autoimmune condition often have one or more family members afflicted with autoimmunity.[24-26] Forty-eight percent of the PV patients in this study (n = 82) reported having a relative with an autoimmune disease, ranging from 1 to 11 affected family members per patient. A total of 172 relatives with autoimmune disease were reported by patients, including 87 (50.6%) first-degree, 59 (34.3%) second-degree, and 26 (15.1%) third-degree relatives.

Five patients in the study had a total of 15 relatives of the first, second, and third degree who had PV themselves (**Fig. 2**). The remaining patients with a family history of autoimmune disease had relatives affected by a wide range of autoimmune diseases, the 3 most common of which were type 1 diabetes (n = 27), thyroid disease (n = 25), and psoriasis (n = 13).

## Subjective Trigger Factors

To shed light on environmental agents potentially relevant for disease induction, patients were asked

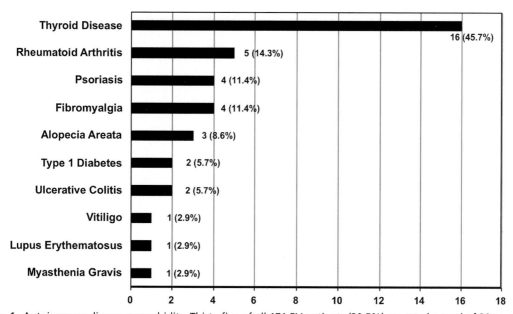

**Fig. 1.** Autoimmune disease comorbidity. Thirty-five of all 171 PV patients (20.5%) reported a total of 39 comorbid autoimmune diseases. The distribution of comorbid autoimmune disease among PV patients is presented as raw numbers of patients and percentage of patients with comorbid autoimmune disease (n = 35).

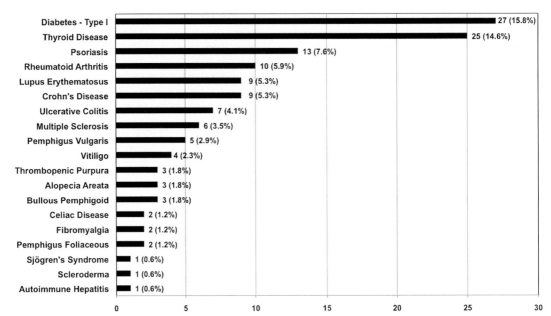

**Fig. 2.** Family history of autoimmune disease. Eighty-two patients (48% of all PV participants) reported a total of 172 relatives with autoimmune disease. Because an individual patient could have one or more relatives with a given autoimmune disease, a total of 133 autoimmune disease affiliations per 82 patients were recorded. Data are presented as number of patients with at least one relative afflicted by the respective autoimmune disease.

to document factors they believed may have triggered the onset of their disease. Sixty-two percent of patients (n = 106) reported subjective trigger factors (**Fig. 3**). Since participants could select more than one trigger, a total of 138 responses were recorded from these 106 patients. Thirty-eight percent (n = 65) of all PV patients reported experiencing a significant emotional trauma/stress before the onset of their disease (including loss of employment, death of a loved one, exposure to violence, neglect, verbal abuse, low self esteem, and depression). Other commonly reported

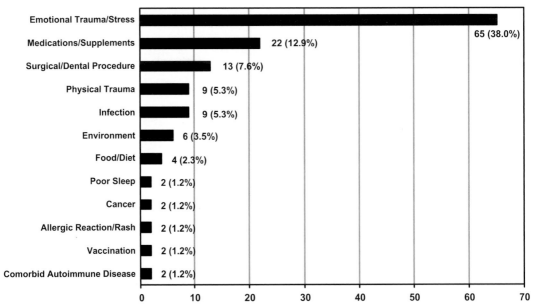

**Fig. 3.** Distribution of subjective trigger factors. One hundred and six patients (62% of all PV participants) reported a total of 138 subjective trigger factors. Data are presented as number of trigger factors reported (percent of all PV patients).

subjective trigger factors were the use of a medication or supplement, a surgical/dental procedure, physical trauma, and illness (mostly infectious in nature). Less commonly mentioned were food/diet, poor sleep, cancer, allergic reaction/rash, vaccination, and climate-associated environmental factors.

When asked whether they had any history of infection before the onset of disease, 64 PV patients reported a total of 76 infections (again, patients could report more than one infection). The most frequently reported infections were of the herpes virus group (n = 35, 46.1% of all reported infections or 20.5% of all participants), including 27 patients with a history of herpes simplex type 1 or 2, 5 with herpes zoster, and 3 with Epstein-Barr virus (EBV) infection (**Fig. 4**).

Food triggers have been described[27,28] but not comprehensively analyzed in PV. Forty percent of all PV study participants (n = 69) indicated that they felt certain food groups precipitate lesion development. The most common food triggers were fruits and vegetables (n = 30, 44.8%), followed by desserts and beverages (n = 13, 18.8%), breads, cereals, and pastas (n = 6, 8.7%), meats, poultry, and fish (n = 5, 7.2%), and milk (n = 4, 5.8%). Sixty-two of 69 patients implicated specific foods such as onions (n = 19) and garlic (n = 22), or general categories such as acidic (n = 29), spicy (n = 21), and hard/crunchy foods (n = 8).

Hormones have also been suggested as possible trigger factors for PV.[9] However, only 18 out of 171 PV patients in the cohort (10.5%) were on hormone replacement therapy (16 female and 2 male). Among the female patients, 11 reported using estrogen, 4 were on nonspecified birth control, 1 took testosterone, and 1 reported thyroid hormone replacement therapy. The 2 male patients were both receiving testosterone.

## DISCUSSION

To date, few large-scale epidemiologic studies have been conducted on PV. This study aimed to fill gaps in knowledge of PV disease characteristics and epidemiology by devising a globally accessible, Internet-based, anonymous survey to comprehensively capture information related to a broad range of disease-associated parameters. This online study was answered predominantly by patients residing in North America, most likely due to the authors' initial announcements through the US-based IPPF. Nevertheless, word of the study spread through online message boards beyond the United States.

Despite the inherent risk of misinterpretation of disease-related parameters in patient self-reporting, and the possibility that patients with severe disease are more likely to join a foundation and/or actively search the Internet for information, overall the survey provides a previously unattainable platform for collecting wide-scale epidemiologic and demographic data relevant to the pathogenesis and clinical expression of complex human diseases, particularly for rare conditions such as pemphigus vulgaris. The authors' approach overcomes recruiting biases of other

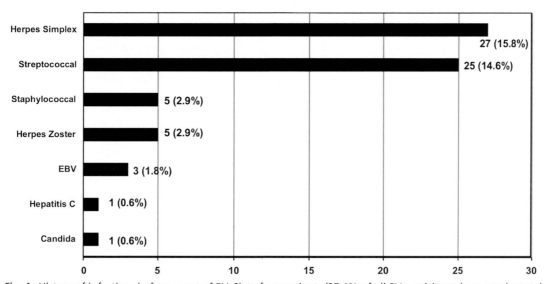

**Fig. 4.** History of infections before onset of PV. Sixty-four patients (37.4% of all PV participants) reported a total of 76 previous infections. Data are presented as number of infections reported (percent of all PV patients). Herpes simplex includes Types 1 and 2; EBV, Epstein-Barr virus.

studies, such as inclusion of patients from restricted geographic areas or availability of insurance coverage to be evaluated by physicians or medical centers performing a certain study. The study is in accordance with the majority of other studies in the literature that report a female predominance in PV, ranging from 1:1.1 to 1:2.25,[1–3,5,9–11,14,29–40] a predominant onset of disease in the fifth decade of life,[9,13,14,35,36] and a predominance of PV in the Ashkenazi Jewish population,[7,8] thus validating the self-reported data collection approach.

The higher number of women versus males with PV echoes the female predominance reported in numerous other autoimmune diseases,[41] although it should be noted that there are a limited number of studies on pemphigus that do not show a female predominance.[12,42–45] An alternative explanation for the predominance of female participants in this study, and the majority of others, may be potentially related in part to the previously documented under-representation of males in survey participation.[46]

Two major morphologic subtypes based on clinical and serologic criteria have been described in PV, the mucosal-dominant and the mucocutaneous types.[47] Correspondingly, in this survey a majority of NAPV and non-NAPV patients reported having a history of one of these two morphologies. While development of mucosal before cutaneous lesions is most common for the mucocutaneous subtype, a sizable portion of PV patients in this study reported the development of cutaneous lesions before developing mucosal lesions, particularly in the non-NAPV population. Also, the non-NAPV population was significantly more likely to report a history of cutaneous-only lesions. A history of cutaneous-only phenotype in PV (ie, never had mucosal lesions) has only rarely been described, but is not unknown. For example, 36.5% of PV patients in a 1998 study conducted in eastern Sicily had initial cutaneous lesions, and 22.2% had exclusively skin manifestations (ie, never had mucosal lesions).[34] Although the desmoglein compensation hypothesis posits that patients with mucosal lesions predominantly have anti-Dsg3 antibodies while patients with the mucocutaneous phenotype additionally have antibodies to Dsg1,[48,49] Yoshida and colleagues[50] reported 4 cases of cutaneous-only PV with an autoantibody profile characterized by high amounts of anti-Dsg1 antibodies but lower anti-Dsg3 levels. These investigators hypothesize that the less frequently seen cutaneous-only phenotype could be produced by pathogenically weak anti-Dsg3 IgG in the presence of potent anti-Dsg1 autoantibodies.[50]

In addition to environmental factors, genetic differences leading to distinct antibody profiles may explain the apparent bias toward cutaneous manifestations in the non-NAPV population in this study. A recent study comparing White European with Indo-Asian PV in patients found a positive association with certain HLA alleles conferring a possible protection against development of Dsg1 antibodies in the former population,[51] which could bias this population toward more mucous membrane manifestations. Because in the present study the non-NAPV population was composed of significantly fewer Caucasian but more Asian participants, possible differences in HLA type could be linked to the differences in lesion morphology and lesion development reported by the patients. In future studies, it will be interesting to correlate the clinical phenotype and the antibody profiles in different populations with their HLA type.

Disorders of autoimmune pathogenesis occur with increased frequency in patients with a history of other autoimmune diseases.[24,25] Twenty percent of participants with PV in the present study also had been diagnosed with additional autoimmune diseases, almost half of which were autoimmune thyroid disease. The percentage of thyroid autoimmune disease reported in this study is similar to the percentage reported in a recent study,[52] in which 8.2% of 1517 patients with a range of systemic autoimmune conditions (including systemic lupus erythematosus, rheumatoid arthritis, and systemic sclerosis) also had Hashimoto thyroiditis or Graves disease. In PV, thyroid conditions have been documented in several case reports.[53,54] In a larger study from Greece, 2.6% of PV patients had thyroid gland problems.[11,55] Of interest, a study from Argentina[55] found that 7 of 15 PV patients examined had detectable levels of thyroid autoantibodies, but only 1 patient presented with clinical evidence of chronic thyroiditis. These data suggest that PV and autoimmune thyroid disease may share common pathogenetic factors.

The genetic basis of autoimmune conditions is reflected in numerous studies indicating that family members of patients with autoimmune diseases are more susceptible to the development of the same or, more frequently, other autoimmune diseases.[44] Apart from a family history of PV itself, participants in the present study reported several other autoimmune diseases affecting their family members, most commonly type 1 diabetes. A study investigating the prevalence of autoimmune diseases in family members of patients with PV[44] found a statistically significant increase in the prevalence of insulin-dependent diabetes ($P<.006$) in

830 relatives of PV patients when compared with a similar number of relatives from random healthy controls. The same study found a significant increase in rheumatoid arthritis ($P<.03$), and a borderline significant increase in autoimmune thyroid disease ($P<.06$). In the present study, thyroid conditions and rheumatoid arthritis were also seen at high rates in family members of PV patients. These results, and those of other published reports suggest a shared genetic background that predisposes individuals to the development of a variety of autoimmune diseases ("autoimmune diathesis"[44]). However, these findings may be reflective of shared environmental (trigger) factors relevant to the pathogenesis of autoimmunity.

In addition to comorbid autoimmune conditions, 11% of the PV participants in the present study reported a history of cancer, which is higher than the reported prevalence of cancer in the general population of the United States (4.1% as of July 1, 2007[56]). While paraneoplastic pemphigus has been described as a distinct entity associated with lymphoproliferative neoplasms,[57] an association between neoplasms and PV has not been established to date. Because the mean age of onset in this study is in the fifth decade of life (similar to other reports worldwide[9,13,14,35,36,39]), the seemingly increased incidence of neoplasms may simply reflect the fact that neoplasms are more common later in life.

Despite numerous case reports and substantial anecdotal data, data directly in support of specific triggering factors in the etiology of pemphigus are sparse. A majority of the study's total patient population subjectively identified triggers for the onset of their disease. The most commonly reported triggers were emotional stress, medication, surgical/dental procedures, physical stress/trauma, and illness. The authors acknowledge that the disadvantage of an anonymous online questionnaire is that patient selection cannot be controlled (ie, patients with more severe disease may be disproportionally included) and that the association of life events with PV may be misinterpreted as trigger factors by patients. Nevertheless, the data are in line with previous studies that implicate stressful life events as a risk factor for initiation or exacerbation of PV.[58,59] Other factors associated with increased risk of developing pemphigus, such as pesticides, metal vapors, and ultraviolet (UV) exposure, have also been described.[39,60,61] However, only 5.7% of the patients who reported subjective triggers in the study indicated environmental factors such as exposure to chemicals, toxins, or UV sun exposure as potentially relevant to the development of their disease. In addition,

influenza, tetanus/diphtheria, hepatitis B, and anti-rabies vaccines have been previously suggested as trigger factors.[62–65] However, in this study only 2 respondents felt that vaccination against poliomyelitis or influenza led to the onset of PV.

The percentage of self-reported herpes virus infection in the study population is well in line with the published prevalence rates for herpes in the general population (21%).[66] Nevertheless, Herpes virus infection in a PV-susceptible host could potentially trigger a nonspecific activation of the immune system, lead to an overproduction of humoral and cellular factors, and thus trigger or perpetuate the autoimmune cascade.[67,68] Although a direct causal link has not been established, an activating or exacerbating role of herpetoviridae has been suggested in PV.[68–72] Various reports have documented the existence of herpes simplex virus (HSV)-1/2, human herpes virus (HHV)-6, HHV-8, and EBV in PV blood and skin,[67,72,73] and, at least for HHV-8, detection via polymerase chain reaction was specific for pemphigus, but not other blistering skin diseases.[72] HSV-1/2 has been associated with perpetuating and slowing the healing of oral lesions.[71,74]

The emergence of the World Wide Web has provided a new avenue for global data collection. The new survey tool described here capitalizes on the possibilities of collecting disease-related information beyond restricted demographic areas. To the authors' knowledge, the present study provides the most comprehensive epidemiologic data and information pertaining to a wide range of defined clinical parameters in PV to date. This survey tool may be additionally useful in future studies for longitudinal data collection, to gather information regarding factors relevant to disease progression and to better address the still unresolved cyclical nature of autoimmune conditions.

## ACKNOWLEDGMENTS

The authors thank the patients who participated in this study for their cooperation, and the International Pemphigus and Pemphigoid Foundation (www.pemphigus.org) for their support of this study.

## REFERENCES

1. Salmanpour R, Shahkar H, Namazi MR, et al. Epidemiology of pemphigus in south-western Iran: a 10-year retrospective study (1991–2000). Int J Dermatol 2006;45(2):103–5.

2. Asilian A, Yoosefi A, Faghini G. Pemphigus vulgaris in Iran: epidemiology and clinical profile. Skinmed 2006;5(2):69–71.

3. Langan SM, Smeeth L, Hubbard R, et al. Bullous pemphigoid and pemphigus vulgaris—incidence and mortality in the UK: population based cohort study. BMJ 2008;337:a180.

4. Bystryn JC, Rudolph JL. Pemphigus. Lancet 2005; 366(9479):61–73.

5. Nanda A, Dvorak R, Al-Saeed K, et al. Spectrum of autoimmune bullous diseases in Kuwait. Int J Dermatol 2004;43(12):876–81.

6. Sinha AA, Lopez MT, McDevitt HO. Autoimmune diseases: the failure of self tolerance. Science 1990;248(4961):1380–8.

7. Sinha AA, Brautbar C, Szafer F, et al. A newly characterized HLA DQ beta allele associated with pemphigus vulgaris. Science 1988;239(4843):1026–9.

8. Lee E, Lendas KA, Chow S, et al. Disease relevant HLA class II alleles isolated by genotypic, haplotypic, and sequence analysis in North American Caucasians with pemphigus vulgaris. Hum Immunol 2006;67(1–2):125–39.

9. Brenner S, Wohl Y. A survey of sex differences in 249 pemphigus patients and possible explanations. Skinmed 2007;6(4):163–5.

10. Chams-Davatchi C, Valikhani M, Daneshpazhooh M, et al. Pemphigus: analysis of 1209 cases. Int J Dermatol 2005;44(6):470–6.

11. Michailidou EZ, Belazi MA, Markopoulos AK, et al. Epidemiologic survey of pemphigus vulgaris with oral manifestations in northern Greece: retrospective study of 129 patients. Int J Dermatol 2007;46(4):356–61.

12. Tallab T, Joharji H, Bahamdan K, et al. The incidence of pemphigus in the southern region of Saudi Arabia. Int J Dermatol 2001;40(9):570–2.

13. Tsankov N, Vassileva S, Kamarashev J, et al. Epidemiology of pemphigus in Sofia, Bulgaria. A 16-year retrospective study (1980–1995). Int J Dermatol 2000;39(2):104–8.

14. Uzun S, Durdu M, Akman A, et al. Pemphigus in the Mediterranean region of Turkey: a study of 148 cases. Int J Dermatol 2006;45(5):523–8.

15. Fox S. Online Health Search 2006. Available at: http://www.pewinternet.org/Reports/2006/Online-Health-Search-2006.aspx. Accessed December 23, 2010.

16. Cumming GP, Currie HD, Moncur R, et al. Web-based survey on the effect of menopause on women's libido in a computer-literate population. Menopause Int 2009;15(1):8–12.

17. Oladimeji O, Farris KB, Urmie JG, et al. Risk factors for self-reported adverse drug events among Medicare enrollees. Ann Pharmacother 2008;42(1):53–61.

18. Dawn A, Papoiu AD, Chan YH, et al. Itch characteristics in atopic dermatitis: results of a web-based questionnaire. Br J Dermatol 2009;160(3):642–4.

19. Kelly MD. Traumatic neuralgia from pressure-point strikes in the martial arts: results from a retrospective online survey. J Am Osteopath Assoc 2008;108(6): 284–7.

20. Anthony J, Heeter C, Reed PL, et al. Longitudinal study engine users manual. Version 1.0. Available at: http://bric.msu.edu/?q=node/26. Accessed January 12, 2010.

21. Harman KE, Gratian MJ, Bhogal BS, et al. A study of desmoglein 1 autoantibodies in pemphigus vulgaris: racial differences in frequency and the association with a more severe phenotype. Br J Dermatol 2000;143(2):343–8.

22. Lee E, Sinha AA. T cell targeted immunotherapy for autoimmune disease. Autoimmunity 2005;38(8): 577–96.

23. Murrell DF, Dick S, Ahmed AR, et al. Consensus statement on definitions of disease, end points, and therapeutic response for pemphigus. J Am Acad Dermatol 2008;58(6):1043–6.

24. Humbert P, Dupond JL, Vuitton D, et al. Dermatological autoimmune diseases and the multiple autoimmune syndromes. Acta Derm Venereol Suppl (Stockh) 1989;148:1–8.

25. Mohan MP, Ramesh TC. Multiple autoimmune syndrome. Indian J Dermatol Venereol Leprol 2003;69(4):298–9.

26. Bordel-Gomez MT, Sanchez-Estella J, Yuste-Chaves M, et al. [Familial pemphigus vulgaris: immunogenetic study of HLA class II antigens]. Actas Dermosifiliogr 2006;97(8):509–13 [in Spanish].

27. Brenner S, Wolf R. Possible nutritional factors in induced pemphigus. Dermatology 1994;189(4): 337–9.

28. Feliciani C, Ruocco E, Zampetti A, et al. Tannic acid induces in vitro acantholysis of keratinocytes via IL-1alpha and TNF-alpha. Int J Immunopathol Pharmacol 2007;20(2):289–99.

29. Aboobaker J, Morar N, Ramdial PK, et al. Pemphigus in South Africa. Int J Dermatol 2001; 40(2):115–9.

30. Golusin Z, Poljacki M, Jovanovic M, et al. Some epidemiological features of pemphigus chronicus in South Vojvodina: a 12-year retrospective study. Int J Dermatol 2005;44(9):792–3.

31. Hahn-Ristic K, Rzany B, Amagai M, et al. Increased incidence of pemphigus vulgaris in southern Europeans living in Germany compared with native Germans. J Eur Acad Dermatol Venereol 2002;16(1):68–71.

32. Heymann AD, Chodick G, Kramer E, et al. Pemphigus variant associated with penicillin use: a case-cohort study of 363 patients from Israel. Arch Dermatol 2007;143(6):704–7.

33. Hietanen J, Salo OP. Pemphigus: an epidemiological study of patients treated in Finnish hospitals between 1969 and 1978. Acta Derm Venereol 1982;62(6):491–6.

34. Micali G, Musumeci ML, Nasca MR. Epidemiologic analysis and clinical course of 84 consecutive cases of pemphigus in eastern Sicily. Int J Dermatol 1998; 37(3):197–200.

35. Seo PG, Choi WW, Chung JH. Pemphigus in Korea: clinical manifestations and treatment protocol. J Dermatol 2003;30(11):782–8.

36. Shamsadini S, Fekri AR, Esfandiarpoor I, et al. Determination of survival and hazard functions for pemphigus patients in Kerman, a southern province of Iran. Int J Dermatol 2006;45(6):668–71.

37. Valikhani M, Kavusi S, Chams-Davatchi C, et al. Pemphigus and associated environmental factors: a case-control study. Clin Exp Dermatol 2007; 32(3):256–60.

38. V'Lckova-Laskoska MT, Laskoski DS, Kamberova S, et al. Epidemiology of pemphigus in Macedonia: a 15-year retrospective study (1990-2004). Int J Dermatol 2007;46(3):253–8.

39. Wohl Y, Brenner S. Pemphigus in Israel—an epidemiologic analysis of cases in search of risk factors. Isr Med Assoc J 2003;5(6):410–2.

40. Simon DG, Krutchkoff D, Kaslow RA, et al. Pemphigus in Hartford County, Connecticut, from 1972 to 1977. Arch Dermatol 1980;116(9):1035–7.

41. McCarthy M. The "gender gap" in autoimmune disease. Lancet 2000;356(9235):1088.

42. Abreu-Velez AM, Hashimoto T, Bollag WB, et al. A unique form of endemic pemphigus in northern Colombia. J Am Acad Dermatol 2003;49(4):599–608.

43. Bastuji-Garin S, Turki H, Mokhtar I, et al. Possible relation of Tunisian pemphigus with traditional cosmetics: a multicenter case-control study. Am J Epidemiol 2002;155(3):249–56.

44. Firooz A, Mazhar A, Ahmed AR. Prevalence of autoimmune diseases in the family members of patients with pemphigus vulgaris. J Am Acad Dermatol 1994; 31(3 Pt 1):434–7.

45. Goon AT, Tan SH. Comparative study of pemphigus vulgaris and pemphigus foliaceus in Singapore. Australas J Dermatol 2001;42(3):172–5.

46. O'Rourke D, Lakner E. Gender bias: analysis of factors causing male underrepresentation in surveys. Int J Publ Opin Res 1989;1(2):164–76.

47. Amagai M, Tsunoda K, Zillikens D, et al. The clinical phenotype of pemphigus is defined by the anti-desmoglein autoantibody profile. J Am Acad Dermatol 1999;40(2 Pt 1):167–70.

48. Mahoney MG, Wang Z, Rothenberger K, et al. Explanations for the clinical and microscopic localization of lesions in pemphigus foliaceus and vulgaris. J Clin Invest 1999;103(4):461–8.

49. Kalish RS. Pemphigus vulgaris: the other half of the story. J Clin Invest 2000;106(12):1433–5.

50. Yoshida K, Takae Y, Saito H, et al. Cutaneous type pemphigus vulgaris: a rare clinical phenotype of pemphigus. J Am Acad Dermatol 2005;52(5):839–45.

51. Saha M, Harman K, Mortimer NJ, et al. Pemphigus vulgaris in White Europeans is linked with HLA class II allele HLA DRB1*1454 but not DRB1*1401. J Invest Dermatol 2010;130:311–4.

52. Biro E, Szekanecz Z, Czirjak L, et al. Association of systemic and thyroid autoimmune diseases. Clin Rheumatol 2006;25(2):240–5.

53. Yalcin B, Tamer E, Toy GG, et al. Development of pemphigus vulgaris in a patient with vitiligo and Hashimoto's thyroiditis. J Endocrinol Invest 2005;28(6): 558–60.

54. Iino Y, Hara H, Suda T, et al. Co-existence of pemphigus vulgaris and Hashimoto's thyroiditis. Eur J Dermatol 2005;15(1):40–2.

55. Pitoia F, Moncet D, Glorio R, et al. Prevalence of thyroid autoimmunity in patients with pemphigus vulgaris. Medicina (B Aires) 2005;65(4):307–10.

56. Altekruse SF, Kosary CL, Krapcho M, et al, editors. SEER cancer statistics review, 1975–2007, National Cancer Institute. Bethesda, MD. Available at: http://seer.cancer.gov/csr/1975_2007/, based on November 2009 SEER data submission, posted to the SEER web site, 2010.

57. Zhu X, Zhang B. Paraneoplastic pemphigus. J Dermatol 2007;34(8):503–11.

58. Cremniter D, Baudin M, Roujeau JC, et al. Stressful life events as potential triggers of pemphigus. Arch Dermatol 1998;134(11):1486–7.

59. Morell-Dubois S, Carpentier O, Cottencin O, et al. Stressful life events and pemphigus. Dermatology 2008;216(2):104–8.

60. Aoki V, Millikan RC, Rivitti EA, et al. Environmental risk factors in endemic pemphigus foliaceus (fogo selvagem). J Investig Dermatol Symp Proc 2004;9(1):34–40.

61. Brenner S, Tur E, Shapiro J, et al. Pemphigus vulgaris: environmental factors. Occupational, behavioral, medical, and qualitative food frequency questionnaire. Int J Dermatol 2001;40(9):562–9.

62. Mignogna MD, Lo Muzio L, Ruocco E. Pemphigus induction by influenza vaccination. Int J Dermatol 2000;39(10):800.

63. Cozzani E, Cacciapuoti M, Parodi A, et al. Pemphigus following tetanus and diphtheria vaccination. Br J Dermatol 2002;147(1):188–9.

64. Berkun Y, Mimouni D, Shoenfeld Y. Pemphigus following hepatitis B vaccination–coincidence or causality? Autoimmunity 2005;38(2):117–9.

65. Yalcin B, Alli N. Pemphigus vulgaris following antirabies vaccination. J Dermatol 2007;34(10):734–5.

66. Xu F, Sternberg MR, Kottiri BJ, et al. Trends in herpes simplex virus type 1 and type 2 seroprevalence in the United States. JAMA 2006;296(8):964–73.

67. Tufano MA, Baroni A, Buommino E, et al. Detection of herpesvirus DNA in peripheral blood mononuclear cells and skin lesions of patients with pemphigus by polymerase chain reaction. Br J Dermatol 1999;141(6):1033–9.

68. Ruocco V, Wolf R, Ruocco E, et al. Viruses in pemphigus: a casual or causal relationship? Int J Dermatol 1996;35(11):782–4.

69. Brenner S, Sasson A, Sharon O. Pemphigus and infections. Clin Dermatol 2002;20(2):114–8.

70. Memar OM, Rady PL, Goldblum RM, et al. Human herpesvirus 8 DNA sequences in blistering skin from patients with pemphigus. Arch Dermatol 1997;133(10):1247–51.

71. Schlupen EM, Wollenberg A, Hanel S, et al. Detection of herpes simplex virus in exacerbated pemphigus vulgaris by polymerase chain reaction. Dermatology 1996;192(4):312–6.

72. Jang HS, Oh CK, Lim JY, et al. Detection of human herpesvirus 8 DNA in pemphigus and chronic blistering skin diseases. J Korean Med Sci 2000;15(4): 442–8.

73. Memar OM, Rady PL, Goldblum RM, et al. Human herpesvirus-8 DNA sequences in a patient with pemphigus vulgaris, but without HIV infection or Kaposi's sarcoma. J Invest Dermatol 1997;108(1): 118–9.

74. Kalra A, Ratho RK, Kaur I, et al. Role of herpes simplex and cytomegalo viruses in recalcitrant oral lesions of pemphigus vulgaris. Int J Dermatol 2005;44(3):259–60.

# Diagnosis and Clinical Features of Pemphigus Foliaceus

Kirk A. James, BS, Donna A. Culton, MD, PhD,
Luis A. Diaz, MD*

## KEYWORDS

- Pemphigus foliaceus • Fogo selvagem • Endemic
- Desmoglein 1 • Diagnosis • History

Pemphigus foliaceus (PF) is an acquired autoimmune blistering disease in which the body's immune system produces IgG autoantibodies that target the intercellular adhesion glycoprotein desmoglein (dsg)-1. The binding of these autoantibodies to dsg-1, which is principally expressed in the granular layer of the epidermis, results in the loss of intercellular connections between keratinocytes (acantholysis) and the formation of subcorneal blisters within the epidermis. The ultimate clinical manifestations of this process are fragile, superficial blisters and bullae of the cutaneous surface that easily rupture to yield erosive lesions.

The pathogenic autoantibodies of PF are of the IgG4 subclass, which has been demonstrated by their passive transfer from human sera to neonatal mice.[1] These IgG4 autoantibodies recognize antigenic epitopes located on the N-terminus of the ectodomain of dsg-1, specifically on extracellular domains 1 and 2.[2,3] The binding of pathogenic IgG to dsg-1 triggers the phosphorylation of p38 mitogen-activated protein kinase, which is thought to induce apoptosis of the affected keratinocyte.[4–6] Although complement component (C) 3 deposition on direct immunofluorescence (DIF) initially suggested that it may play a role in acantholysis in PF, both C5-deficient mice and total complement-depleted mice develop subcorneal vesicles upon passive transfer of pathogenic human sera.[7] The pathogenesis of PF is covered elsewhere in this issue in more detail by Valeria Aoki.

There are two predominant types of PF: idiopathic PF, which is found universally and occurs sporadically, and fogo selvagem (FS), an endemic variety linked exclusively to multiple distinct geographic areas. Other, albeit rarer, variants of PF have been described, including pemphigus erythematosus (PE, Senear-Usher syndrome) and drug-induced PF. IgA pemphigus and pemphigus herpetiformis (PH) have previously been described in the literature as variants of PF, but appear to be distinct subtypes of the general pemphigus category, both clinically and histopathologically.[8]

## CLINICAL FEATURES
### Epidemiology

The worldwide incidence and prevalence of PF is very low, making it a rare disease. Because of the presence of endemic areas, however, these figures may vary considerably based on the specific geographic area being studied. For instance, the incidence of PF in Tunisia has been found to be as high as 6.7 new cases per million per year.[9] In Brazil, which has multiple foci of endemic PF, there is a region located in the state of Mato Grosso do Sul that has a prevalence equal to approximately 3% of its population.[10,11] Other

Financial disclosure and conflict of interest statement: The authors have no financial disclosures or conflicts of interest to express.

Department of Dermatology, University of North Carolina at Chapel Hill, 405 Mary Ellen Jones Building, CB#7287, Chapel Hill, NC 27599–7287, USA

* Corresponding author.

E-mail address: luis_diaz@med.unc.edu

Dermatol Clin 29 (2011) 405–412

doi:10.1016/j.det.2011.03.012

endemic areas are found within Colombia and Peru.[12–14] The average age of nonendemic PF symptom onset ranges from 40 to 60 years of age. FS affects a larger number of children and young adults as symptoms usually begin during the second or third decade of life.[14] Both sporadic and endemic PF are typically seen equally in men and women and affect those of all races and ethnicities. However, there are populations of FS that may deviate from the norm. For example, epidemiologic studies in Tunisia found the female-to-male ratio of incidence rates to be approximately 4 to 1.[9]

### Patient History

Patients usually report a history of blister formation on the skin (**Fig. 1**). Lesions commonly begin on the trunk, but may also originate as localized lesions on the face or scalp. The patient may be unaware of the blisters because they rupture very easily. In these cases, there may only be a history of superficial sores or areas of crusting. Pain and/or a burning sensation localized to the areas of the lesions may be noted. Unlike pemphigus vulgaris (PV), there is typically no history of oral or other mucosal lesions. The lesions may become widespread. Patients with the mildest form of PF may only report a history of a small, solitary, recurrent scaly and crusty lesion of the face (**Fig. 2**). In these cases, it may be years before the patient is correctly diagnosed. In cases of PE, patients report the development of lesions in sun-exposed areas of the face, scalp, and upper chest and back—similar to the distribution of lesions seen in lupus erythematosus.

Because multiple drugs have been found to be associated with the development of PF, it is important to thoroughly review the patient's current medications. The most commonly implicated drug is penicillamine, which is a chelating agent

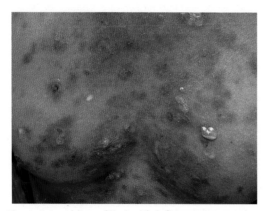

**Fig. 1.** Intact blister filled with inflammatory exudate on left side of chest.

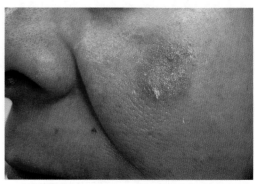

**Fig. 2.** Isolated scaly, erythematous plaque with peripheral erosion on left cheek.

used to treat Wilson disease, lead and arsenic poisoning, and severe active rheumatoid arthritis.[15] Drug-associated cases may persist or quickly clear after the offending agent is withdrawn. Various angiotensin-converting enzyme (ACE) inhibitors have also been found to induce pemphigus. **Box 1** shows other drugs that have been associated with PF. Most of these drugs contain thiol (-SH) functional groups in their chemical structure, whereas others have disulfide bonds that are cleaved during metabolism to yield thiol groups.[16] PF can also be either induced or exacerbated by exposure to ultraviolet light and ionizing radiation.[17–20]

A growing number of diseases have been associated with PF, including bullous pemphigoid, myasthenia gravis, and other autoimmune diseases.[29–32] A complete past medical history should also be obtained to identify all pre-existing medical

| Box 1 |
|---|
| **Drugs associated with PF** |
| ACE inhibitors |
|     Captopril[21] |
|     Lisinopril[22] |
|     Enalapril[23] |
|     Fosinopril[24] |
| Disease-modifying antirheumatic drugs |
|     Penicillamine |
|     Bucillamine[25] |
| Angiotensin-II receptor blockers |
|     Candesartan[26] |
|     Antibiotics |
|     Rifampicin[27] |
|     Orphan drugs |
|     Tiopronin[28] |

conditions of the patient. PF has been associated with certain neoplasms, including B-cell lymphoma, T-cell lymphoma, prostate cancer, and cutaneous squamous cell carcinoma.[33–36] Transition from PF to other forms of pemphigus and vice versa may occur. There have been a few documented cases of patients with clinical, histopathological, and serologic features of PV who subsequently underwent a confirmed transition to PF.[37,38] Although both are rare, this is found more commonly than a shift from PF to PV.[39]

Nonendemic PF may occur in the neonate via transplacental transit of pathogenic IgG anti–dsg-1 autoantibodies from a mother with active disease.[40–42] These cases are uncommon and most neonates born of mothers with PF will not develop active disease.[43] A study of 19 mothers with documented FS revealed that all respective babies were born with normal skin.[44] Given that the sera of all of the mothers showed high titers of FS autoantibodies, the placenta may act as an immunoadsorbant of unwanted autoantibodies.[45] Additionally, dsg-3 has been found to be present in all layers of the epidermis in neonates, including the superficial layer, in contrast to adults, who express dsg-1 superficially and dsg-3 intermediately and basally.[46] This expression of dsg-3 in the superficial epidermis is thought to be protective against the formation of blisters induced by PF antibodies in neonates.[46]

FS, which has been extensively studied in Brazil, is thought to be triggered by an environmental factor, perhaps from an antigen transmitted by the bite of a hematophagous insect, in genetically-susceptible individuals. The antibodies produced against this unidentified antigen may cross-react with dsg-1, leading to the development of FS. This theory is based on the following observations from endemic areas of Brazil: (1) Specific HLA genes have been associated with increased FS susceptibility,[47] (2) FS displays geographic and familial clustering, (3) the families typically share a common bedroom in poor living conditions, (4) the living dwellings tend to be infested with blood-feeding arthropods,[48] (5) a spike in FS cases occurs after the end of the rainy season when insect breeding conditions are optimal,[48] and (6) FS cases tend to decrease as the living conditions improve in endemic areas of Brazil.[10] Recent research has focused on the study of a protein transmitted from the saliva of *Simulium nigrimanum*, a type of black fly.[49]

## Physical Exam

The endemic and nonendemic forms of PF typically share the same clinical findings.[50] The primary lesions are flaccid, superficial vesicles and bullae of the skin. These lesions may not be seen on examination because of their fragile and subsequent transient nature. More often, only secondary lesions, such as shallow erosions, are seen. Scaling of these lesions is commonly seen, representing the detachment of the overlying stratum corneum from the area of intraepidermal acantholysis, the stratum granulosum. Most lesions appear on the chest, back, and shoulders (**Fig. 3**). On certain areas of the body such as the face and scalp, the exudate from the erosive lesions dries quickly, leaving areas of crusting over an erythematous base.

A common clinical finding in PF is a positive Nikolsky sign. This is performed by applying shear stress to the affected skin, usually by rubbing the periphery of existing primary or secondary lesions. If positive, this tangentially-applied force will result in the separation of the upper epidermal layers from the underlying lower layers. This finding has been shown to be moderately sensitive, but highly specific in diagnosing pemphigus.[51]

In its most severe form, PF can produce an exfoliative erythroderma characterized by generalized erythema and diffuse scaling of the cutaneous surface (**Fig. 4**). In these cases, it may also lead to alopecia. These patients require prompt hospitalization to prevent serious and sometimes fatal complications from metabolic instability.

The variant PE combines features of PF and lupus erythematosus. Small, flaccid vesicles and

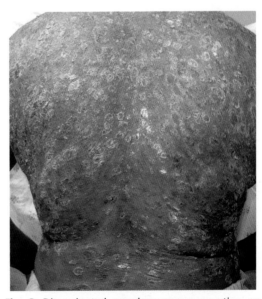

**Fig. 3.** Disseminated papulosquamous eruption on back evolving from the preceding superficial blisters and secondary erosions of PF.

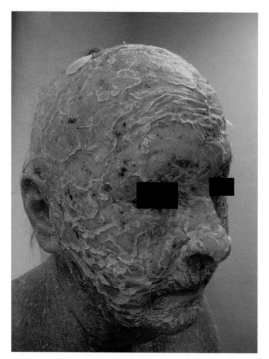

**Fig. 4.** Severe exfoliative erythroderma.

bullae may be seen in a butterfly-distribution on the face, involving the cheeks and nose. Photo-distributed lesions of the scalp, and upper chest and back are also common. Ruptured blisters reveal an erythematous base, and lesions on the face and scalp may have think, greasy scales and yellow crusts. Many patients test positive for antinuclear antibodies in their serum.[52]

Unusual presentations of PF have previously been described. Several cases have been documented of PF presenting as an acute eruption of multiple hyperpigmented and hyperkeratotic lesions that closely resemble the appearance of seborrheic keratoses.[53,54] In cases of sporadic PF in children, patients present with the same primary and secondary lesions, but they often have a distinct configuration having been described as arcuate, circinate, and/or polycyclic.[55]

### Differential Diagnosis

The differential diagnosis of endemic and nonendemic PF includes bullous impetigo, IgA pemphigus, PH, drug eruption, subcorneal pustular dermatosis, and lupus erythematosus. If lesions are localized to the face or scalp with abundant scaling and yellow crusting, seborrheic dermatitis may be considered. Papulosquamous diseases, including psoriasis, pityriasis rubra pilaris, and drug hypersensitivity, should be additional

diagnostic considerations for patients presenting with exfoliative erythroderma.

### Diagnosis

There are varieties of diagnostic studies that can be used to support clinical suspicion of PF. Histology and DIF require tissue samples from the patient. Biopsy for DIF should be taken from perilesional skin—normal-appearing skin immediately adjacent to a lesion—since inflamed and blistered skin may lead to the destruction of immune deposits and result in a false-negative study.[56] Indirect immunofluorescence (IIF) and ELISA studies require patient serum. Ultimately, the diagnosis of PF is based on three criteria: (1) the overall clinical picture, including patient history and physical examination; (2) the histopathological findings of the biopsy; and (3) the presence of autoantibodies as detected by DIF and IIF studies. None of these alone is diagnostic of PF.

### Histopathology

The earliest preacantholytic findings in PF are the formation of vacuoles within the intercellular spaces of the granular and/or upper spinous layers of the epidermis.[57] Eosinophilic spongiosis of the epidermis may also be seen.[58] As PF lesions progress, the vacuoles become larger and eventually lead to subcorneal blister formation within the upper epidermis (**Fig. 5**). There are variable amounts of acantholytic keratinocytes, neutrophils, and fibrin within the blisters.[59] Older PF lesions show evidence of chronic inflammation, including papillomatosis, acanthosis, hyperkeratosis, parakeratosis, and follicular plugging. Keratinocytes of the granular layer display dyskeratotic

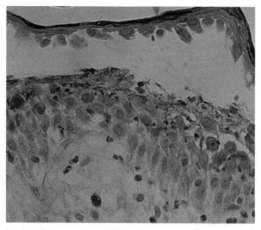

**Fig. 5.** Biopsy of PF lesion. Subcorneal blister formation due to acantholysis of keratinocytes.

changes. There is an increase in pigment formation of basal melanocytes. The capillaries of the papillary dermis become dilated. Upper dermal edema may be present to varying degrees. An inflammatory infiltrate composed of small amounts of neutrophils, eosinophils, and lymphocytes may be present in a variable distribution.[60]

## DIF

DIF is a special immunostaining procedure that is used to detect antibody and complement deposition within the tissue sample. For diagnosis of any pemphigus disease, its sensitivity has been found to range from 80% to 95%.[61] DIF becomes positive earlier in the course of disease than IIF and is, therefore, considered slightly more reliable in detecting the initial presentations of PF.[62] PF shows a DIF pattern characterized by fluorescent staining around keratinocytes, which is known as the intercellular space (ICS) staining pattern—representative of all pemphigus disease. In PF, this is a result of dsg-1–bound antibody on the desmosomes at the keratinocyte cell surface. The intensity of this fluorescent stain in PF may be greater in the upper epidermis due to the increased density of dsg-1 and subsequent antibody deposition in the superficial epidermis.[63] C3 may also stain at the ICS in PF.[64] PE may show staining of both the ICS and the basement membrane zone.[65]

## IIF

IIF is a staining technique that uses patient serum to identify antibodies directed against an antigen on a specific type of tissue substrate. It has been found to have a sensitivity ranging between 79% and 90% for diagnosing pemphigus disease.[61] Human skin is commonly used as substrate for IIF staining in patients suspected of having PF since it has been found to be more sensitive (greater density of dsg-1) whereas monkey esophagus is preferentially used to detect PV because of heightened sensitivity (greater density of dsg-3, the autoantigen target of PV).[66,67] However, the use of both has been found to improve sensitivity to 100%.[68] Like DIF, IIF will show ICS staining in PF with a potential greater fluorescent intensity in the upper epidermis (**Fig. 6**).[69] IgG subclass staining for PF shows both IgG1 and IgG4 subclasses are produced against dsg-1, with IgG4 being the predominant autoantibody subclass.[70,71] IIF titers can be used as an approximate estimate of disease activity in patients.[72] For instance, patients with severe disease will typically have high titers and patients with mild disease will

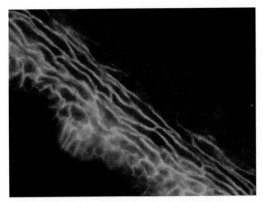

**Fig. 6.** Positive IIF staining using PF patient serum on human skin substrate. This staining pattern directed against the ICS is characteristic of pemphigus.

have low titers. The direct correlation of disease extent with the level of circulating IgG autoantibody as measured by IIF has been best demonstrated by mouse models of pemphigus.[73]

## ELISA

ELISA studies have been found to be a sensitive and specific tool for pemphigus diagnosis. This method uses purified recombinant human dsg-1 to detect PF IgG autoantibodies in patient serum.[74] ELISA also provides a quantitative way to measure the amount of circulating autoantibodies,[75] which can be used to monitor a patient's response to treatment. One study found that the sensitivity of diagnosing untreated cases of PF was 100%, whereas in treated cases it was 92%.[76] However, the negative cases could represent a successful response to treatment. The threshold for a positive result in this study was chosen to give a specificity of 98%. A larger study found the sensitivity and specificity of detecting dsg-1 autoantibodies in PF patients to be 97.9% and 98.9%, respectively.[77] In endemic regions of FS, the specificity of ELISA is relatively lower because more normal individuals in these areas test positive (increase in false positives) for total IgG anti–dsg-1 autoantibodies.[11] However, a positive ELISA result for IgG4 anti–dsg-1 autoantibodies in normal individuals from endemic areas can be used to predict those with preclinical FS who could develop clinical manifestations in the future.[78] Unlike the rough estimate of disease severity that IIF provides in humans, ELISA titers have been found to consistently correlate with disease activity throughout the patient's clinical course.[79–82] Therefore, it can be considered the best laboratory analysis for monitoring a patient's response to therapy.

## REFERENCES

1. Rock B, Martins CR, Theofilopoulos AN, et al. The pathogenic effect of IgG4 autoantibodies in endemic pemphigus foliaceus (fogo selvagem). N Engl J Med 1989;320:1463–9.

2. Sekiguchi M, Futei Y, Fujii Y. Dominant autoimmune epitopes recognized by pemphigus antibodies map to the N-terminal adhesive region of desmogleins. J Immunol 2001;167:5439–48.

3. Li N, Aoki V, Hans-Filho G, et al. The role of intramolecular epitope spreading in the pathogenesis of endemic pemphigus foliaceus (fogo selvagem). J Exp Med 2003;197:1501–10.

4. Rubenstein DS, Diaz LA. Pemphigus antibody induced phosphorylation of keratinocyte proteins. Autoimmunity 2006;39:577–86.

5. Berkowitz P, Chua M, Liu Z, et al. Autoantibodies in the autoimmune disease pemphigus foliaceus induce blistering via p38 mitogen-activated protein kinase-dependent signaling in the skin. Am J Pathol 2008;173:1628–36.

6. Lee HE, Berkowitz P, Jolly PS, et al. Biphasic activation of p38MAPK suggests that apoptosis is a downstream event in pemphigus acantholysis. J Biol Chem 2009;284:12524–32.

7. España A, Diaz LA, Mascaró JM Jr. Mechanisms of acantholysis in pemphigus foliaceus. Clin Immunol Immunopathol 1997;85:83–9.

8. Robinson ND, Hashimoto T, Amagai M, et al. The new pemphigus variants. J Am Acad Dermatol 1999;40:649–71.

9. Bastuji-Garin S, Souissi R, Blum L, et al. Comparative epidemiology of pemphigus in Tunisia and France unusual incidence of pemphigus foliaceus in young Tunisian women. J Invest Dermatol 1995; 104:302–5.

10. Culton DA, Qian Y, Li N, et al. Advances in pemphigus and its endemic pemphigus foliaceus. J Autoimmun 2008;31:311–24.

11. Warren SJ, Lin MS, Giudice GJ, et al. The prevalence of antibodies against desmoglein 1 in endemic pemphigus foliaceus in Brazil. Cooperative Group on Fogo Selvagem Research. N Engl J Med 2000;343:23–30.

12. Abreu-Velez AM, Hashimoto T, Bollag WB, et al. A unique form of endemic pemphigus in northern Colombia. J Am Acad Dermatol 2003;49:599–608.

13. Robledo MA, Prada S, Jaramillo D, et al. South American pemphigus foliaceus: study of an epidemic in El Bagre and Nechi, Colombia 1982 to 1986. Br J Dermatol 1988;118:737–44.

14. Meyer N, Misery L. Geoepidemiologic considerations of auto-immune pemphigus. Autoimmun Rev 2010;9:A379–82.

15. Penas PF, Buezo GF, Carvajal I, et al. D-Penicillamine-induced pemphigus foliaceus with autoantibodies to desmoglein-1 in a patient with mixed connective tissue disease. J Am Acad Dermatol 1997;37:121–3.

16. Brenner S, Bialy-Golan A, Ruocco V. Drug-induced pemphigus. Clin Dermatol 1998;16:393–7.

17. Perry HO, Brunsting LA. Pemphigus foliaceus. Further observations. Arch Dermatol 1965;91:10–23.

18. Cram DL, Winkelmann RK. Ultraviolet-induced acantholysis in pemphigus. Arch Dermatol 1965; 92:7–13.

19. Aghassi D, Dover JS. Pemphigus foliaceus induced by psoralen-UV-A. Arch Dermatol 1998;134: 1300–1.

20. Low GJ, Keeling JH. Ionizing radiation-induced pemphigus. Case presentations and literature review. Arch Dermatol 1990;126:1319–23.

21. Kaplan RP, Potter TS, Fox JN. Drug-induced pemphigus related to angiotensin-converting enzyme inhibitors. J Am Acad Dermatol 1992;26: 364–6.

22. Patterson CR, Davies MG. Pemphigus foliaceus: an adverse reaction to lisinopril. J Dermatolog Treat 2004;15:60–2.

23. Shelton RM. Pemphigus foliaceus associated with enalapril. J Am Acad Dermatol 1991;24:503–4.

24. Ong CS, Cook N, Lee S. Drug-related pemphigus and angiotensin converting enzyme inhibitors. Australas J Dermatol 2000;41:242–6.

25. Fujita H, Iguchi M, Watanabe R, et al. Pemphigus foliaceus induced by bucillamine. Eur J Dermatol 2007;17:98–9.

26. Bae YI, Yun SJ, Lee SC, et al. Pemphigus foliaceus induced by an angiotensin II receptor blocker. Clin Exp Dermatol 2008;33:721–3.

27. Lee CW, Lim JH, Kang HJ. Pemphigus foliaceus induced by rifampicin. Br J Dermatol 1984;111: 619–22.

28. Lucky PA, Skovby F, Thier SO. Pemphigus foliaceus and proteinuria induced by alpha-mercapto-propionylglycine. J Am Acad Dermatol 1983;8: 667–72.

29. Korman NJ, Stanley JR, Woodley DT. Coexistence of pemphigus foliaceus and bullous pemphigoid. Arch Dermatol 1991;127:387–90.

30. Ishiko A, Hashimoto T, Shimizu H, et al. Combined features of pemphigus foliaceus and bullous pemphigoid: immunoblot and immunoelectron microscopic studies. Arch Dermatol 1995;131:732–4.

31. Imamura S, Takigawa M, Ikai K, et al. Pemphigus foliaceus, myasthenia gravis, thymoma and red cell aplasia. Clin Exp Dermatol 1978;3:285–91.

32. Ng PP, Ng SK, Chng HH. Pemphigus foliaceus and oral lichen planus in a patient with systemic lupus erythematosus and thymoma. Clin Exp Dermatol 1998;23:181–4.

33. Cowley NC, Neill SM, Staughton RC. Pemphigus foliaceus and non-Hodgkin's lymphoma. Int J Dermatol 1994;33:510–1.

34. Rybojad M, Leblanc T, Flageul B, et al. Paraneoplastic pemphigus in a child with a T-cell lymphoblastic lymphoma. Br J Dermatol 1993;128:418–22.

35. Ota M, Sato-Matsumura KC, Matsumura T, et al. Pemphigus foliaceus and figurate erythema in a patient with prostate cancer. Br J Dermatol 2000; 142:816–8.

36. Inaoki M, Kaji K, Furuse S, et al. Pemphigus foliaceus developing after metastasis of cutaneous squamous cell carcinoma to regional lymph nodes. J Am Acad Dermatol 2001;45:767–70.

37. Kawana S, Hashimoto T, Nishikawa T, et al. Changes in clinical features, histologic findings, and antigen profiles with development of pemphigus foliaceus from pemphigus vulgaris. Arch Dermatol 1994;130: 1534–8.

38. Tsuji Y, Kawashima T, Yokota K, et al. Clinical and serological transition from pemphigus vulgaris to pemphigus foliaceus demonstrated by desmoglein ELISA system. Arch Dermatol 2002;138: 95–6.

39. Ishii K, Amagai M, Ohata Y, et al. Development of pemphigus vulgaris in a patient with pemphigus foliaceus: antidesmoglein antibody profile shift confirmed by enzyme-linked immunosorbent assay. J Am Acad Dermatol 2000;42:859–61.

40. Walker DC, Kolar KA, Hebert AA, et al. Neonatal pemphigus foliaceus. Arch Dermatol 1995;131: 1308–11.

41. Avalos-Díaz E, Olague-Marchan M, López-Swiderski A, et al. Transplacental passage of maternal pemphigus foliaceus autoantibodies induces neonatal pemphigus. J Am Acad Dermatol 2000;43:1130–4.

42. Hirsch R, Anderson J, Weinberg JM, et al. Neonatal pemphigus foliaceus. J Am Acad Dermatol 2003;49: S187–9.

43. Eyre RW, Stanley JR. Maternal pemphigus foliaceus with cell surface antibody bound in neonatal epidermis. Arch Dermatol 1988;124:25–7.

44. Rocha-Alvarez R, Friedman H, Campbell IT, et al. Pregnant women with endemic pemphigus foliaceus (Fogo Selvagem) give birth to disease-free babies. J Invest Dermatol 1992;99:78–82.

45. Swinburne LM. Leucocyte antigens and placental sponge. Lancet 1970;2:592–4.

46. Wu H, Wang ZH, Yan A, et al. Protection against pemphigus foliaceus by desmoglein 3 in neonates. N Engl J Med 2000;343:31–5.

47. Moraes ME, Fernandez-Vina M, Lazaro A, et al. An epitope in the third hypervariable region of the DRB1 gene is involved in the susceptibility to endemic pemphigus foliaceus (fogo selvagem) in three different Brazilian populations. Tissue Antigens 1997;49:35–40.

48. Eaton DP, Diaz LA, Hans-Filho G, et al. Comparison of black fly species on an American reservation with a high prevalence of fogo selvage to neighboring disease-free sites in the state of Mato Grosso do Sul, Brazil. J Med Entomol 1998;35:120–31.

49. Ribeiro JM, Valenzuela JG, Pham VM, et al. An insight into the sialotranscriptome of *Simulium nigrimanum*, a black fly associated with fogo selvagem in South America. Am J Trop Med Hyg 2010;82: 1060–75.

50. Diaz LA, Sampaio SA, Rivitti EA, et al. Endemic pemphigus foliaceus (fogo selvagem): II current and historic epidemiologic studies. J Invest Dermatol 1989;92:4–12.

51. Uzun S, Durdu M. The specificity and sensitivity of Nikolsky sign in the diagnosis of pemphigus. J Am Acad Dermatol 2006;54(3):411–5.

52. Steffen C, Thomas D. The men behind the eponym: Francis E. Senear, Barney Usher, and the Senear-Usher syndrome. Am J Dermatopathol 2003;25: 432–6.

53. Bruckner N, Katz RA, Hood AF. Pemphigus foliaceus resembling eruptive seborrheic keratoses. Arch Dermatol 1980;116:815–6.

54. Kahana M, Trau H, Schewach-Millet M, et al. Pemphigus foliaceus presenting as multiple giant seborrheic keratoses. J Am Acad Dermatol 1984; 11:299–300.

55. Metry DW, Hebert AA, Jordon RE. Nonendemic pemphigus foliaceus in children. J Am Acad Dermatol 2002;46:419–22.

56. Mutasim DF, Adams BB. Immunofluorescence in dermatology. J Am Acad Dermatol 2001;45: 803–22.

57. Kouskoukis CE, Ackerman AB. Vacuoles in the upper part of the epidermis as a clue to eventuation of superficial pemphigus and bullous impetigo. Am J Dermatopathol 1984;6:183–6.

58. Osteen FB, Wheeler CE Jr, Briggaman RA, et al. Pemphigus foliaceus. Early clinical appearance as dermatitis herpetiformis with eosinophilic spongiosis. Arch Dermatol 1976;112:1148–52.

59. Kouskoukis CE, Ackerman AB. What histologic finding distinguishes superficial pemphigus and bullous impetigo? Am J Dermatopathol 1984;6: 179–81.

60. Furtado T. Histopathology of pemphigus foliaceus. Arch Dermatol 1959;80:66.

61. Harrist TJ, Mihm MC Jr. Cutaneous immunopathology. The diagnostic use of direct and indirect immunofluorescence techniques in diagnostic dermatopathology. Hum Pathol 1979;10:625.

62. Judd KP, Lever WF. Correlation of antibodies in skin and serum with disease severity in pemphigus. Arch Dermatol 1979;115:428–32.

63. Rodriguez J, Bystryn JC. Pemphigus foliaceus associated with absence of intercellular antigens in lower layers of epidermis. Arch Dermatol 1977;113: 1696–9.

64. Bhogal B, Wojnarowska F, Black MM, et al. The distribution of immunoglobulins and the C3 component of complement in multiple biopsies from the uninvolved and perilesional skin in pemphigus. Clin Exp Dermatol 1986;11:49–53.

65. Chorzelski TP, Jablonska S, Blaszczyk M. Immunopathological investigations in the Senear-Usher syndrome (coexistence of pemphigus and lupus erythematosus). Br J Dermatol 1968;80:211–7.

66. Feibleman C, Stolzner G, Provost TT. Pemphigus: superiority of monkey esophagus in the determination of pemphigus antibody. Arch Dermatol 1981; 117:561–2.

67. Shirakata Y, Amagai M, Hanakawa Y, et al. Lack of mucosal involvement in pemphigus foliaceus may be due to low expression of desmoglein 1. J Invest Dermatol 1998;110:76–8.

68. Harman KE, Gratian MJ, Bhogal BS, et al. The use of two substrates to improve the sensitivity of indirect immunofluorescence in the diagnosis of pemphigus. Br J Dermatol 2000;142:1135–9.

69. Bystryn JC, Abel FL, DeFeo D. Pemphigus foliaceus: subcorneal intercellular antibodies of unique specificity. Arch Dermatol 1974;110:857–61.

70. Futei Y, Amagai M, Ishii K, et al. Predominant IgG4 subclass in autoantibodies of pemphigus vulgaris and foliaceus. J Dermatol Sci 2001;26:55–61.

71. Hacker MK, Janson M, Fairley JA, et al. Isotypes and antigenic profiles of pemphigus foliaceous and pemphigus vulgaris autoantibodies. Clin Immunol 2002;105:64–74.

72. Fitzpatrick RE, Newcomer VD. The correlation of disease activity and antibody titers in pemphigus. Arch Dermatol 1980;116:285–90.

73. Anhalt GJ, Labib RS, Voorhees JJ, et al. Induction of pemphigus in neonatal mice by passive transfer of IgG from patients with the disease. N Engl J Med 1982;306:1189–96.

74. Ishii K, Amagai M, Hall RP, et al. Characterization of autoantibodies in pemphigus using antigen-specific enzyme-linked immunosorbent assays with baculovirus-expressed recombinant desmogleins. J Immunol 1997;159:2010–7.

75. Crowther JR. ELISA. Theory and practice. Methods Mol Biol 1995;42:1–218.

76. Harman KE, Gratian MJ, Seed PT, et al. Diagnosis of pemphigus by ELISA: a critical evaluation of two ELISAs for the detection of antibodies to the major pemphigus antigens, desmoglein 1 and 3. Clin Exp Dermatol 2000;25:236–40.

77. Amagai M, Komai A, Hashimoto T, et al. Usefulness of enzyme-linked immunosorbent assay (ELISA) using recombinant desmogleins 1 and 3 for serodiagnosis of pemphigus. Br J Dermatol 1999;140:351–7.

78. Qaqish BF, Prisayanh P, Qian Y, et al. Development of an IgG4-based predictor of endemic pemphigus foliaceus (fogo selvagem). J Invest Dermatol 2009; 129:110–8.

79. Aoyama Y, Tsujimura Y, Funabashi M, et al. An experience for ELISA for desmoglein 1, suggesting a possible diagnostic help to determine the initial therapy for pemphigus foliaceus. Eur J Dermatol 2000;10:18–21.

80. Cheng SW, Kobayashi M, Kinoshita-Kuroda K, et al. Monitoring disease activity in pemphigus with enzyme-linked immunosorbent assay using recombinant desmogleins 1 and 3. Br J Dermatol 2002;147:261–5.

81. Abasq C, Mouquet H, Gilbert D, et al. ELISA testing of anti-desmoglein 1 and 3 antibodies in the management of pemphigus. Arch Dermatol 2009; 145:529–35.

82. Schmidt E, Dähnrich C, Rosemann A, et al. Novel ELISA systems for antibodies to desmoglein 1 and 3: correlation of disease activity with serum autoantibody levels in individual pemphigus patients. Exp Dermatol 2010;19:458–63.

# Pathogenesis of Endemic Pemphigus Foliaceus

Valeria Aoki, MD[a],*, Joaquim Xavier Sousa Jr, MD[a],
Luis A. Diaz, MD[b], The Cooperative Group on Fogo
Selvagem Research

## KEYWORDS

• Autoimmunity • Pemphigus • Desmoglein

Pemphigus refers to a group of human autoimmune blistering diseases involving skin and/or mucous membranes.[1,2] Circulating and in situ autoantibodies against epithelial transmembrane glycoproteins of the desmosome, mostly desmoglein 1 (Dsg1) and desmoglein 3 (Dsg3), are found in pemphigus patients. Immunoglobulin-G (IgG) autoantibodies against the extracellular domain of Dsg1 and Dsg3 proved to be pathogenic when passively transferred into experimental mouse models.[3,4] Endemic pemphigus foliaceus (EPF), also known as fogo selvagem (FS) is an organ-specific autoimmune blistering disease, first reported in the beginning of the 20th century (1903) in Brazil. Interestingly, the skin condition was thought to be one of the clinical variants of a superficial mycosis, known as tinea imbricata or tokelau.[5] FS occurs in rural areas of Brazil, following the course of streams and creeks, and vanishes after urbanization of the endemic areas. The disease is observed in other countries of South America, such as Colombia, Venezuela, Peru, Ecuador and Paraguay, and also in Northern Africa (Tunisia).[6,7]

The skin lesions are characterized by subcorneal blisters that result from the autoimmune aggression, with no mucosal involvement. Although EPF shares clinical, histologic and immunologic features with the classic form, described by Cazenave in1844, its epidemiologic profile is unique, including endemic geographic areas, familial cases, and disease onset at earlier ages, with no differences in gender distribution.[1,2,5,8]

## DISEASE PRESENTATION

The primary lesion is a superficial blister that easily ruptures, leaving superficial, denuded areas. Predominant sites occur in seborrheic areas, such as head (scalp and face), neck, and upper trunk. Nikolsky sign is present in most FS patients with active disease. The skin lesions may be worsened by sun exposure and progress in weeks or months. Acute and fulminant FS is seldom reported, with extensive bullae erupting over a period of 1 to 3 weeks.[1] FS most reported clinical presentations are below described.[1,2,5]

### Localized Form (Forme Fruste)

Small vesicles that easily rupture, leaving erosions and crusts are seen on seborrheic areas of the face and trunk. Individual lesions may appear as round or oval keratotic plaques with a yellow–brown surface. Discoid lupus erythematous (DLE)-like lesions, characterized by erythematous-violaceus

This work was partially supported by Conselho Nacional de Pesquisa-CNPq-471,257/2008-7 (VA). NIH grants R01-AR30281, RO1-AR32599, T32 AR07369 (LAD).

Conflict of interest: none declared.

[a] Department of Dermatology, University of São Paulo Medical School, Avenida Doutor Eneas de Carvalho Aguiar, 255 Sala 3016 ICHC, São Paulo, CEP 05403-002, Brazil
[b] Department of Dermatology, University of North Carolina at Chapel Hill, 405 Mary Ellen Jones Building CB#7287, Chapel Hill, NC 27599-7287, USA
* Corresponding author.
E-mail address: valeria.aoki@gmail.com

Dermatol Clin 29 (2011) 413–418
doi:10.1016/j.det.2011.03.014

derm.theclinics.com

or hyperpigmented papules and plaques, distributed in the same seborrheic areas, are also described (**Fig. 1**). However, FS lesions lack the follicular prominence (carpet tack sign), the epidermal atrophic changes, and hypopigmentation, which are usually seen in DLE lesions. Localized FS may remain unchanged for months or years; its course may lead to spontaneous remission, or to acral spreading, involving the trunk and extremities, culminating in generalized disease.[5,9,10]

### Generalized Forms of FS

#### Bullous invasion

Patients will present with acute, aggressive disease, in which there is a predominance of widespread, blistering lesions. The lesions are usually confluent on the trunk, and remain isolated in the arms and legs (**Fig. 2**). Fever, arthralgia, and general malaise are associated with the onset of the vesicular eruption, but bacteremia and sepsis are seldom observed. Occasionally vesicles form circinate or annular patterns, and after rupturing, produce exfoliation resembling the superficial mycosis, tinea imbricata.[5]

#### Exfoliative erythroderma

Superficial blisters appear on erythematous base, and after their rupture, the skin surface becomes eroded and moist. Keratin maceration leads to

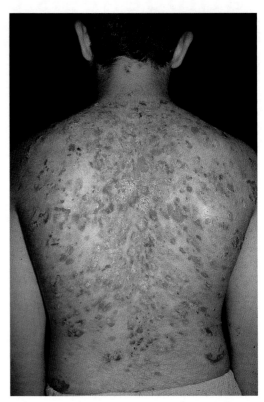

**Fig. 2.** Fogo selvagem: generalized form—bullous invasion: superficial blistering all over the trunk.

a characteristic smell (rat's nest). Other causes of exfoliative dermatitis must be eliminated before diagnosing FS. Confluent superficial erosions with crusting and serum exudate are the prominent features of the disease (**Fig. 3**).[5]

#### Keratotic

Disseminated, keratotic plaques and nodular lesions, similar to the ones present in chronic and localized forms of the disease will be present. These patients may comprise a small cohort of FS who are resistant to therapy.

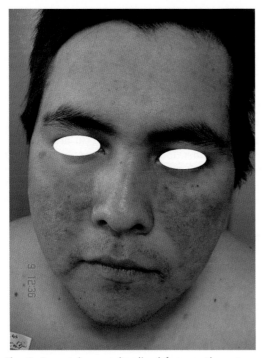

**Fig. 1.** Fogo selvagem: localized form-erythematous-erosive lesions on the malar regions of the face.

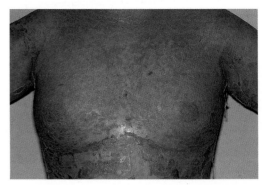

**Fig. 3.** Fogo selvagem: generalized form—erythroderma.

### Hyperpigmented

This form is often seen in patients undergoing remission. It may be restricted to areas of previous lesions, or be disseminated. Before the introduction of systemic treatment with corticosteroids, diffuse hyperpigmentation was considered an early indicator of spontaneous remission or cure. Several patients undergoing clinical remission would experience dramatic changes in their skin color, with marked skin darkening.

### Pemphigus herpetiformis

This form is characterized by vesicles or pustules in herpetiform arrangement, and eosinophilic spongiosis. Lesions may either precede or follow typical FS lesions.[8] Immunochemical analysis of pemphigus herpetiformis autoantigens demonstrates reactivity against either Dsg1 or Dsg3.

Before the steroid era, some complications such as growth retardation and dwarfism in children, and azoospermia in adults were described.

## DISEASE PATHOGENESIS

FS is an autoimmune disease with intermingled environmental, immunologic, and genetic influences triggering its onset.

### Environmental Factors

FS shows unique and remarkable features such as the geographic and temporal clustering of cases, the increased frequency of cases among young adults and children, the increased frequency of familial cases, and an association with certain distinct HLA-DR alleles.[1,2,5,6,9,11] Another striking observation is the decreasing prevalence of FS in some geographic areas that follows urban development.[2] Settlements of native Brazilians, especially the Terena Reservation of Limao Verde, in Mato Grosso do Sul, Brazil,[11] exhibit a high prevalence (3.2%) of FS, and an incidence of 1 to 4 new cases per year.

A possible role of hematophagous black flies (Simuliid) has been hypothesized for many years. In a hospital-based epidemiologic case–control study, it was reported that black fly bites were 4.7 times more frequent in individuals developing FS than in control individuals.[10] Interestingly, a predominant black fly species (Simulium nigrimanum) in the Terena Reservation of Limao Verde was found, which is rarely seen in nonendemic areas of Brazil.[12] A case–control study performed in the Terena village suggested (**Fig. 4**) that individuals living in this endemic area might be at risk of developing FS, considering their housing (thatched roofs, adobe walls) and exposure to hematophagous insect bites (kissing bugs or bed bugs).[10]

The same ecological systems found in the 'pemphigus country overlap with those described in Chagas disease and leishmaniasis. Interestingly, many patients with diseases transmitted by hematophagous vectors (ie, onchocerciasis [black flies], leishmaniasis [sandflies], and Chagas disease [kissing bugs]) possess antibodies against the extracellular domain 5 of Dsg1.[13] It is possible

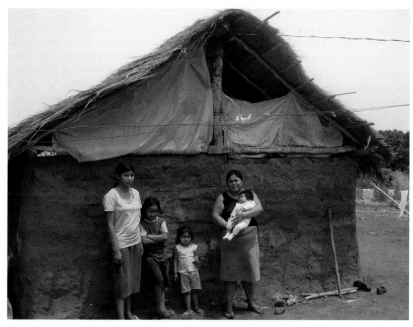

**Fig. 4.** Typical house (adobe and thatch roof) of an endemic site of fogo selvagem.

that these vectors carry a molecule that triggers the anti-Dsg1 EC5 antibody response (antigen mimicry or cross-reactivity). Recently, the sialo-transcriptome of adult female *S nigrimanum* flies, the most seen black fly in endemic FS areas has been isolated, comprising over 70 distinct genes within over 30 protein families, including several novel families. The sialotranscriptome provides an infinite platform for testing pemphigus patient sera against recombinant salivary proteins from *S nigrimanum*.[14]

## Genetics

Previous studies in FS documented genetic influence in the etiopathogenesis of FS. Classic Brazilian studies from the 19702 (n = 2686 FS patients from Goiania, Brazil)[10,11] reported that 18% of the patients were blood relatives, and 93% of these familial cases were found in genetically related family members. Further publications revealed that the expression of DRB1-0404, 1402, or 1406 alleles is linked to FS, with a relative risk of 14.[15] The hypervariable region of the DRB1 gene of these alleles at the level of residues 67 to 74 shares the same sequence: LLEQRRAA, which may confer susceptibility to FS.

## Autoimmunity

### FS autoantigen

Eyre and Stanley[16] demonstrated by immunoprecipitation techniques that sera of patients with either classic PF or FS recognize Dsg1, a 160kDa glycoprotein that belongs to the cadherin family of calcium-dependent cell adhesion molecules (CAMs). Dsg3, a 130kDa cadherin, and the major autoantigen for pemphigus vulgaris (mainly with mucous involvement) is seldom recognized by PF or FS patients (7%).[17] Desmosomal cadherins share extensive homology with other members of this gene superfamily of CAMs, such as desmocollins and E and P cadherins. Dsg1 and Dsg3 are glycoproteins with an ectodomain that contains 6 putative calcium-binding sites, a transmembrane region, and an intracellular domain that is linked to the keratinocyte cytoskeleton via desmosomal plaque proteins.[10,18]

### FS autoimmune response

**IgG anti-Dsg1** The autoantibody response in FS is based on IgG, and is predominantly of the IgG4 subclass. Total IgG4, F(ab)2, and Fab fragments of FS IgG are all pathogenic in the FS mouse model.[3] Anti-Dsg1 antibodies are detected not only in the sera of FS patients, but also in normal controls that live in endemic areas.[9,19] Moreover, the percentage of enzyme-linked immunosorbent assay (ELISA)-positive sera among the normal control population is inversely related to the distance from the endemic FS focus. At the molecular level, FS immunopathogenesis presents as an epitope-spreading model (**Fig. 5**). When using domain-swapped Dsg1 and Dsg3, anti-Dsg1 antibodies from healthy controls and FS, patients on remission show an exclusive response to the extracellular domain (EC-5) of the molecule, whereas FS patients with active disease reveal a major reactivity against the extracellular domains 1 and 2 (EC1-2) of Dsg1.[20] When analyzing preclinical stages of FS, EC-5 remains the major domain involved in the autoimmune response; however, intramolecular spreading may occur at the disease onset, leading to an EC1-2 oriented IgG response.[20] IgG4 is a novel classifier/predictor that identifies donors with immunologic features of FS and is highly sensitive (92% [95% confidence interval, CI: 82–95]) and specific (97% [95% CI: 89–100]). In an FS-prone population, with a prevalence of 3% of the disease, it has a positive predictive value (PPV) of 49% and a negative predictive value (NPV) of 99.7%.[21]

**IgM anti-Dsg1 response** Continuous exposure to an environmental antigen that may share epitopes to Dsg1 is a strong stimulus to nonpathogenic anti-IgM and -IgG production in areas at high risk for FS. In counterpart, FS patients who moved away from their original home and live in the urban areas show a marked decrease in the IgM anti-Dsg1 response, suggesting that the environment does interfere with the immune response, and indicating IgM as a possible serologic marker for FS.[22]

**IgE anti-Dsg1 response** A recent report[23] reveals significant distinct IgE anti-Dsg1levels between FS and PF from the northern hemisphere, indicating that it may also be a serologic marker for FS. Moreover, it reinforces the environmental influence on the disease, once IgE antibodies are detected in individuals who are chronically exposed to allergens or to immunotherapy.[23]

**T cell response** T cells from patients with FS recognize epitopes on the ectodomain of Dsg1. The proliferation of FS T cells to Dsg1 is antigen-specific and restricted to HLA-DR. T cells are CD4 memory T cells and produce interleukin (IL)-4, IL-5, and IL-6, but not $\gamma$-interferon (g-IFN), suggesting a Th2-like cytokine profile.[24]

## Acantholysis

Epidermal cell detachment in FS remains under investigation. Hypotheses include impairment of Dsg1 or Dsg3 adhesive function; binding of

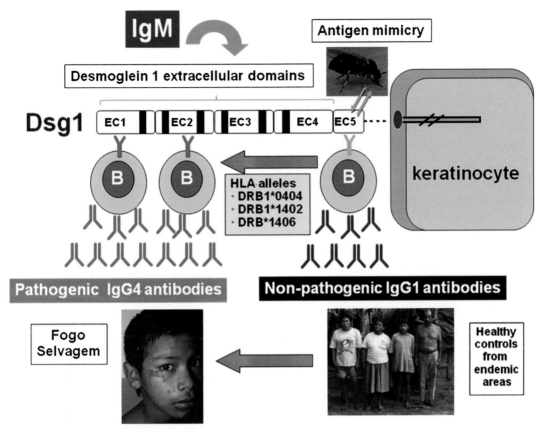

**Fig. 5.** Etiopathogenesis of fogo selvagem.

pemphigus autoantibodies to the epidermis, either leading to alteration of the normal distribution of Dsg1 and Dsg3 (compensation theory), or triggering phosphorylation and activation of transmembrane signaling pathways (release of effector molecules–plasminogen activator).[6,25]

In summary, FS is a unique model of skin disease that encompasses break of tolerance, leading to autoimmunity, which may be activated by the combination of multiple triggering factors, such as genetic predisposition and environment. Further studies concerning its etiopathogenesis are relevant, once they can be extended to other autoimmune conditions.

## REFERENCES

1. Diaz LA, Sampaio SA, Rivitti EA, et al. Endemic pemphigus foliaceus (fogo selvagem). I. Clinical features and immunopathology. J Am Acad Dermatol 1989;20(4):657–69.
2. Diaz LA, Sampaio SA, Rivitti EA, et al. Endemic pemphigus foliaceus (fogo selvagem). II. Current and historic epidemiologic studies. J Invest Dermatol 1989;92(1):4–12.
3. Roscoe JT, Diaz L, Sampaio SA, et al. Brazilian pemphigus foliaceus autoantibodies are pathogenic to BALB/c mice by passive transfer. J Invest Dermatol 1985;85(6):538–41.
4. Warren SJ, Lin MS, Giudice GJ, et al. The prevalence of antibodies against desmoglein 1 in endemic pemphigus foliaceus in Brazil. Cooperative Group on Fogo Selvagem Research. N Engl J Med 2000;343(1):23–30.
5. Sampaio SA, Rivitti EA, Aoki V, et al. Brazilian pemphigus foliaceus, endemic pemphigus foliaceus, or fogo selvagem (wild fire). Dermatol Clin 1994;12(4):765–76.
6. Culton DA, Qian Y, Li N, et al. Advances in pemphigus and its endemic pemphigus foliaceus (fogo selvagem) phenotype: a paradigm of human autoimmunity. J Autoimmun 2008;31(4):311–24.
7. Morini JP, Jomaa B, Gorgi Y, et al. Pemphigus foliaceus in young women. An endemic focus in the Sousse area of Tunisia. Arch Dermatol 1993;129(1): 69–73.
8. Santi CG, Maruta CW, Aoki V, et al. Pemphigus herpetiformis is a rare clinical expression of nonendemic pemphigus foliaceus, fogo selvagem, and pemphigus vulgaris. Cooperative Group on Fogo

Selvagem Research. J Am Acad Dermatol 1996; 34(1):40–6.

9. Hans-Filho G, dos Santos V, Katayama JH, et al. An active focus of high prevalence of fogo selvagem on an Amerindian reservation in Brazil. Cooperative Group on Fogo Selvagem Research. J Invest Dermatol 1996;107(1):68–75.

10. Aoki V, Millikan RC, Rivitti EA, et al. Environmental risk factors in endemic pemphigus foliaceus (fogo selvagem). J Investig Dermatol Symp Proc 2004; 9(1):34–40.

11. Auad A, Castro RM, Fraga S, et al. The treatment of Brazilian pemphigus foliaceus (fogo selvagem). Int J Dermatol 1970;9(2):130–6.

12. Eaton DP, Diaz LA, Hans-Filho G, et al. Comparison of black fly species (Diptera simuliidae) on an Amerindian reservation with a high prevalence of fogo selvagem to neighboring disease-free sites in the State of Mato Grosso do Sul, Brazil. The Cooperative Group on Fogo Selvagem Research. J Med Entomol 1998;35(2):120–31.

13. Diaz LA, Arteaga LA, Hilario-Vargas J, et al. Antidesmoglein-1 antibodies in onchocerciasis, leishmaniasis and Chagas disease suggest a possible etiological link to fogo selvagem. J Invest Dermatol 2004;123(6):1045–51.

14. Ribeiro JM, Valenzuela JG, Pham VM, et al. An insight into the sialotranscriptome of Simulium nigrimanum, a black fly associated with fogo selvagem in South America. Am J Trop Med Hyg 2010;82(6):1060–75.

15. Moraes ME, Fernandez-Vina M, Lazaro A, et al. An epitope in the third hypervariable region of the DRB1 gene is involved in the susceptibility to endemic pemphigus foliaceus (fogo selvagem) in three different Brazilian populations. Tissue Antigens 1997;49(1):35–40.

16. Eyre RW, Stanley JR. Identification of pemphigus vulgaris antigen extracted from normal human epidermis and comparison with pemphigus foliaceus antigen. J Clin Invest 1988;81(3):807–12.

17. Hilario-Vargas J, Dasher DA, Li N, et al. Prevalence of antidesmoglein-3 antibodies in endemic regions of fogo selvagem in Brazil. J Invest Dermatol 2006; 126(9):2044–8.

18. Wheelock MJ, Johnson KR. Cadherins as modulators of cellular phenotype. Annu Rev Cell Dev Biol 2003;19:207–35.

19. Warren SJ, Arteaga LA, Rivitti EA, et al. The role of subclass switching in the pathogenesis of endemic pemphigus foliaceus. J Invest Dermatol 2003; 120(1):104–8.

20. Li N, Aoki V, Hans-Filho G, et al. The role of intramolecular epitope spreading in the pathogenesis of endemic pemphigus foliaceus (fogo selvagem). J Exp Med 2003;197(11):1501–10.

21. Qaqish BF, Prisayanh P, Qian Y, et al. Development of an IgG4-based predictor of endemic pemphigus foliaceus (fogo selvagem). J Invest Dermatol 2009; 129(1):110–8.

22. Diaz LA, Prisayanh PS, Dasher DA, et al. The IgM anti-desmoglein 1 response distinguishes Brazilian pemphigus foliaceus (fogo selvagem) from other forms of pemphigus. J Invest Dermatol 2008; 128(3):667–75.

23. Qian Y, Prisayanh P, Andracca E, et al. IgE, IgM, and IgG4 antidesmoglein 1 autoantibody profile in endemic pemphigus foliaceus (fogo selvagem). Available at: www.jidonline. Accessed December 30, 2010.

24. Lin MS, Fu CL, Aoki V, et al. Desmoglein-1-specific T lymphocytes from patients with endemic pemphigus foliaceus (fogo selvagem). J Clin Invest 2000;105: 203–17.

25. Espana A, Diaz LA, Mascaro JM Jr, et al. Mechanisms of acantholysis in pemphigus foliaceus. Clin Immunol Immunopathol 1997;85(1):83–9.

# Paraneoplastic Pemphigus (Paraneoplastic Autoimmune Multiorgan Syndrome): Clinical Presentations and Pathogenesis

John W. Frew, MBBS, M. Clin Epi[a,b],
Dédée F. Murrell, MA, BMBCh, FAAD, MD, FACD[c,*]

## KEYWORDS

- Paraneoplastic pemphigus
- Paraneoplastic autoimmune multiorgan syndrome
- Lymphoproliferative disorders

Paraneoplastic pemphigus (PNP) is a life-threatening autoimmune blistering disease, which is commonly associated with lymphoproliferative neoplasms.[1] It was first described in a case series in 1990 by Anhalt and colleagues[2] and approximately 250 case reports of PNP have been documented since that time.[1,3] PNP has a wide geographic distribution and equal predominance across both genders with an average age of onset of 51 years.[3] It is characterized by painful mucosal erosions with a polymorphous skin eruption (not always defined by bullae) in association with an occult or verified neoplasm.[1,3–5] These neoplasms are typically of a lymphoproliferative type (chronic lymphocytic leukemia, lymphoma, Castleman's disease, thymoma, and so forth) although case reports have described rare occurrences of the condition in other neoplasms, such as metastatic melanoma.[4] Mortality due to the disease has been reported to be as high as 90%.[5] Response to therapy is highly variable, with an incomplete knowledge of the pathogenesis of the disease making targeted therapies a challenge.[5–7] This article reviews the varied clinical presentations and pathologic characteristics pertaining to PNP. Management of PNP will be covered in the next issue of this journal.

## PRESENTATIONS OF PNP

PNP has a variety of clinical presentations, with painful mucosal and skin lesions presenting a wide variation in morphology (**Fig. 1**).[1,3–5] There has also been well-documented evidence of involvement of internal organs, such as lungs, thyroid, kidney, smooth muscle, and gastrointestinal tract.[5] Such internal organ involvement has led to the proposal that the term, *paraneoplastic pemphigus*, should be replaced

[a] Department of Dermatology, St George Hospital, Gray Street, Kogarah, Sydney, NSW, Australia
[b] Faculty of Medicine, University of New South Wales, High Street, Kensington, Sydney, NSW, Australia
[c] Department of Dermatology, St George Hospital, University of New South Wales, Gray Street, Kogarah, Sydney, NSW 2217, Australia
* Corresponding author.
*E-mail address:* d.murrell@unsw.edu.au

Dermatol Clin 29 (2011) 419–425
doi:10.1016/j.det.2011.03.018

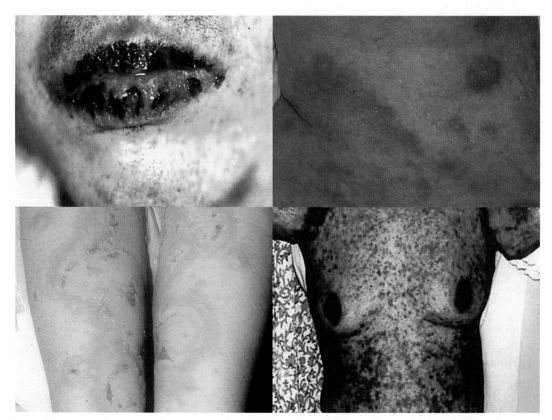

**Fig. 1.** Clinical manifestations of paraneoplastic pemphigus. (*Top left*) Severe stomatitis in PNP/PAMS. (*Top right*) Pemphigus-like PNP/PAMS with vesicles on background erythema. (*Bottom left*) Erythema multiforme–like lesions associated with paraneoplastic pemphigus/PAMS. (*Bottom right*) Lichen planus–like violaceus papules in PNP/PAMS. (*From* Gardiner J, Evans K, Goldstein S, et al. Vorinostat for the treatment of bullous pemphigoid in the setting of advanced refractory cutaneous T cell Lymphoma. Arch Dermatol 2009;145:983–8; with permission; and Wang J, Zhu X, Li R, et al. Paraneoplastic pemphigus associated with Castleman's tumour: a commonly reported subtype of paraneoplastic pemphigus in China. Arch Dermatol 2005;141:1285–93; with permission.)

by the term, *paraneoplastic autoimmune multiorgan syndrome (PAMS)*, to more accurately describe the full spectrum of presentations and pathologic findings associated with this condition,[5] although this proposed change has been met with mixed reaction by professionals in the field.

Currently, no consensus definitions exist as to the precise characteristics that define PNP/PAMS. Three different definitions have been put forward by various investigators[2,6,8] and are presented in **Table 1**. Examples of common aspects present in all proposed definitions of PNP/PAMS include initial mucosal involvement, detection of circulating autoantibodies against envoplakin and/or periplakin, and detection of a neoplasm.[1]

The clinical presentation of PNP, although highly varied, typically begins with a florid, painful eruption of mucous membrane lesions, which may involve the oropharynx, nasopharynx, tongue, vermillion of the lips, conjunctiva, anogenital region, or esophagus.[1,3–5] The onset of cutaneous

lesions has a variable delay after the appearance of mucous membrane lesions, ranging from days to months.[1–3] The heterogeneity in the presentation of the cutaneous manifestations of this disease has led to a stratification of PNP/PAMS based on their similarity to other dermatologic conditions into 5 different clinical variants[5] (**Table 2**). These cutaneous manifestations often present in waves of lesions and, in contrast to pemphigus vulgaris, blisters in PNP/PAMS do not arise from normal skin but typically develop from inflammatory papules or macules, which greatly outnumber bullous eruptions in PNP/PAMS on individual patients.[7]

Common causes of mortality in PNP include overwhelming sepsis and complications due to treatment for the underlying neoplasm.[3,5] A more common cause of mortality in children and those where the underlying malignant condition in Castleman's disease is bronchiolitis obliterans.[5] This condition is characterized by the sloughing of

**Table 1**
**Three different proposed definitions for paraneoplastic pemphigus**

| Proposed Consensus Definitions | Zhu and Zhang[8] | Anhalt et al[2] | Joly et al[6] |
|---|---|---|---|
| Year | 2007 | 1990 | 2000 |
| Clinical Characteristics | Painful mucosal involvement and polymorphic cutaneous eruption | Painful mucosal erosions with a polymorphous skin eruption culminating in vesicles/bullae in the context of an occult/confirmed neoplasm | Presence of painful oral erosions |
| Histopathology | Intraepidermal acatholysis, keratinocyte necrosis, and vacuolar interface dermatitis | Intraepidermal acantholysis, vascular interfacial dermatoses, and keratinocyte necrosis | Suprabasal acantholysis with keratinocyte necrosis or vacuolar interface dermatitis or lichenoid infiltrate |
| DIF | Not specified | Deposition of complement and IgG in intracellular epidermal spaces and in the basement membrane zone in linear granular lesions | Presence of circulating or in vivo bound antiepithelial cell surface and anti–basement membrane zone antibodies |
| IIF | IIF of patient serum with rat bladder epithelia shows intercellular staining | Not specified | Labeling of rat bladder |
| Circulating Autoantibodies | Not specified | Detection in the serum similar to that of pemphigus. | Confirmation of autoantibodies to periplakin and/or envoplakin |
| Presence of a neoplasm | Occult or confirmed | Occult or confirmed | Association with lymphoproliferative disorders |

*Data from* Refs.[2,6,8]

the epithelial lining of the bronchioles, which can lead to complete obstructions of terminal bronchioles and individual alveoli. This aspect of the disease is the only commonly reported internal manifestation of PNP/PAMS, and although other internal organs have reported autoantibody reactivity, no clinical manifestations or complications have been directly attributed to the disease process.[4,5]

## PATHOLOGIC FINDINGS
### Histopathology

As outlined in **Table 2**, since the original description of PNP by Anhalt and colleagues[2] in 1990, clinical-pathologic correlation has prompted investigators to define PNP as one presentation in the spectrum of disorders known as PAMS. The histologic findings from patients with different clinical presentations of PNP/PAMS have shown similarities with other known dermatologic conditions (**Fig. 2**), perhaps indicating commonalities in pathogenesis. This has led to hypotheses regarding the degree of humoral or cell-mediated immunologic involvement in different subtypes of PNP/PAMS.[5]

Anhalt and colleagues' original description of PNP showed histologic changes, including intraepidermal or subepidermal blistering with no or few mononuclear cells.[1] This original PNP (otherwise classified as pemphigus-like PAMS) is seen at the humoral-mediated end of the spectrum of PNP/PAMS. The bullous pemphigoid–like subtype presents with dyskeratosis and mild mononuclear infiltrate at the dermal-epidermal junction (see **Fig. 2**). Progressing toward the cell-mediated end of the spectrum, erythema multiforme–like and graft-versus-host disease–like PNP/PAMS

**Table 2**
Clinical, histologic, and immunofluorescence findings in the 5 proposed subtypes of PNP/PAMS

| PNP/PAMS Subtype | Pemphigus-like | Bullous Pemphigoid–like | Erythema Multiforme–like | Graft-versus-Host Disease–like | Lichen Planus–like |
|---|---|---|---|---|---|
| Clinical Presentation | Superficial vesicles with occasional erythema | Scaling erythematous papules without bullous lesions | Scaling erythematous papules with occasional ulceration or erosions | Scaled, dusky red papules | Violaceus papules |
| Common Sites of Cutaneous Lesions | Head, trunk, and proximal extremlties | More commonly seen on extremities | Mucosae, trunk, and extremities | Trunk and extremities | Trunk and extremities, which may include acral regions |
| Histologic Findings | Intraepidermal and/or subepidermal bullae | Dyskeratosis and mild mononuclear infiltrate at the dermal-epidermal junction | Dyskeratosis with areas of epidermal separation due to disintegration of the basal layer and perivascular infiltrate | No detachment, hyperparakeratosis, orthoparakeratosis, parakeratosis, and dyskeratosis and pronounced interface dermatitis | No blisters, hyperkeratosis, dyskeratosis, or lichenoid infiltrate |
| DIF Findings | Epidermal intracellular as well as intercellular/linear deposits of IgG and complement C3 | | | | |
| IIF Findings | IgG and complement C3 reaction with stratified squamous, transitional and simple columnar epithelium (typically rate bladder and myocardial tissue) | | | | |

*Data from* Sehgal VN, Srivastava G. Paraneoplastic pemphigus/ paraneoplastic autoimmune multiorgan syndrome. Int J Dermatol 2009;48:162–9; and Nguyen VT, Ndoye A, Bassler KD, et al. Classification, clinical manifestations and immunopathological mechanisms of the epithelial variant of paraneoplastic autoimmune multiorgan syndrome. Arch Dermatol 2001;137:193–206.

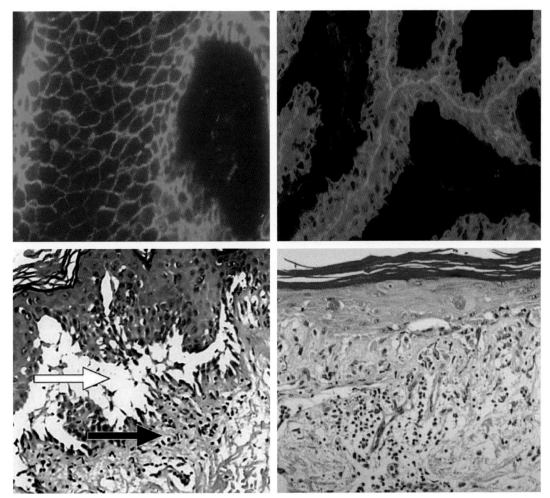

**Fig. 2.** Pathologic findings in PNP/PAMS. (*Top left*) DIF of PNP/PAMS lesion showing intracellular deposition of IgG in the epidermis as well as intercellular staining (magnfication ×400). (*Top right*) Indriect IF on rat bladder shows intercellular antihuman IgG staining (magnification ×400). (*Bottom left*) Hematoxylin-eosin stain of PNP/PAMS lesion showing suprabasilar cleft (*white arrow*) and lymphocytic infiltrate (*black arrow*) (magnification ×200). (*Bottom right*) Lichenoid pattern of histopathology in PNP/PAMS (magnification ×200). (*From* Nguyen VT, Ndoye A, Bassler KD, et al. Classification, clinical manifestations and immunopathological mechanisms of the epithelial variant of paraneoplastic autoimmune multiorgan syndrome. Arch Dermatol 2001;137:193–206; with permission; and Wang J, Zhu X, Li R, et al. Paraneoplastic pemphigus associated with Castleman's tumour: a commonly reported subtype of paraneoplastic pemphigus in China. Arch Dermatol 2005;141:1285–93; with permission.)

show increasing vascularity and lymphoid infiltrates.[5] At the far end of the cell-mediated end of the spectrum, the lichen planus–like PNP subtype shows no blisters but a diffuse lichenoid infiltrate with dyskeratosis.[5]

Nguyen and colleagues[5] have demonstrated that the CD8+, cytotoxic T lymphocytes, CD56+, natural killer cells, and CD68+ monocytes/macrophages found in the dermal-epidermal junction in lichen planus, graft-versus-host disease, and erythema multiforme are also present in PNP/PAMS, an interesting observation as to the

contribution of cellular autoimmunity in the spectrum of PNP/PAMS.

## Immunofluorescence

Immunofluorescence is considered one of the main diagnostic criteria for PNP/PAMS. Direct IF (DIF) of cutaneous or mucosal lesions reveals IgG and complement C3 deposits in an intercellular and/or linear pattern (see **Fig. 2**). Joly and colleagues[6] documented that positive DIF had only a 41% sensitivity but specificity above

87% when compared with pemphigus patients with and without concurrent neoplasm. Patient serum testing using indirect IF (IIF) demonstrates the above IgG and complement C3 intercellular and/or linear pattern on stratified squamous epithelium. Unlike other autoimmune blistering diseases, PNP/PAMS antibodies also stain simple columnar and transitional epithelial tissue substrates (typically rat bladder and cardiac muscle [see **Fig. 2**]).[4,5] IIF has higher sensitivity and specificity than DIF, 86% and 98%, respectively.[6]

### Multiple Antigenic Targets

Autoantibodies to plakins are characteristic and diagnostic of PNP/PAMS.[2] As structural components of desmosomal and hemodesmosomal plaques, their interaction with the keratin cytoskeleton of keratinocytes can result in the suprabasal clefting seen in PNP/PAMS if affected by autoantibodies.

The specific autoantibodies to plakins correlated with PNP/PAMS include periplakin, envoplakin, desmoplakins 1 and 2, plectin, and a 170-kDa protein that has not yet been molecularly characterized.[1,7] Of those, periplakin and envoplakin are most specific to PNP/PAMS.[6] Based on Joly and colleagues'[6] study of 22 PNP/PAMS patients, the presence of autoantibodies to periplakin or envoplakin (as measured by immunoblotting) was the most specific and sensitive test for PNP, with 82% sensitivity and 100% specificity.

### Underlying Neoplasm

Lymphoproliferative neoplasms comprise the majority of neoplasms associated with PNP/PAMS. The most frequently documented is non-Hodgkin lymphoma (38.6%), followed by chronic lymphocytic leukemia (18.4%) and Castleman's disease (18.4%).[7] Rarely, nonhematologic neoplasms are involved in PNP/PAMS and include epithelial-origin carcinomas (pancreas, colon, breast prostate, squamous cell carcinoma, basal cell carcimona, and bronchogenic carcinomas) (8.6%) and mesenchymal-origin sarcomas (reticulum cell sarcomas, liposarcomas, leiomyosarcomas, and dendritic cell sarcomas) (6.2%).[7] One case of PNP has been associated with malignant melanoma.[9] Simultaneous recognition of the neoplasm and diagnosis of PNP/PAMS is a common occurrence; however, some cases of PNP without any obvious underlying tumor have been reported.[10]

## PATHOGENESIS OF PNP/PAMS

The exact mechanisms by which neoplasia induces PNP/PAMS are incompletely understood.[1,3–7] Circulating autoantibodies to the plakin proteins responsible in the pathogenesis of PNP/PAMS have been shown in several studies to be produced directly by coexisting neoplasms.[11,12] Several hypotheses have been put forward, and Vezzoli and colleagues[7] classify them into 5 broad categories:

- Epitope spreading: the tumor induces a cell-mediated lichenoid interface dermatitis that uncovers previously hidden antigens
- Antigen mimicry: humoral immune responses against the tumor cross-reacting with normal epithelial proteins
- Cytotoxicity: autoreactive cellular cytotoxicity mediated by CD8$^+$ cytotoxic T lymphocytes, CD56$^+$ natural killer cells, and CD68$^+$ macrophages
- Autoantibodies: production of autoantibodies reacting to epidermal proteins by the cells from the associated tumors
- Interleukin 6: dysregulation of cytokine production by tumor cells, with secretion of massive amounts of interleukin 6.

## SUMMARY

PNP is a rare condition with high rates of mortality. Although its pathogenesis is incompletely understood, its pathologic findings have significant overlap with other autoimmune blistering diseases, such as pemphigus vulgaris and pemphigus foliaceus. A universally accepted consensus definition is needed to firmly define the condition. This would aid in identification of PNP and the institution of timely and appropriate treatment to avoid rapid patient deterioration as well as recruitment for trials to further examine the pathogenesis and new therapeutic modalities.

## REFERENCES

1. Zimmerman J, Bahmer F, Rose C, et al. [Clinical and immunopathological spectrum of paraneoplastic pemphigus]. J Dtsch Dermatol Ges 2010;8: 598–605 [in German].
2. Anhalt GJ, Kim SC, Stanley GR, et al. Paraneoplastic pemphigus. An autoimmune mucocutaneous disease associated with neoplasia. N Engl J Med 1990;323:1729–35.
3. Robinson ND, Hashimoto T, Amagai M, et al. The new pemphigus variants. J Am Acad Dermatol 1999;40:649–71.

4. Sehgal VN, Srivastava G. Paraneoplastic pemphigus/ paraneoplastic autoimmune multiorgan syndrome. Int J Dermatol 2009;48:162–9.

5. Nguyen VT, Ndoye A, Bassler KD, et al. Classification, clinical manifestations and immunopathological mechanisms of the epithelial variant of paraneoplastic autoimmune multiorgan syndrome. Arch Dermatol 2001;137:193–206.

6. Joly P, Richard C, Gilbert D, et al. Sensitivity and specificity of clinical, histologic, and immunologic features in the diagnosis of paraneoplastic pemphigus. J Am Acad Dermatol 2000;43:619–26.

7. Vezzoli P, Berti E, Marzano AV. Rationale and efficacy for the use of rituximab in paraneoplastic pemphigus. Expert Rev Clin Immunol 2008;4(3): 351–64.

8. Zhu X, Zhang B. Paraneoplastic pemphigus. J Dermatol 2007;34:503–11.

9. Schaeppi H, Bauer JW, Hametner R, et al. Localised variant of paraneoplastic pemphigus: acantholysis associated with malignant melanoma. Br J Dermatol 2001;144:1249–54.

10. Park GT, Lee JH, Yun SJ, et al. Paraneoplastic pemphigus without an underlying neoplasm. Br J Dermatol 2007;156:725–32.

11. Wang L, Bu D, Yang Y. Castleman's tumours and production of autoantibody in paraneoplastic pemphigus. Lancet 2004;363:525–31.

12. Wang L, Bu D, Li T, et al. Autoantibody production from a thymom and dendritic cell sarcoma associated with paraneoplastic pemphigus. Br J Dermatol 2005;153:558–64.

# Clinical Features and Practical Diagnosis of Bullous Pemphigoid

Enno Schmidt, MD, PhD[a,b,*], Rocco della Torre, MD[c],
Luca Borradori, MD[c]

## KEYWORDS

- Autoantibody • BP180 • BP230 • ELISA
- Immunofluorescence microscopy

Bullous pemphigoid (BP) belongs to the group of autoimmune subepidermal blistering diseases, which are characterized by an autoantibody response directed against distinct components of the dermoepidermal junction of skin and adjacent mucous membranes. Besides BP, this group, which has overlapping clinical and immunopathologic features, also comprises pemphigoid gestationis (also called gestational pemphigoid), mucous membrane pemphigoid, linear IgA disease, anti-p200/laminin γ1 pemphigoid, and epidermolysis bullosa acquisita.

Pemphigoid diseases were first differentiated from pemphigus in 1953 by Lever[1] who described intraepidermal split formation and loss of cell adherence between keratinocytes (acantholysis) as the histopathologic hallmark of pemphigus, whereas he coined the term pemphigoid for conditions in which a subepidermal split formation was typically present. A decade later, Jordon and colleagues[2] showed that patients with BP had tissue-bound and circulating autoantibodies directed against the dermoepidermal junction. Further milestones in the understanding of BP included the immunochemical characterization of the hemidesmosomal target proteins BP180 (also called BPAG2 or type XVII collagen) and BP230 (BPAG1-e), the cloning of their genes, and the demonstration that autoantibodies to BP180 are pathogenic.[3–7]

## EPIDEMIOLOGY

The incidence of BP has been estimated at between 4.5 and 14 new cases per million per year.[8–13] In a recent prospective study encompassing the entire Swiss population, the incidence was found to be 12.7 new cases per million per year.[14] These data are consistent with a recent prospective study in Lower Franconia, a well-defined region in southern Germany, where the incidence of BP was estimated to be 13.4/1 million/y.[15] A higher incidence of 42.8/1 million/y has recently been reported in Great Britain based on a data registry established on the general practitioner level. However, the British study, in which the immunopathologic criteria used were not specified, did not differentiate the various pemphigoid diseases and most likely also included bullous drug eruptions.[10] In Lower Franconia,

The work is dedicated to Leonie and Justus, who came into being during the preparation of this manuscript, thereby changing the life of E.S.

Conflict of Interest: E.S. has a scientific cooperation with Euroimmun AG, Lübeck. R.d.S. and L.B. have nothing to disclose.

Funding: This work was in part supported by the Schleswig-Holstein Cluster of Excellence in Inflammation Research (DFG EXC 306/1, to E.S.), by grants of the European Community's FP7 (Coordination Theme 1 HEALTH-F2-2008-200515) and the Swiss National Foundation for Scientific Research (31003A-121966 and 31003A-09811, to L.B.).

[a] Department of Dermatology, University of Lübeck, Ratzeburger Allee 160, 23538 Lübeck, Germany
[b] Comprehensive Center for Inflammation Medicine, University of Lübeck, Ratzeburger Allee 160, 23538 Lübeck, Germany
[c] Department of Dermatology, Inselspital, University Hospital of Bern, Freiburgstrasse, 3010 Bern, Switzerland
* Corresponding author.
*E-mail address:* enno.schmidt@uk-sh.de

Germany, and Great Britain the incidence of BP has considerably increased within the last 10 years (twofold and 4.8-fold, respectively),[10,15,16] an observation that may be related to either the increasing age of the general population or a better knowledge of the disease with proper diagnosis.

BP is probably the only autoimmune diseases of which the incidence increases with age. BP is typically a disease of the elderly and its diagnosis is usually made in patients aged between 75 and 81 years.[9,14,15,17–19] In the population older than 80 years of age, the incidence is 150 to 180 new patients/1 million/y.[14,15]

## CLINICAL FEATURES

The name BP itself is a pleonasm. Pemphigoid is derived from Greek and means a form of blister (pemphix, blister, and eidos, form). Hence, from a purely etymologic point of view, the adjective bullous should not be added to designate the blistering in pemphigoid. However, the spectrum of clinical presentations is extremely broad (**Boxes 1** and **2**).

Characteristically, BP is an intensely pruritic eruption with widespread blister formation. In this bullous stage, vesicles and bullae develop on apparently normal or erythematous skin together with urticated and infiltrated plaques with an occasionally annular or figurate pattern (**Fig. 1**). The blisters are tense with a clear, sometimes hemorrhagic, exudate; the Nikolsky sign is negative. Pruritus, which may be invalidating, is almost constantly present.[17] Blisters are typically symmetrically distributed and may persist for several days, leaving eroded and crusted areas. Predilection sites involve the flexural aspects of the limbs and abdomen. In our own prospective Swiss cohort of patients encompassing 164 patients with BP for a 2-year period, the clinical presentation at time of diagnosis consisted of typical blisters localized on the trunk and on the extremities in about 80% of cases. In the intertriginous spaces, vegetating plaques may occur, and oral lesions develop in

---

**Box 1**
**Clinical manifestations suggestive of BP in elderly patients with chronic pruritic skin eruptions**

- Papular and/or urticarial lesions
- Eczematous lesions
- Prurigo-like lesions
- Excoriations, hemorrhagic crusts
- Localized vesicles or erosions

---

**Box 2**
**Unusual clinical variants of BP**

- Dyshidrosiform pemphigoid
- Intertrigo-like pemphigoid
- Prurigo-nodularis-like pemphigoid
- Papular pemphigoid
- Lymphomatoid papulosis–like
- Vesicular/eczematous pemphigoid
- Erythrodermic pemphigoid
- Localized forms

  ○ pretibial
  ○ peristomal
  ○ umbilical
  ○ stump pemphigoid
  ○ on paralyzed body sites
  ○ on irradiated/traumatized body sites

- Brunsting-Perry form (variant of cicatricial pemphigoid)

---

10% to 20% of cases.[20] The mucosae of eyes, nose, pharynx, esophagus, and anogenital areas are rarely affected (reviewed in Refs.[21,22]).

However, before the development of tense generalized blisters, BP is typically preceded by a prodromal nonbullous phase. In this stage, diagnosis is difficult. Mild to intractable pruritus, alone or in association with excoriated, eczematous, popular, and/or urticarial lesions are found that may persist for several weeks or even months (see **Box 1**; **Fig. 2**). These unspecific skin findings may remain the only signs of the disease. In this same context, several clinical variants of BP (see **Box 2**) (reviewed in Ref.[22]) have been described with a variety of different denominations, such as prurigo nodularis–like, prurigo-like,[23] erythrodermalike, ecthyma gangrenosum–like,[24] intertrigolike, and toxic epidermolysis–like lesions. Localized forms have been described confined to areas affected by radiotherapy, surgery, trauma, and burns, as well as lesions limited around stomata, hemodialysis fistulae,[25] the pretibial (**Fig. 3**) or umbilical area,[26] the palmoplantar region (mimicking dyshidrotic eczema), and the genital area.

## TRIGGER FACTORS AND ASSOCIATED DISEASES

Several triggers have been implicated in the disease onset of individual patients, including

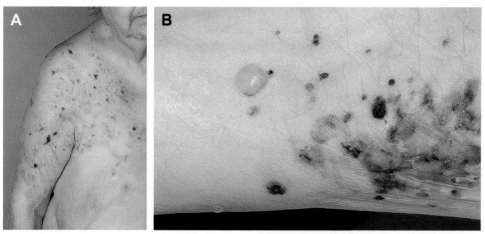

Fig. 1. Bullous pemphigoid. (*A*) Confluent urticated plaques and eczematous lesions with tense blisters on the trunk and right arm. (*B*) Close-up view.

trauma, burns, radiotherapy, and ultraviolet radiation. In addition, various autoimmune disorders, psoriasis, and neurologic disorders have also been described in association with BP. A large variety of drugs have been anecdotally reported to induce BP. A weak association with aldosterone antagonists and neuroleptics was found[27] and,

most recently, with spironolactone and phenothiazines with aliphatic side chains.[28] Based on these data, the use of latter drugs should be carefully evaluated in BP. In 2 case-control studies including more than 1700 patients with BP and age-matched controls in Sweden and Japan, a low association with gastric cancer was identified in the Japanese

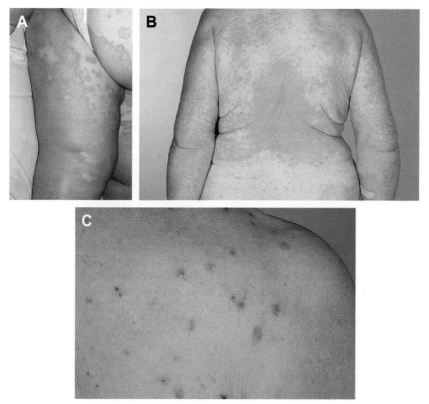

Fig. 2. Bullous pemphigoid. (*A*) Erythematous urticarial infiltrated plaques on the abdomen and legs with a figurate distribution. (*B*) Extensive eczematous and urticarial lesions on the trunk and arms. (*C*) Prurigo nodularis–like lesions and excoriated lesions on the shoulder.

leading to autoimmunity against the target antigens of BP (epitope-spreading phenomenon).

Most recently, the association between BP and neurologic disorders has been highlighted, such as stroke (odds ratio 2.1), Parkinson disease (odds ratio 3.0 and 2.2), major cognitive impairment (odds ratio 2.2), psychiatric disorders such unipolar and bipolar disorders (odds ratio 5.3), epilepsy (odds ratio 1.7), and most strongly with multiple sclerosis (odds ratio 6.7 and 10.7).[28,35–37] These findings are particularly intriguing because some evidence has been provided suggesting that both antigens BP180 and BP230 are expressed in the central nervous system,[38–40] and mice with either target disruption of or inherited mutations in the dystonin (DST) gene encoding for various isoforms of BPAG1 (including the epithelial isoform BP230/BPAG1-e) develop severe dystonia and sensory nerve degeneration.[41]

## TARGET ANTIGENS

In BP, autoantibodies recognize BP180 (also known as type XVII collagen or BP antigen 2) and BP230 (also known as BPAG1-e or BP antigen 1). These proteins are components of junctional adhesion complexes called hemidesmosomes, which are expressed in stratified and complex epithelia, such as skin, mucous membranes, and the ear, nose, and throat area. BP180 is a transmembrane glycoprotein of about 1500 amino acids. Ultrastructurally, it spans the lamina lucida before kinking back from the lamina densa into the lamina lucida (reviewed in Refs.[42,43]). The juxta-membrane domain of the extracellular portion of BP180 called NC16A was identified as the immunodominant region of BP180 in BP.[44,45] BP180 interacts with the β4 chain of α6β4 integrin, plectin, BP230, and most likely with laminin 332[46]). It provides a structural link between the intermediate filaments of the cytoskeleton and dermal collagen fibers. The importance of BP180 for the structural integrity of the skin is attested to by the observation that pathogenic mutations in its gene, COLXVII, lead to nonlethal junctional epidermolysis bullosa.[47]

In contrast, BP230 is an intracellular constituent of the hemidesmosomal plaque and belongs to the plakin family of cytolinkers. Its globular C-terminal domain mediates the anchorage of keratin filaments to the cell membrane.[46] Targeted inactivation of the DST gene encoding BP230 in mice resulted in mild skin fragility. Unexpectedly, affected mice developed neurologic defects with sensory neuron degeneration.[41] The phenotype was identical to those observed in mice suffering

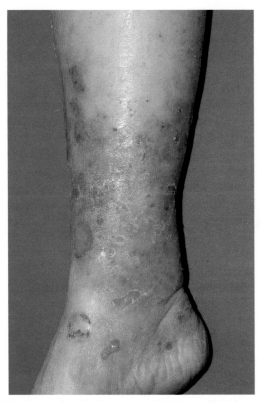

**Fig. 3.** Localized bullous pemphigoid: pretibial form. Postbullous erosions and eczematous lesions on the right lower leg.

cohort.[29,30] The previously described higher incidence of malignancies in patients with BP was probably biased by the lack of appropriate age-matched controls and the intensive work-up of affected patients in an hospital setting. Nevertheless, patients who develop BP at less than 60 years of age may be at higher risk for an underlying malignancy.[31] We usually perform an age-related cancer screen based on patient's history and clinical examination without a systematic and extensive cancer screening.

Several autoimmune disorders, such as rheumatoid arthritis, Hashimoto thyroiditis, dermatomyositis, lupus erythematosus, and autoimmune thrombocytopenia, have been reported in BP. However, a case-control study did not find any increased risk for autoimmune disorders in BP,[32] but a genetically determined susceptibility to develop autoimmune diseases is likely. BP has also been found in association with certain inflammatory dermatoses, such as psoriasis and lichen planus[33,34]; a statistically significant link has not been provided. It is conceivable that the inflammatory process at the dermoepidermal junction in these disorders raises a secondary immune response

from dystonia musculorum, with a spontaneous mutation in the so called DST gene.[48–50] Better understanding of the phenotype of these animals has led to characterization of several tissue-specific isoforms of BP230, including at least a neuronal and a muscle-specific variant. These findings, together with the recently highlighted increased association between BP and neurologic disorders,[28,35–37] may suggest that autoimmunity to BP230 is involved in the development of neurologic diseases. Recently, mutations in the DST gene have been identified in a patient with epidermolysis bullosa exhibiting mild, localized blistering.[51]

## DIAGNOSIS

Diagnosis of BP is based on a combination of clinical features and immunopathologic findings (**Fig. 4**).[43,52] In atypical and nonbullous variants, diagnosis of BP critically relies on the findings of direct immunofluorescence (IF) microscopy together with the characterization of the specificity of circulating autoantibodies and/or findings from other approaches (**Fig. 4**).

### Clinical Criteria

The typical patient with BP is older than 75 years and presents with a pruritic eczematous, urticarial eruption with or without frank blistering. Mucous membranes and the face and neck region are usually not affected. In many patients, there are simply excoriated lesions. Knowledge of the wide spectrum of clinical presentations and atypical variants is important to consider the diagnosis of BP. Vaillant and colleagues[53] showed that the diagnosis of BP can be made with high specificity and sensitivity in patients with linear immunoglobulin G (IgG) and/or C3 deposits along the dermoepidermal junction when 3 of the 4 clinical criteria are present: age greater than 70 years, absence

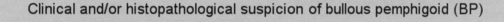

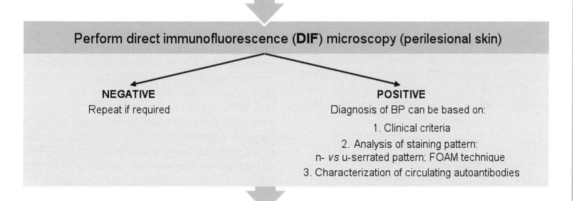

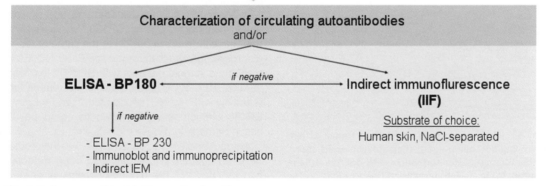

**Fig. 4.** Bullous pemphigoid. Diagnostic algorithm.

of atrophic scars, absence of mucosal involvement, and absence of predominant bullous lesions on the neck and head.[53]

### Histopathology and Immunohistochemistry

Histopathology is not essential for the diagnosis of BP. Findings may be either typical or suggestive, or at least useful, for the differential diagnosis. When BP is suspected, the biopsy specimen should ideally include a macroscopically visible vesicle, a bulla, or at least the edge of a larger bulla. Light microscopy studies of an early bulla typically reveal a subepidermal blister formation with a superficial dermal inflammatory infiltrate rich in eosinophils (**Fig. 5**) In early nonbullous phases, subepidermal clefts and eosinophilic spongiosis can be found. Recently, immunohistochemical studies have suggested that the detection of C3d deposits at the dermoepidermal junction in formalin-fixed tissue is useful for the diagnosis.[54,55]

### Direct IF Microscopy

Studies of a biopsy specimen obtained from perilesional skin still represent the diagnostic gold standard. They show the presence of deposits of IgG and/or C3 along the dermoepidermal junction (**Fig. 6**A). IgM, IgE and fibrinogen may also be detected with variable frequency. The proper choice of the site for the skin biopsy is critical because lesional biopsies may give false-positive or false-negative results. Close analysis of the linear fluorescence pattern at the BMZ (n-serrated vs u-serrated pattern)[56] as well as examination of patient's skin after treatment with 1 M NaCl (referred to as salt-split skin of autologous skin)

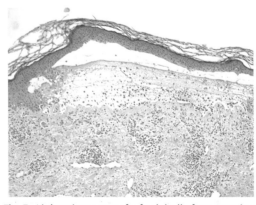

**Fig. 5.** Light microscopy of a fresh bulla from a patient with bullous pemphigoid (hematoxylin-eosin stain): subepidermal blister formation with discrete inflammatory infiltrate (eosinophils and neutrophils) in the blister cavity and in the dermis by light microscopy.

is also helpful for the diagnosis[57]: In patients with BP, IgG localizes to the epidermal side of the split, whereas a dermal staining is seen in patients with anti-laminin 332 mucous membrane pemphigoid, anti-p200/laminin γ1 pemphigoid, and epidermolysis bullosa acquisita, respectively. The distribution of C3 seems less reliable than that of IgG.[58]

### Indirect IF Microscopy

In up to 80% to 85% of patients, indirect IF microscopy studies show the presence of circulating IgG autoantibodies that typically bind to the epidermal side of 1M NaCl-split normal human skin, the substrate of reference (see **Fig. 6**B), differentiating BP sera from sera from patients with anti-laminin 332 mucous membrane pemphigoid, anti-p200/laminin γ1 pemphigoid, and epidermolysis bullosa acquisita, which all bind to the dermal side.[59,60] Additional circulating autoantibodies of the IgA, IgE, and IgM class can also be found. Isotype reactivity with the epidermal side of the artificial split appeared to be associated with age: sera from younger patients contained significantly more IgA reactivity, whereas IgG reactivity was predominantly found in older patients.[61]

### Enzyme-linked Immunosorbent Assays

Enzyme-linked immunosorbent assays (ELISAs) using recombinant proteins of various portions of BP180 (such as the NC16A domain, the C-terminal portion, or its entire ectodomain) have been found to be highly specific and sensitive.[62–73] The NC16A domain of BP180 has been identified as an immunodominant stretch in BP IgG. These anti-BP180 NC16A antibodies were found in between 75% and 90% of patients with BP[44,45,68,69,71–73] and their level correlates with the disease activity of patients with BP.[20,71,73–76] Two highly sensitive and specific ELISA systems for serum anti-BP180 antibodies are commercially available (Euroimun, Lübeck, Germany and MBL, Nagoya, Japan).[72,73]

Most patients with BP also develop, beside IgG, IgA anti-BP180 reactivity.[77] Sera from patients with linear IgA bullous disease also contain IgG and IgA antibodies against BP180,[61,77] suggesting that these 2 diseases belong to the same group of disorders. IgE reactivity against BP180 NC16A is also found in most patients with BP.[78–80] In recent studies, 10% of BP sera contained IgE but no IgG reactivity with the NC16A domain,[80] and IgE anti-BP180 antibodies were shown to contribute to tissue damage in mouse models.[81,82]

Autoantibodies against BP230, the other targeted antigen in BP, can also been detected by ELISA.[70,83–85] The globular C-terminal domain of BP230 is targeted by about 80% of the

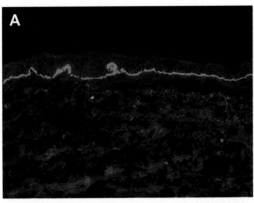
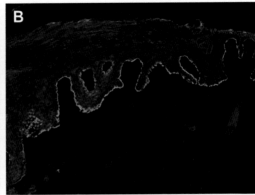

Fig. 6. (A) Direct immunofluorescence microscopy study of perilesional skin from a patient with bullopus pemphigoid revealed linear, continuous deposits of C3 along the dermoepidermal junction. (B) Indirect immunofluorescence microscopy study using NaCl-split normal human skin as a substrate. Staining of the epidermal side of the split typical for autoantibodies in bullous pemphigoid.

BP230-reactive BP sera.[20,86] Two ELISA kits have been commercialized (Euroimun and MBL) and use a recombinant C-terminal stretch of BP230, whereas, in the MBL ELISA, an N-terminal fragment is also included. Both ELISA systems are less sensitive compared with the BP180 ELISA, with anti-BP230 reactivity in only 50% to 70% of BP sera.[70,83–85] For routine analysis, a search for anti-BP230 antibodies is only helpful in patients with positive direct IF microcopy but negative BP180 ELISA reactivity.

### Immunoblot and Immunoprecipitation

In the past, detection of anti-BP180 and anti-BP230 reactivity relied on immunoblot and immunoprecipitation studies using extracts of cultured keratinocytes or human epidermis,[3,5,87,88] conditioned medium of cultured human keratinocytes, as well as various recombinant forms of BP180 and BP230 produced in different expression systems.[45,66,77,78,89–91] The combination of various ELISAs with immunoblotting, as well as cell-based IF studies, allows the detection of autoantibodies in virtually all BP sera.[20,90] Currently, immunoblotting and immunoprecipitation studies are only used for investigative studies.

### REACTIVITY WITH BP180 AND BP230 IN INDIVIDUALS WITHOUT BP

In a large cohort of 337 patients with various dermatologic disorders, 4.2% of the tested sera showed low positive values for BP180 (range between 9.2 and 33.1; normal, <9.0) and BP230 (range between 9.1 and 15.2; normal, <9.0), independently of age or sex.[92] Foureur and colleagues[93] confirmed this finding in a group of 138 dermatologic patients without evidence for

BP. However, anti-BP180 reactivity has also been reported in patients with a variety of pruritic disorders.[94–96] At present, the detection of low-level anti-BP180 and anti-BP230 serum antibodies in patients without clinical signs of BP does not require further investigations. In patients with pruritic disorders and ELISA reactivity against BP180 or BP230, direct IF microscopy is required to differentiate between unspecific autoantibody reactivity and BP.

### DIFFERENTIAL DIAGNOSIS

In our experience, BP is a great imitator. In either the nonbullous prodromal stage or in atypical presentations, it can bear close resemblance to a variety of dermatoses including localized or generalized drug reactions, contact and allergic dermatitis, prurigo, fixed urticaria, urticarial vasculitis, arthropod reactions, scabies, ecthyma, or even pityriasis lichenoides. Detailed patient history, clinical evaluation, histopathologic features, and, above all, direct immunofluorescence microscopy studies are essential to distinguish these disorders from BP. The development of specific and sensitive ELISA systems in recent years may now allow the serologic diagnosis of BP in most patients.

Diseases of the pemphigus group can be easily differentiated by distinctive clinical (positive Nikolski sign) and immunopathologic features. Mucous membrane pemphigoid is differentiated form BP by its predominant involvement of mucosal surfaces.[97] In contrast, the distinction of BP from linear IgA disease, epidermolysis bullosa acquisita, and anti-p200/laminin γ1 pemphigoid based simply on clinical and histopathologic features is usually impossible and requires direct IF microscopy (for linear IgA disease) and serologic analyses (for the last 2 entities). Lichen planus pemphigoides is clinically characterized by the presence of lichen planus lesions on otherwiese unaffected skin in addition to tense blisters. In dermatitis herpetiformis, direct IF microscopy findings, and particularly the serologic profile (presence of anti-tissue and anti-epidermal transglutaminase as well as anti-gliadin IgA antibodies) are characteristic.

## PROGNOSIS AND MORTALITY

BP frequently has a chronic evolution with remissions and relapses. It is associated with significant morbidity, such as severe itch, bullous and eroded lesions, and impetiginization. The impact on the quality of life is significant. In a recent prospective study encompassing, at entry, 114 patients with BP, 47% of the 96 evaluable patients experienced a disease relapse within 1 year after cessation of therapy, confirming the recurring nature of the disease. There have been some controversies about the prognosis and mortality of BP.[98–104] It is likely that the reported diverging mortalities are related to the inclusion of populations of different mean age, in different general conditions (outpatients vs inpatients), and the use of different treatment protocols (oral corticosteroids, immunosuppressants) as well as diagnostic accuracy. For example, the 1-year mortality in 62 patients with a median age of 76 years, who were treated with methylprednisolone, dapsone, and clobetasol propionate cream, was as low as 6%,[98] whereas in a study of 312 patients with an average age of 82 years and treated by clobetasol propionate cream alone, the 1-year mortality was 39%.[104] The 1-year mortality after diagnosis of BP was reported to be 29%, 26%, 23%, and 19% in 369, 341, 223, and 869 patients with BP from Germany, France, the United States and the United Kingdom respectively.[10,18,19,103] Langan and colleagues[10] reported a 2.3-fold higher 1-year mortality risk for patients with BP compared with age-matched and sex-matched controls. In 2 large studies encompassing 369 and 177 patients, the following risk factors for lethal outcome in the first year after diagnosis were identified: (1) age greater than 82 and 80 years, respectively; (2) daily prednisolone dose of more than 37 mg after hospitalization; (3) serum albumin levels of less than 3.6 g/dL; (4) an erythrocyte sedimentation rate greater than 300 mm/h; and (5) a Karnofsky score of 40 or less.[19,102]

## CONCLUDING REMARKS

Recent animal models of BP have provided unequivocal evidence for the pathogenic effect of autoantibodies to BP180 as well as novel insights into the cascade of events leading to tissue damage in BP. Despite these advances, BP still represents a clinical, diagnostic, and therapeutic challenge in our practice. The protean clinical features, the difficult diagnosis of early and atypical forms of BP, and the advanced age of affected patients with multiple comorbidities require a high degree of expertise and caution with the management of affected patients. Better knowledge of the pathophysiology of BP will hopefully facilitate the development of new immunomodulatory treatments with fewer side effects for this debilitating disease. The joint efforts by all international experts are required to improve the evaluation and treatment of these patients.

## REFERENCES

1. Lever WF. Pemphigus. Medicine 1953;32:1–123.
2. Jordon RE, Beutner EH, Witebsky E, et al. Basement zone antibodies in bullous pemphigoid. JAMA 1967;200:751–6.
3. Labib RS, Anhalt GJ, Patel HP, et al. Molecular heterogeneity of the bullous pemphigoid antigens as detected by immunoblotting. J Immunol 1986; 136:1231–5.
4. Diaz LA, Ratrie H 3rd, Saunders WS, et al. Isolation of a human epidermal cDNA corresponding to the 180-kD autoantigen recognized by bullous pemphigoid and herpes gestationis sera. Immunolocalization of this protein to the hemidesmosome. J Clin Invest 1990;86:1088–94.
5. Stanley JR, Hawley-Nelson P, Yuspa SH, et al. Characterization of bullous pemphigoid antigen: a unique basement membrane protein of stratified squamous epithelia. Cell 1981;24:897–903.
6. Liu Z, Diaz LA, Troy JL, et al. A passive transfer model of the organ-specific autoimmune disease, bullous pemphigoid, using antibodies generated against the hemidesmosomal antigen, BP180. J Clin Invest 1993;92:2480–8.
7. Nishie W, Sawamura D, Goto M, et al. Humanization of autoantigen. Nat Med 2007;13:378–83.
8. Bernard P, Vaillant L, Labeille B, et al. Incidence and distribution of subepidermal autoimmune bullous skin diseases in three French regions. Bullous Diseases French Study Group. Arch Dermatol 1995;131:48–52.
9. Jung M, Kippes W, Messer G, et al. Increased risk of bullous pemphigoid in male and very old patients: a population-based study on incidence. J Am Acad Dermatol 1999;41:266–8.
10. Langan SM, Smeeth L, Hubbard R, et al. Bullous pemphigoid and pemphigus vulgaris–incidence and mortality in the UK: population based cohort study. BMJ 2008;337:a180.
11. Gudi VS, White MI, Cruickshank N, et al. Annual incidence and mortality of bullous pemphigoid in the Grampian Region of North-east Scotland. Br J Dermatol 2005;153:424–7.

12. Cozzani E, Parodi A, Rebora A, et al. Bullous pemphigoid in Liguria: a 2-year survey. J Eur Acad Dermatol Venereol 2001;15:317–9.

13. Serwin AB, Bokiniec E, Piascik M, et al. Epidemiological and clinical analysis of pemphigoid patients in northeastern Poland in 2000-2005. Med Sci Monit 2007;13:CR360–4.

14. Marazza G, Pham HC, Scharer L, et al. Incidence of bullous pemphigoid and pemphigus in Switzerland: a 2-year prospective study. Br J Dermatol 2009;161:861–8.

15. Bertram F, Brocker EB, Zillikens D, et al. Prospective analysis of the incidence of autoimmune bullous disorders in Lower Franconia, Germany. J Dtsch Dermatol Ges 2009;7:434–40.

16. Zillikens D, Wever S, Roth A, et al. Incidence of autoimmune subepidermal blistering dermatoses in a region of central Germany. Arch Dermatol 1995;131:957–8.

17. Kippes W, Schmidt E, Roth A, et al. [Immunopathologic changes in 115 patients with bullous pemphigoid]. Hautarzt 1999;50:866–72 [in German].

18. Parker SR, Dyson S, Brisman S, et al. Mortality of bullous pemphigoid: an evaluation of 223 patients and comparison with the mortality in the general population in the United States. J Am Acad Dermatol 2008;59:582–8.

19. Joly P, Benichou J, Lok C, et al. Prediction of survival for patients with bullous pemphigoid: a prospective study. Arch Dermatol 2005;141:691–8.

20. Di Zenzo G, Thoma-Uszynski S, Fontao L, et al. Multicenter prospective study of the humoral autoimmune response in bullous pemphigoid. Clin Immunol 2008;128:415–26.

21. Liu HN, Su WP, Rogers RS 3rd. Clinical variants of pemphigoid. Int J Dermatol 1986;25:17–27.

22. Korman N. Bullous pemphigoid. J Am Acad Dermatol 1987;16:907–24.

23. Schmidt E, Sitaru C, Schubert B, et al. Subacute prurigo variant of bullous pemphigoid: autoantibodies show the same specificity compared with classic bullous pemphigoid. J Am Acad Dermatol 2002;47:133–6.

24. Geiss Steiner J, Trueb RM, Kerl K, et al. Ecthyma-gangrenosum-like bullous pemphigoid. Dermatology 2010;221:142–8.

25. Tran JT, Mutasim DF. Localized bullous pemphigoid: a commonly delayed diagnosis. Int J Dermatol 2005;44:942–5.

26. Schmidt E, Benoit S, Brocker EB. Bullous pemphigoid with localized umbilical involvement. Acta Derm Venereol 2009;89:419–20.

27. Bastuji-Garin S, Joly P, Picard-Dahan C, et al. Drugs associated with bullous pemphigoid. A case-control study. Arch Dermatol 1996;132:272–6.

28. Bastuji-Garin S, Joly P, Lemordant P, et al. Risk factors for bullous pemphigoid in the elderly: a prospective case-control study. J Invest Dermatol 2011;131:637–43.

29. Lindelof B, Islam N, Eklund G, et al. Pemphigoid and cancer. Arch Dermatol 1990;126:66–8.

30. Ogawa H, Sakuma M, Morioka S, et al. The incidence of internal malignancies in pemphigus and bullous pemphigoid in Japan. J Dermatol Sci 1995;9:136–41.

31. Bourdon-Lanoy E, Roujeau JC, Joly P, et al. [Bullous pemphigoid in young patients: a retrospective study of 74 cases]. Ann Dermatol Venereol 2005;132:115–22 [in French].

32. Taylor G, Venning V, Wojnarowska F, et al. Bullous pemphigoid and autoimmunity. J Am Acad Dermatol 1993;29:181–4.

33. Wilczek A, Sticherling M. Concomitant psoriasis and bullous pemphigoid: coincidence or pathogenic relationship? Int J Dermatol 2006;45:1353–7.

34. Shipman AR, Cooper S, Wojnarowska F. Autoreactivity to bullous pemphigoid 180: is this the link between subepidermal blistering diseases and oral lichen planus? Clin Exp Dermatol 2011;36:267–9.

35. Langer-Gould A, Albers KB, Van Den Eeden SK, et al. Autoimmune diseases prior to the diagnosis of multiple sclerosis: a population-based case-control study. Mult Scler 2010;16:855–61.

36. Jedlickova H, Hlubinka M, Pavlik T, et al. Bullous pemphigoid and internal diseases - A case-control study. Eur J Dermatol 2010;20:96–101.

37. Langan SM, Groves RW, West J. The relationship between neurological disease and bullous pemphigoid: a population-based case-control study. J Invest Dermatol 2011;131:631–6.

38. Seppanen A, Suuronen T, Hofmann SC, et al. Distribution of collagen XVII in the human brain. Brain Res 2007;1158:50–6.

39. Chen J, Li L, Zeng Y, et al. Sera of elderly bullous pemphigoid patients with associated neurological diseases recognize bullous pemphigoid antigens in the human brain. Gerontology 2010. [Epub ahead of print].

40. Leung CL, Zheng M, Prater SM, et al. The BPAG1 locus: alternative splicing produces multiple isoforms with distinct cytoskeletal linker domains, including predominant isoforms in neurons and muscles. J Cell Biol 2001;154:691–7.

41. Guo L, Degenstein L, Dowling J, et al. Gene targeting of BPAG1: abnormalities in mechanical strength and cell migration in stratified epithelia and neurologic degeneration. Cell 1995;81:233–43.

42. Zillikens D, Giudice GJ. BP180/type XVII collagen: its role in acquired and inherited disorders or the dermal-epidermal junction. Arch Dermatol Res 1999;291:187–94.

43. Di Zenzo G, Marazza G, Borradori L. Bullous pemphigoid: physiopathology, clinical features and management. Adv Dermatol 2007;23:257–88.

44. Giudice GJ, Emery DJ, Zelickson BD, et al. Bullous pemphigoid and herpes gestationis autoantibodies recognize a common non-collagenous site on the BP180 ectodomain. J Immunol 1993; 151:5742–50.

45. Zillikens D, Rose PA, Balding SD, et al. Tight clustering of extracellular BP180 epitopes recognized by bullous pemphigoid autoantibodies. J Invest Dermatol 1997;109:573–9.

46. Borradori L, Sonnenberg A. Structure and function of hemidesmosomes: more than simple adhesion complexes. J Invest Dermatol 1999;112:411–8.

47. Fine JD, Eady RA, Bauer EA, et al. The classification of inherited epidermolysis bullosa (EB): report of the third international consensus meeting on diagnosis and classification of EB. J Am Acad Dermatol 2008;58:931–50.

48. Goryunov D, Adebola A, Jefferson JJ, et al. Molecular characterization of the genetic lesion in dystonia musculorum (dt-Alb) mice. Brain Res 2007; 1140:179–87.

49. Brown A, Lemieux N, Rossant J, et al. Human homolog of a mouse sequence from the dystonia musculorum locus is on chromosome 6p12. Mamm Genome 1994;5:434–7.

50. Dalpe G, Leclerc N, Vallee A, et al. Dystonin is essential for maintaining neuronal cytoskeleton organization. Mol Cell Neurosci 1998;10:243–57.

51. Groves RW, Liu L, Dopping-Hepenstal PJ, et al. A homozygous nonsense mutation within the dystonin gene coding for the coiled-coil domain of the epithelial isoform of BPAG1 underlies a new subtype of autosomal recessive epidermolysis bullosa simplex. J Invest Dermatol 2010;130:1551–7.

52. Schmidt E, Zillikens D. Modern diagnosis of autoimmune blistering skin diseases. Autoimmun Rev 2010;10:84–9.

53. Vaillant L, Bernard P, Joly P, et al. Evaluation of clinical criteria for diagnosis of bullous pemphigoid. French Bullous Study Group. Arch Dermatol 1998;134:1075–80.

54. Pfaltz K, Mertz K, Rose C, et al. C3d immunohistochemistry on formalin-fixed tissue is a valuable tool in the diagnosis of bullous pemphigoid of the skin. J Cutan Pathol 2010;37:654–8.

55. Magro CM, Dyrsen ME. The use of C3d and C4d immunohistochemistry on formalin-fixed tissue as a diagnostic adjunct in the assessment of inflammatory skin disease. J Am Acad Dermatol 2008; 59:822–33.

56. Vodegel RM, Jonkman MF, Pas HH, et al. U-serrated immunodeposition pattern differentiates type VII collagen targeting bullous diseases from other subepidermal bullous autoimmune diseases. Br J Dermatol 2004;151:112–8.

57. Domloge-Hultsch N, Bisalbutra P, Gammon WR, et al. Direct immunofluorescence microscopy of 1

58. Gammon WR, Kowalewski C, Chorzelski TP, et al. Direct immunofluorescence studies of sodium chloride-separated skin in the differential diagnosis of bullous pemphigoid and epidermolysis bullosa acquisita. J Am Acad Dermatol 1990;22: 664–70.

59. Gammon WR, Briggaman RA, Inman AO 3rd, et al. Differentiating anti-lamina lucida and anti-sublamina densa anti-BMZ antibodies by indirect immunofluorescence on 1.0 M sodium chloride-separated skin. J Invest Dermatol 1984;82:139–44.

60. Kelly SE, Wojnarowska F. The use of chemically split tissue in the detection of circulating anti-basement membrane zone antibodies in bullous pemphigoid and cicatricial pemphigoid. Br J Dermatol 1988;118:31–40.

61. Mulyowa GK, Jaeger G, Kabakyenga J, et al. Autoimmune subepidermal blistering diseases in Uganda: correlation of autoantibody class with age of patients. Int J Dermatol 2006;45:1047–52.

62. Giudice GJ, Wilske KC, Anhalt GJ, et al. Development of an ELISA to detect anti-BP180 autoantibodies in bullous pemphigoid and herpes gestationis. J Invest Dermatol 1994;102:878–81.

63. Ide A, Hashimoto T, Amagai M, et al. Detection of autoantibodies against bullous pemphigoid and pemphigus antigens by an enzyme-linked immunosorbent assay using the bacterial recombinant proteins. Exp Dermatol 1995;4:112–6.

64. Zillikens D, Mascaro JM, Rose PA, et al. A highly sensitive enzyme-linked immunosorbent assay for the detection of circulating anti-BP180 autoantibodies in patients with bullous pemphigoid. J Invest Dermatol 1997;109:679–83.

65. Nakatani C, Muramatsu T, Shirai T. Immunoreactivity of bullous pemphigoid (BP) autoantibodies against the NC16A and C-terminal domains of the 180 kDa BP antigen (BP180): immunoblot analysis and enzyme-linked immunosorbent assay using BP180 recombinant proteins. Br J Dermatol 1998; 139:365–70.

66. Haase C, Budinger L, Borradori L, et al. Detection of IgG autoantibodies in the sera of patients with bullous and gestational pemphigoid: ELISA studies utilizing a baculovirus-encoded form of bullous pemphigoid antigen 2. J Invest Dermatol 1998; 110:282–6.

67. Hofmann S, Thoma-Uszynski S, Hunziker T, et al. Severity and phenotype of bullous pemphigoid relate to autoantibody profile against the NH2- and COOH-terminal regions of the BP180 ectodomain. J Invest Dermatol 2002;119:1065–73.

68. Mariotti F, Grosso F, Terracina M, et al. Development of a novel ELISA system for detection of

anti-BP180 IgG and characterization of autoantibody profile in bullous pemphigoid patients. Br J Dermatol 2004;151:1004–10.

69. Sakuma-Oyama Y, Powell AM, Oyama N, et al. Evaluation of a BP180-NC16a enzyme-linked immunosorbent assay in the initial diagnosis of bullous pemphigoid. Br J Dermatol 2004;151:126–31.

70. Thoma-Uszynski S, Uter W, Schwietzke S, et al. BP230- and BP180-specific auto-antibodies in bullous pemphigoid. J Invest Dermatol 2004;122: 1413–22.

71. Tsuji-Abe Y, Akiyama M, Yamanaka Y, et al. Correlation of clinical severity and ELISA indices for the NC16A domain of BP180 measured using BP180 ELISA kit in bullous pemphigoid. J Dermatol Sci 2005;37:145–9.

72. Sitaru C, Dahnrich C, Probst C, et al. Enzyme-linked immunosorbent assay using multimers of the 16th non-collagenous domain of the BP180 antigen for sensitive and specific detection of pemphigoid autoantibodies. Exp Dermatol 2007;16: 770–7.

73. Kobayashi M, Amagai M, Kuroda-Kinoshita K, et al. BP180 ELISA using bacterial recombinant NC16a protein as a diagnostic and monitoring tool for bullous pemphigoid. J Dermatol Sci 2002;30:224–32.

74. Schmidt E, Obe K, Brocker EB, et al. Serum levels of autoantibodies to BP180 correlate with disease activity in patients with bullous pemphigoid. Arch Dermatol 2000;136:174–8.

75. Feng S, Wu Q, Jin P, et al. Serum levels of autoantibodies to BP180 correlate with disease activity in patients with bullous pemphigoid. Int J Dermatol 2008;47:225–8.

76. Amo Y, Ohkawa T, Tatsuta M, et al. Clinical significance of enzyme-linked immunosorbent assay for the detection of circulating anti-BP180 autoantibodies in patients with bullous pemphigoid. J Dermatol Sci 2001;26:14–8.

77. Kromminga A, Scheckenbach C, Georgi M, et al. Patients with bullous pemphigoid and linear IgA disease show a dual IgA and IgG autoimmune response to BP180. J Autoimmun 2000;15:293–300.

78. Dopp R, Schmidt E, Chimanovitch I, et al. IgG4 and IgE are the major immunoglobulins targeting the NC16A domain of BP180 in bullous pemphigoid: serum levels of these immunoglobulins reflect disease activity. J Am Acad Dermatol 2000;42: 577–83.

79. Iwata Y, Komura K, Kodera M, et al. Correlation of IgE autoantibody to BP180 with a severe form of bullous pemphigoid. Arch Dermatol 2008;144: 41–8.

80. Messingham KA, Noe MH, Chapman MA, et al. A novel ELISA reveals high frequencies of BP180-specific IgE production in bullous pemphigoid. J Immunol Methods 2009;346:18–25.

81. Zone JJ, Taylor T, Hull C, et al. IgE basement membrane zone antibodies induce eosinophil infiltration and histological blisters in engrafted human skin on SCID mice. J Invest Dermatol 2007;127: 1167–74.

82. Fairley JA, Burnett CT, Fu CL, et al. A pathogenic role for IgE in autoimmunity: bullous pemphigoid IgE reproduces the early phase of lesion development in human skin grafted to nu/nu mice. J Invest Dermatol 2007;127:2605–11.

83. Kromminga A, Sitaru C, Hagel C, et al. Development of an ELISA for the detection of autoantibodies to BP230. Clin Immunol 2004;111: 146–52.

84. Yoshida M, Hamada T, Amagai M, et al. Enzyme-linked immunosorbent assay using bacterial recombinant proteins of human BP230 as a diagnostic tool for bullous pemphigoid. J Dermatol Sci 2006;41:21–30.

85. Tampoia M, Lattanzi V, Zucano A, et al. Evaluation of a new ELISA assay for detection of BP230 autoantibodies in bullous pemphigoid. Ann N Y Acad Sci 2009;1173:15–20.

86. Skaria M, Jaunin F, Hunziker T, et al. IgG autoantibodies from bullous pemphigoid patients recognize multiple antigenic reactive sites located predominantly within the B and C subdomains of the COOH-terminus of BP230. J Invest Dermatol 2000;114:998–1004.

87. Mueller S, Klaus-Kovtun V, Stanley JR. A 230-kD basic protein is the major bullous pemphigoid antigen. J Invest Dermatol 1989;92:33–8.

88. Bernard P, Didierjean L, Denis F, et al. Heterogeneous bullous pemphigoid antibodies: detection and characterization by immunoblotting when absent by indirect immunofluorescence. J Invest Dermatol 1989;92:171–4.

89. Marinkovich MP, Taylor TB, Keene DR, et al. LAD-1, the linear IgA bullous dermatosis autoantigen, is a novel 120-kDa anchoring filament protein synthesized by epidermal cells. J Invest Dermatol 1996; 106:734–8.

90. Schmidt E, Kromminga A, Mimietz S, et al. A highly sensitive and simple assay for the detection of circulating autoantibodies against full-length bullous pemphigoid antigen 180. J Autoimmun 2002;18:299–309.

91. Tanaka M, Hashimoto T, Amagai M, et al. Characterization of bullous pemphigoid antibodies by use of recombinant bullous pemphigoid antigen proteins. J Invest Dermatol 1991;97:725–8.

92. Wieland CN, Comfere NI, Gibson LE, et al. Anti-bullous pemphigoid 180 and 230 antibodies in a sample of unaffected subjects. Arch Dermatol 2010;146:21–5.

93. Foureur N, Mignot S, Senet P, et al. [Correlation between the presence of type-2 anti-pemphigoid antibodies and dementia in elderly subjects with no clinical signs of pemphigoid]. Ann Dermatol Venereol 2006;133:439–43 [in French].

94. Jedlickova H, Racovska J, Niedermeier A, et al. Anti-basement membrane zone antibodies in elderly patients with pruritic disorders and diabetes mellitus. Eur J Dermatol 2008;18:534–8.

95. Feliciani C, Caldarola G, Kneisel A, et al. IgG auto-antibody reactivity against bullous pemphigoid (BP) 180 and BP230 in elderly patients with pruritic dermatoses. Br J Dermatol 2009;161:306–12.

96. Hofmann SC, Tamm K, Hertl M, et al. Diagnostic value of an enzyme-linked immunosorbent assay using BP180 recombinant proteins in elderly patients with pruritic skin disorders. Br J Dermatol 2003;149:910–2.

97. Chan LS, Ahmed AR, Anhalt GJ, et al. The first international consensus on mucous membrane pemphigoid: definition, diagnostic criteria, pathogenic factors, medical treatment, and prognostic indicators. Arch Dermatol 2002;138:370–9.

98. Schmidt E, Kraensel R, Goebeler M, et al. Treatment of bullous pemphigoid with dapsone, methylprednisolone, and topical clobetasol propionate: a retrospective study of 62 cases. Cutis 2005;76:205–9.

99. Colbert RL, Allen DM, Eastwood D, et al. Mortality rate of bullous pemphigoid in a US medical center. J Invest Dermatol 2004;122:1091–5.

100. Joly P, Benichou J, Saiag P, et al. Response to: mortality rate of bullous pemphigoid in a US medical center. J Invest Dermatol 2005;124:664–5.

101. Bystryn JC, Rudolph JL. Why is the mortality of bullous pemphigoid greater in Europe than in the US? J Invest Dermatol 2005;124:xx–xxi.

102. Roujeau JC, Lok C, Bastuji-Garin S, et al. High risk of death in elderly patients with extensive bullous pemphigoid. Arch Dermatol 1998;134:465–9.

103. Rzany B, Partscht K, Jung M, et al. Risk factors for lethal outcome in patients with bullous pemphigoid: low serum albumin level, high dosage of glucocorticosteroids, and old age. Arch Dermatol 2002;138:903–8.

104. Joly P, Roujeau JC, Benichou J, et al. A comparison of two regimens of topical corticosteroids in the treatment of patients with bullous pemphigoid: a multicenter randomized study. J Invest Dermatol 2009;129:1681–7.

# Pathogenesis of Bullous Pemphigoid

Hideyuki Ujiie, MD, PhD*, Wataru Nishie, MD, PhD,
Hiroshi Shimizu, MD, PhD

## KEYWORDS

- Bullous pemphigoid • Pathogenesis • Type XVII collagen
- NC16A • Animal model • IgE autoantibody

Bullous pemphigoid (BP), the most common autoimmune blistering disorder, is induced by autoantibodies against the components of the skin basement membrane zone (BMZ).[1,2] Clinically, tense blisters and erosions with itchy urticarial plaques and erythema develop on the whole body (**Fig. 1A**). Histologic examination of lesional skin reveals subepidermal blisters with inflammatory infiltration consisting of eosinophils and lymphocytes (see **Fig. 1B**). Direct immunofluorescence (IF) shows linear deposition of IgG and complement C3 at the dermal-epidermal junction (DEJ) (see **Fig. 1C**). In addition, indirect IF using the patient's sera shows linear deposition of IgG at the DEJ of normal human skin, and the autoantibodies usually deposit on the roof side of the artificial split-skin blister induced by 1M sodium chloride (see **Fig. 1D**). Immunoblotting reveals that the autoantibodies usually react with 180-kDa or 230-kDa proteins in epidermal extractions of normal human skin as candidate autoantigens. The 230-kDa protein, called BP230 or BPAG1, is a plakin family protein that was originally identified as the major antigen for BP.[3,4] BP230 is a cytoplasmic component of hemidesmosomes that enhances the linkage of keratin intermediate filaments to hemidesmosomes.[5] Although several studies have indicated that BP230 is pathogenic,[6,7] it remains unclear whether the autoantibodies against BP230 are pathogenic. The 180-kDa protein is considered to be the main pathogenic antigen in BP.

## THE MAJOR PATHOGENIC ANTIGEN IN BP: TYPE XVII COLLAGEN (COL17)

Autoantibodies against the hemidesmosomal antigen of type XVII collagen (COL17, also called BP180 or BPAG2), a 180-kDa protein, are believed to induce the inflammatory process, resulting in dermal-epidermal separation. COL17 is a type II transmembrane protein that spans the lamina lucida and projects into the lamina densa of the BMZ (**Fig. 2A**).[8–10] COL17 has 15 collagenous domains in the extracellular domain (see **Fig. 2B**).[11] The noncollagenous 16A (NC16A) domain in the juxtamembranous extracellular part is considered to have the major pathogenic epitope for BP (see **Fig. 2B**).[12,13] The extracellular part of COL17 is constitutively shed from the cell surface within the NC16A domain.[14]

Epitope mapping using several fragments of COL17 and enzyme-linked immunosorbent assay analysis has elucidated that sera from most patients with BP recognize NC16A.[12,15] The titer of anti-COL17 NC16A antibodies has been shown to correlate with the disease severity of BP.[16] Autoantibodies against COL17 other than its NC16A domain are also detected in BP sera. About half of the BP sera recognize the C-terminal regions of the extracellular domain of COL17, and the presence of autoantibodies against both NC16A and the C-terminal portions of COL17 seems to be associated with the clinical involvement of mucosal lesions in patients with BP.[17] Epitope spreading has been suggested as

Financial disclosures and conflicts of interest: The authors have nothing to disclose.
Department of Dermatology, Hokkaido University Graduate School of Medicine, N-15 W-7, Kita-ku, Sapporo 060-8638, Japan
* Corresponding author.
*E-mail address:* h-ujiie@med.hokudai.ac.jp

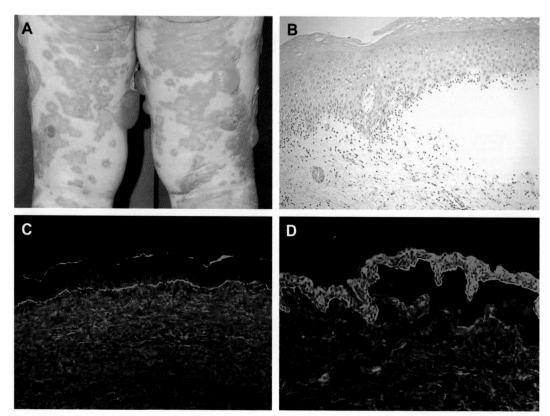

Fig. 1. Clinical, histologic, and direct IF features of BP. Tense blisters and erosions develop in itchy edematous erythema on the thighs (*A*). Histopathologic finding in a skin specimen taken from a tense bulla. Subepidermal blister formation associated with dermal inflammatory cell infiltration mainly of eosinophils and lymphocytes (*B*). Direct IF of lesional skin shows linear deposition of IgG at the DEJ (*C*). Indirect IF using 1M sodium chloride split skin as a substrate shows linear deposition of IgG on the roof side of the separation at the DEJ (*D*).

a mechanism for the generation of autoantibodies against various parts of COL17 in patients with BP.[18] Intramolecular epitope spreading within COL17 has been shown in an animal model developed by grafting human COL17-expressing transgenic (Tg) mice skin on to wild-type mice.[19] The pathogenic role of autoantibodies against COL17 other than its NC16A domain has not been fully elucidated.

Recently, precise cleavage sites within the NC16A domain of COL17 have been reported.[20] Cleavage of collagen XVII was shown to generate neoepitopes around aminoterminal cleavage sites on the shed ectodomain. It is well known that autoantibodies from patients with BP[21] as well as from patients with linear IgA bullous dermatosis[22] preferentially recognize the shed ectodomain of COL17, 1 explanation for which could be that these autoantibodies recognize shedding-generating neoepitopes.[20]

The pathogenicity of anti-COL17 IgG antibodies from patients with BP (BP-IgG) has been shown in vitro. BP-IgG against recombinant COL17 NC16A caused dermal-epidermal separation in cryosections of human skin when the skin was incubated with leukocytes from healthy volunteers.[23] In addition, polyclonal rabbit antibodies that target the shedding-generating neoepitopes also showed the potential to induce dermal-epidermal separation in human skin cryosections.[20] Furthermore, antibodies reacted with the nonblistering regions at the periphery of blister in patients with BP, suggesting the presence of neoepitopes in the early stage of BP that are likely to be involved in the pathogenesis of BP.[20]

Although some previous studies mentioned the pathogenic role of complement activation in BP, Iwata and colleagues[24] have reported that only BP-IgG is able to deplete the expression of COL17 in cultured normal human keratinocytes and reduce the attachment of cells from the dish in a complement-independent manner. This finding suggests that BP-IgG could reduce the content of hemidesmosomal COL17, resulting in weakness of the adhesion of hemidesmosomes to the lamina lucida.

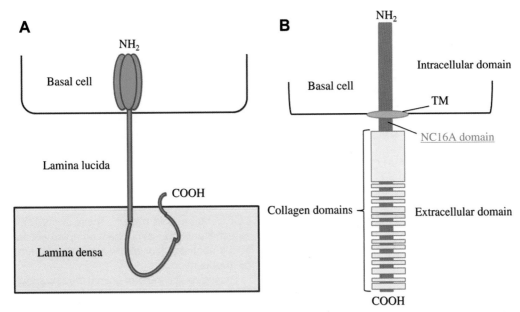

**Fig. 2.** The COL17 molecule in vivo. COL17 is a type II transmembrane protein that spans the lamina lucida and projects into the lamina densa of the epidermal BMZ. The extracellular domain of COL17 has at least 1 loop structure in the lamina densa in vivo (*A*). The extracellular region of COL17 involves 15 collagenous domains separated from one another by noncollagenous domains. The noncollagenous 16A (NC16A) domain, located at the membrane-proximal region of COL17, is considered to be the major pathogenic epitope for BP (*B*).

## IN VIVO STUDIES ON BP

The pathogenic role of antibodies against COL17 has been shown in a passive transfer mouse model using rabbit IgG antibodies against the murine homolog of human COL17 NC16A (murine COL17 NC14A).[25] The injected neonatal mice show skin fragility associated with the linear deposition of rabbit IgG and mouse C3 at the DEJ of their skin, and subepidermal separation with inflammatory cell infiltration; these correspond to the clinical, histologic, and immunopathologic features of BP.[25] Using this experimental BP model, Liu and colleagues revealed that subepidermal blister formation in their neonatal mouse model depends on complement activation,[26] mast cell degranulation,[27] and neutrophil infiltration.[28] These investigators also showed that the degradation of COL17 in that model depends on neutrophil elastase secreted by infiltrating neutrophils.[29]

Passive transfer of BP-IgG fails to induce a BP-like phenotype in mice, which is explained by the low similarity of the NC16A amino acid sequence between humans and mice. To further investigate the pathogenic roles of antihuman COL17 antibodies, a Tg mouse expressing human COL17 (hCOL17) cDNA driven under the control of a keratin 14 promoter was generated.[30] Olasz and colleagues[30] reported that wild-type mice grafted with hCOL17 Tg skin produce a high level

of anti-hCOL17 IgG and lose the Tg skin grafts with the deposition of IgG and C3 at the DEJ and with a neutrophil infiltration, resulting in the microscopic subepidermal blisters that are observed in BP. These findings show that the anti-hCOL17 IgG induced by Tg skin grafting is pathogenic against Tg skin that expresses hCOL17 antigens. These investigators also showed that major histocompatibility complex (MHC) class II$^{-/-}$ mice grafted with Tg skin develop neither anti-hCOL17 IgG nor graft loss, indicating that MHC II and CD4$^+$ T-cell interactions are crucial for these responses.

Although these studies strongly supported the hypothesis that anti-hCOL17 IgG autoantibodies in patients with BP have pathogenic activity, such activity had not been directly shown in vivo. In 2007, Nishie and colleagues[31] confirmed this hypothesis by using the unique technique of humanization of autoantigen. First, they generated murine *Col17*-knockout (m*Col17*$^{-/-}$) mice that developed blisters and erosions on the skin, symptoms that reproduce the human disease non-Herlitz epidermolysis bullosa, which is caused by null mutations in the *COL17A1* gene. By crossing Col17 knockout mice with hCOL17-expressing Tg mice, COL17-humanized (hCOL17$^{+/+}$, mCol17$^{-/-}$) mice were generated. Those COL17-humanized mice lack mCol17 but express hCOL17. Neonatal COL17-humanized mice were passively transferred with

BP-IgG, which produced diffuse erythema and epidermal detachment by gentle skin friction associated with dermal-epidermal separation and inflammatory cell infiltration of neutrophils and lymphocytes (**Fig. 3**A, B). Direct IF showed linear deposition of human IgG and murine C3 at the DEJ (see **Fig. 3**C, D), which simulates the human BP phenotype. This passive transfer neonatal mouse model was the first to directly show the pathogenicity of BP-IgG in vivo.

Some studies focusing on complement activation have been performed using a neonatal COL17-humanized BP mouse model. Wang and colleagues[32] generated recombinant Fab fragments against hCOL17 NC16A from antibody repertoires of patients with BP using a phage display method. Complement activation is considered to be critical for blister formation in neonatal BP model mice.[27] Some of the recombinant Fab fragments showed marked ability to inhibit the binding of BP autoantibodies to hCOL17 and to

inhibit subsequent complement activation in vitro. Those recombinant Fabs also prevented the binding of anti-COL17 NC16A antibodies to the NC16A domain in neonatal COL17-humanized mice and inhibited complement activation. Li and colleagues[33] recently generated a recombinant IgG1 monoclonal antibody against hCOL17 NC16A that can reproduce the BP phenotype in the neonatal COL17-humanized mice. These investigators introduced alanine substitutions at various C1q binding sites of the Fc region of the monoclonal antibody. Those mutated IgG antibodies failed to activate the complement in vitro and drastically lost pathogenic activity in neonatal COL17-humanized mice.[33] These 2 studies indicate that antibody-dependent complement activation is necessary for blister formation in neonatal BP model mice.

Those passive transfer animal models show only transient disease activity. Recently, an active BP mouse model that continuously produces

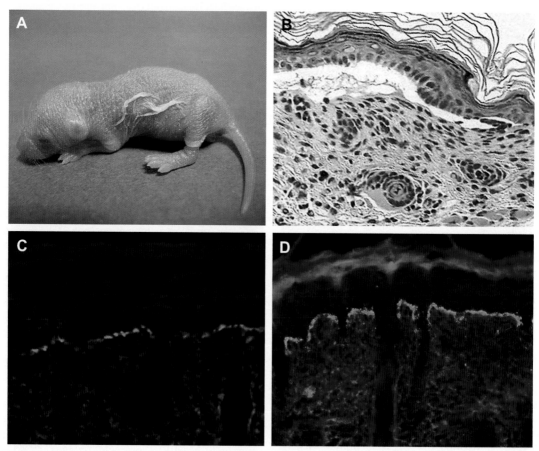

**Fig. 3.** A passive transfer neonatal BP model using the COL17-humanized mouse. The neonatal COL17-humanized mouse that was passively transferred with IgG affinity-purified against hCOL17 NC16A from patients with BP shows epidermal detachment by gentle skin friction at 48 hours after transfer (*A*). Lesional skin specimen shows dermal-epidermal separation and infiltration of inflammatory cells, including neutrophils and lymphocytes (*B*). Direct IF reveals linear deposition of human IgG (*C*) and murine C3 (*D*) at the DEJ.

pathogenic IgG in vivo and that stably shows the BP phenotype has been developed using immunodeficient $Rag\text{-}2^{-/-}$/COL17-humanized mice.[34] Adoptive transfer of splenocytes from wild-type mice immunized by the grafting of hCOL17-expressing Tg mouse skin into $Rag\text{-}2^{-/-}$/COL17-humanized mice induced continuous production of anti-hCOL17 IgG and blister formation corresponding to the clinical, histologic, and immunopathologic features of BP (**Fig. 4**). This study also showed that CD4[+] T cells are crucial for the development of the BP phenotype in the active BP model.[34] In human BP, the presence of autoreactive CD4[+] T cells has been reported, indicating the pathogenic role of CD4[+] T cells in producing BP.[35–37] High frequencies of particular MHC class II alleles have been also reported.[38] These findings indicate that the autoreactive CD4[+] T cells may be activated through the interaction of the specific MHC class II molecule in BP.

## STUDIES ON IGE ANTIBODIES AGAINST COL17

Not only IgG but also IgE autoantibodies against COL17 are considered to be pathogenic in patients with BP.[39] The early urticarial phase of the eruptions seen in BP seems to be associated with IgE, which is based on the common knowledge of IgE-mediated degranulation of mast cells in allergic forms of urticaria.[40] Total IgE levels are increased in 70% of untreated patients with BP and IgE autoantibodies against COL17 are detected in 86% of untreated patients with BP.[41] Iwata and colleagues[42] reported that the existence of IgE autoantibodies against COL17 relates to a severe form of BP. Patients with BP with IgE against COL17 require a longer period of treatment of remission, greater amounts of corticosteroids, and more intensive treatments for remission.[42] These findings suggest that IgE autoantibodies against COL17 are associated with BP pathogenesis and disease activity.

The passive transfer models for BP using IgG against COL17 do not induce the eosinophil infiltration that is a characteristic finding in human BP.[25,31] Zone and colleagues[43] successfully reproduced the itchy erythematous lesions in engrafted human skin in SCID (severe combined immunodeficiency) mice using IgE antibodies against LABD97, a component of the shed ectodomain of hCOL17, which are generated with IgE hybridoma to the LABD97 antigen. The hybridoma was injected subcutaneously in

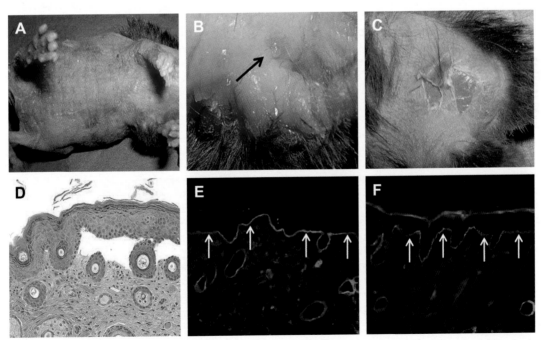

**Fig. 4.** Clinical, histologic, and direct IF features of an active BP mouse model. $Rag\text{-}2^{-/-}$/COL17-humanized mice given immunized splenocytes show large patches of hair loss associated with erythema, and erosions and crusts on the trunk and paws (*A*). Spontaneously developing blisters are also observed in the recipients (*arrow*) (*B*). Epidermal detachment by gentle friction on the trunk is observed (*C*). Histologic examination of diseased mice reveals separation between dermis and epidermis with mild inflammatory cell infiltration (*D*). Direct IF of lesional skin biopsy reveals linear deposition of mouse IgG (*arrows*) (*E*) and mouse C3 (*arrows*) (*F*) at the DEJ.

SCID mice engrafted with human skin, and they produced IgE antibodies against LABD97 in vivo. The IgE bound to the DEJ of the engrafted human skin and induced erythema. Then, all the injected mice developed severe eosinophil infiltration and mast cell degranulation within the grafts and most of them developed histologic, but not clinically detectable, subepidermal blisters. This BP model induced by IgE antibodies reproduces the clinical and histologic findings of human BP lesions including eosinophil infiltration.

Fairley and colleagues[44] developed an experimental BP mouse model using IgE autoantibodies from patients with BP. They isolated total IgE from BP sera and injected it into human skin grafted onto athymic nude mice. Increased erythematous plaques similar to early-stage BP lesions developed in all the human skin grafts after injection of the BP IgE. Histologic examination of the lesions revealed the engorgement of blood vessels and a dermal inflammatory infiltrate composed of neutrophils, eosinophils, and degranulated mast cells. Higher doses of BP IgE autoantibodies induced histologic dermal-epidermal separation in the grafts. This study provided direct evidence of a pathogenic role for IgE autoantibodies in BP. More recently, these investigators[45] reported a case of steroid-unresponsive BP that was successfully treated with omalizumab, a humanized monoclonal antibody that inhibits IgE binding to the high-affinity receptor FcεRI, suggesting that IgE autoantibodies could be a new therapeutic target in BP.

## SUMMARY

Recent studies using animal models have shown the pathogenicity of IgG and IgE antibodies against COL17 as well as the subsequent immune responses, such as complement activation, mast cell degranulation, and infiltration of inflammatory cells, including of neutrophils and/or eosinophils, although some of these responses seem to remain controversial. Moreover, in vitro studies of COL17 protein reveal the precise mechanisms of dermal-epidermal separation. The autoreactive CD4+ T lymphocytes that probably serve as a commander of autoimmune reactions in BP should be further investigated, because they are a potential therapeutic target in BP.

## REFERENCES

1. Bernard P, Vaillant L, Labeille B, et al. Incidence and distribution of subepidermal autoimmune bullous skin diseases in three French regions. Bullous Diseases French Study Group. Arch Dermatol 1995;13:48–52.
2. Marazza G, Pham HC, Scharer L, et al. Incidence of bullous pemphigoid and pemphigus in Switzerland: a 2-year prospective study. Br J Dermatol 2009;161: 861–8.
3. Stanley JR, Hawley-Nelson P, Yuspa SH, et al. Characterization of bullous pemphigoid antigen: a unique basement membrane protein of stratified squamous epithelia. Cell 1981;24:897–903.
4. Stanley JR, Tanaka T, Mueller S, et al. Isolation of complementary DNA for bullous pemphigoid antigen by use of patients' autoantibodies. J Clin Invest 1988;82:1864–70.
5. Guo L, Degenstein L, Dowling J, et al. Gene targeting of BPAG1: abnormalities in mechanical strength and cell migration in stratified epithelia and neurologic degeneration. Cell 1995;81:233–43.
6. Hall RP 3rd, Murray JC, McCord MM, et al. Rabbits immunized with a peptide encoded for by the 230-kD bullous pemphigoid antigen cDNA develop an enhanced inflammatory response to UVB irradiation: a potential animal model for bullous pemphigoid. J Invest Dermatol 1993;101: 9–14.
7. Kiss M, Husz S, Janossy T, et al. Experimental bullous pemphigoid generated in mice with an antigenic epitope of the human hemidesmosomal protein BP230. J Autoimmun 2005;24:1–10.
8. Diaz LA, Ratrie H 3rd, Saunders WS, et al. Isolation of a human epidermal cDNA corresponding to the 180-kD autoantigen recognized by bullous pemphigoid and herpes gestationis sera. Immunolocalization of this protein to the hemidesmosome. J Clin Invest 1990;86:1088–94.
9. Bedane C, McMillan JR, Balding SD, et al. Bullous pemphigoid and cicatricial pemphigoid autoantibodies react with ultrastructurally separable epitopes on the BP180 ectodomain: evidence that BP180 spans the lamina lucida. J Invest Dermatol 1997;108:901–7.
10. Ishiko A, Shimizu H, Kikuchi A, et al. Human autoantibodies against the 230-kD bullous pemphigoid antigen (BPAG1) bind only to the intracellular domain of the hemidesmosome, whereas those against the 180-kD bullous pemphigoid antigen (BPAG2) bind along the plasma membrane of the hemidesmosome in normal human and swine skin. J Clin Invest 1993;91:1608–15.
11. Giudice GJ, Emery DJ, Diaz LA. Cloning and primary structural analysis of the bullous pemphigoid autoantigen BP180. J Invest Dermatol 1992; 99:243–50.
12. Giudice GJ, Emery DJ, Zelickson BD, et al. Bullous pemphigoid and herpes gestationis autoantibodies recognize a common non-collagenous site on the BP180 ectodomain. J Immunol 1993;151:5742–50.

13. Zillikens D, Rose PA, Balding SD, et al. Tight clustering of extracellular BP180 epitopes recognized by bullous pemphigoid autoantibodies. J Invest Dermatol 1997;109:573–9.

14. Franzke CW, Bruckner-Tuderman L, Blobel CP. Shedding of collagen XVII/BP180 in skin depends on both ADAM10 and ADAM9. J Biol Chem 2009; 284:23386–96.

15. Zillikens D, Mascaro JM, Rose PA, et al. A highly sensitive enzyme-linked immunosorbent assay for the detection of circulating anti-BP180 autoantibodies in patients with bullous pemphigoid. J Invest Dermatol 1997;109:679–83.

16. Haase C, Budinger L, Borradori L, et al. Detection of IgG autoantibodies in the sera of patients with bullous and gestational pemphigoid: ELISA studies utilizing a baculovirus-encoded form of bullous pemphigoid antigen 2. J Invest Dermatol 1998;110:282–6.

17. Hofmann S, Thoma-Uszynski S, Hunziker T, et al. Severity and phenotype of bullous pemphigoid relate to autoantibody profile against the NH2- and COOH-terminal regions of the BP180 ectodomain. J Invest Dermatol 2002;119:1065–73.

18. Di Zenzo G, Grosso F, Terracina M, et al. Characterization of the anti-BP180 autoantibody reactivity profile and epitope mapping in bullous pemphigoid patients. J Invest Dermatol 2004;122:103–10.

19. Di Zenzo G, Calabresi V, Olasz EB, et al. Sequential intramolecular epitope spreading of humoral responses to human BPAG2 in a transgenic model. J Invest Dermatol 2009;130:1040–7.

20. Nishie W, Lamer S, Schlosser A, et al. Ectodomain shedding generates Neoepitopes on collagen XVII, the major autoantigen for bullous pemphigoid. J Immunol 2010;185:4938–47.

21. Schumann H, Baetge J, Tasanen K, et al. The shed ectodomain of collagen XVII/BP180 is targeted by autoantibodies in different blistering skin diseases. Am J Pathol 2000;156:685–95.

22. Hofmann SC, Voith U, Schonau V, et al. Plasmin plays a role in the in vitro generation of the linear IgA dermatosis antigen LADB97. J Invest Dermatol 2009;129:1730–9.

23. Sitaru C, Schmidt E, Petermann S, et al. Autoantibodies to bullous pemphigoid antigen 180 induce dermal-epidermal separation in cryosections of human skin. J Invest Dermatol 2002;118:664–71.

24. Iwata H, Kamio N, Aoyama Y, et al. IgG from patients with bullous pemphigoid depletes cultured keratinocytes of the 180-kDa bullous pemphigoid antigen (type XVII collagen) and weakens cell attachment. J Invest Dermatol 2009;129:919–26.

25. Liu Z, Diaz LA, Troy JL, et al. A passive transfer model of the organ-specific autoimmune disease, bullous pemphigoid, using antibodies generated against the hemidesmosomal antigen, BP180. J Clin Invest 1993;92:2480–8.

26. Liu Z, Giudice GJ, Swartz SJ, et al. The role of complement in experimental bullous pemphigoid. J Clin Invest 1995;95:1539–44.

27. Chen R, Ning G, Zhao ML, et al. Mast cells play a key role in neutrophil recruitment in experimental bullous pemphigoid. J Clin Invest 2001;108:1151–8.

28. Liu Z, Giudice GJ, Zhou X, et al. A major role for neutrophils in experimental bullous pemphigoid. J Clin Invest 1997;100:1256–63.

29. Liu Z, Shapiro SD, Zhou X, et al. A critical role for neutrophil elastase in experimental bullous pemphigoid. J Clin Invest 2000;105:113–23.

30. Olasz EB, Roh J, Yee CL, et al. Human bullous pemphigoid antigen 2 transgenic skin elicits specific IgG in wild-type mice. J Invest Dermatol 2007;127:2807–17.

31. Nishie W, Sawamura D, Goto M, et al. Humanization of autoantigen. Nat Med 2007;13:378–83.

32. Wang G, Ujiie H, Shibaki A, et al. Blockade of autoantibody-initiated tissue damage by using recombinant fab antibody fragments against pathogenic autoantigen. Am J Pathol 2010;176:914–25.

33. Li Q, Ujiie H, Shibaki A, et al. Human IgG1 monoclonal antibody against human collagen L17 noncollagenous 16A domain induces blisters via complement activation in experimental bullous pemphigoid model. J Immunol 2010;185:7746–55.

34. Ujiie H, Shibaki A, Nishie W, et al. A novel active mouse model for bullous pemphigoid targeting humanized pathogenic antigen. J Immunol 2010; 184:2166–74.

35. Budinger L, Borradori L, Yee C, et al. Identification and characterization of autoreactive T cell responses to bullous pemphigoid antigen 2 in patients and healthy controls. J Clin Invest 1998; 102:2082–9.

36. Lin MS, Fu CL, Giudice GJ, et al. Epitopes targeted by bullous pemphigoid T lymphocytes and autoantibodies map to the same sites on the bullous pemphigoid 180 ectodomain. J Invest Dermatol 2000; 115:955–61.

37. Thoma-Uszynski S, Uter W, Schwietzke S, et al. Autoreactive T and B cells from bullous pemphigoid (BP) patients recognize epitopes clustered in distinct regions of BP180 and BP230. J Immunol 2006;176:2015–23.

38. Delgado JC, Turbay D, Yunis EJ, et al. A common major histocompatibility complex class II allele HLA-DQB1* 0301 is present in clinical variants of pemphigoid. Proc Natl Acad Sci U S A 1996;93: 8569–71.

39. Provost TT, Tomasi TB Jr. Immunopathology of bullous pemphigoid. Basement membrane deposition of IgE, alternate pathway components and fibrin. Clin Exp Immunol 1974;18:193–200.

40. Friedmann PS. Assessment of urticaria and angiooedema. Clin Exp Allergy 1999;29(Suppl 3):109–12.

41. Dimson OG, Giudice GJ, Fu CL, et al. Identification of a potential effector function for IgE autoantibodies in the organ-specific autoimmune disease bullous pemphigoid. J Invest Dermatol 2003;120: 784–8.

42. Iwata Y, Komura K, Kodera M, et al. Correlation of IgE autoantibody to BP180 with a severe form of bullous pemphigoid. Arch Dermatol 2008;144:41–8.

43. Zone JJ, Taylor T, Hull C, et al. IgE basement membrane zone antibodies induce eosinophil infiltration and histological blisters in engrafted human skin on SCID mice. J Invest Dermatol 2007;127: 1167–74.

44. Fairley JA, Burnett CT, Fu CL, et al. A pathogenic role for IgE in autoimmunity: bullous pemphigoid IgE reproduces the early phase of lesion development in human skin grafted to nu/nu mice. J Invest Dermatol 2007;127:2605–11.

45. Fairley JA, Baum CL, Brandt DS, et al. Pathogenicity of IgE in autoimmunity: successful treatment of bullous pemphigoid with omalizumab. J Allergy Clin Immunol 2009;123:704–5.

# Pemphigoid Gestationis: Pathogenesis and Clinical Features

Lizbeth R.A. Intong, MD, DPDS,
Dédée F. Murrell, MA, BMBCh, FAAD, MD, FACD*

## KEYWORDS

- Pregnancy • Pemphigoid gestationis • Blistering
- Dermatoses • Autoimmunity

Pemphigoid gestationis (PG), formerly known as herpes gestationis, is a rare autoimmune blistering disease (AIBD) of pregnancy. It was first described in 1872 by Dr John Laws Milton, founder of the St John's Hospital for Diseases of the Skin in London, stemming a team of subsequent experts in the condition from this institution, in particular Dr Martin Black.[1,2] Recent advances have shown this disease to be similar to the pemphigoid group of diseases in terms of clinical and immunologic features. The specific dermatoses of pregnancy have since been reclassified and pemphigoid gestationis is the current terminology used.[3,4] Since then, there have been a number of case reports and large case series on this disease.[5–8]

## EPIDEMIOLOGY

The incidence of PG is very low, estimated at approximately 1 case per 50,000 pregnancies.[4,6] Reports are variable, but the disease commonly presents in the second or third trimester of pregnancy. In a review of 505 women with specific dermatoses of pregnancy, 21 were diagnosed with PG, with 48% of cases occurring in primigravid women. Disease onset was typically during the third trimester (71%), and less commonly during the second trimester (29%).[4] In another case series of 117 patients with PG, the mean age of patients was 28 years, with 17.9% presenting in the first trimester, 34.2% in the second trimester, 34.2% in the third trimester, and 13.7% during the postpartum period. There are also reports of this disease occurring in women with trophoblastic tumors, hydatidiform mole, or choriocarcinoma.[5]

## IMMUNOPATHOGENESIS

In normal pregnancies, there is a state of homeostasis between the mother and the fetus, whereby the mother tolerates the genetically and immunologically different fetal tissue growing inside her.[9,10] Changes to this tightly regulated immune state of the mother during pregnancy may lead to the development of various autoimmune diseases, one of which is PG. Fetal trophoblastic cells are typically devoid of major histocompatibility complex (MHC) class 1 and 2 molecules, and this is to ensure that the maternal immune system does not mount an immune response against the growing fetus.[10] The major target antigen in PG is collagen XVII (BP180), a transmembrane hemidesmosomal glycoprotein, which is found in the basement membranes of the skin and the amniotic epithelium of placental tissues. In a recent immunohistochemical study of the basement membrane zone and dermal extracellular matrix of normal amnion, BP180 was found to be greatly reduced in comparison with nonreproductive epithelium.[11] This self-antigen is presented to the maternal immune system by

Department of Dermatology, St George Hospital, University of New South Wales, Gray Street, Kogarah, Sydney, NSW 2217, Australia
* Corresponding author.
E-mail address: d.murrell@unsw.edu.au

Dermatol Clin 29 (2011) 447–452
doi:10.1016/j.det.2011.03.002

abnormally expressed HLA class 2 molecules in the placenta.[9–16] Antibodies, mainly immunoglobulin-G (IgG) and complement C3, are formed against the extracellular noncollagenous 16A (NC16A) domain of the 180-kd target antigen. This is the same immunodominant region of BP180 that is involved in bullous pemphigoid. Earlier reports state that the main IgG subclasses involved are IgG1 and IgG3,[9,14] but more recently, with the use of sandwich double antibody immunofluorescence (SDAI), the predominant subclass identified is IgG4.[15] IgG4 is the subclass that can cross the placenta, so if the infant had gradually developed an immune response to the mother's different BP180 sequence, this might explain why it only develops several months into pregnancy and why it would disappear after delivery. A more recent paper has identified IgE antibodies reactive against the NC16A domain of BP180.[16] The epitope profile of PG includes other target sites on the BP180 molecule outside of the NC16A domain. In a paper by Zambruno and colleagues,[13] PG sera bound to a total of 8 epitopes in the intracellular domain (ICD) and extracellular domain (ECD) by immunologic screening analyses and enzyme-linked immunosorbent assay (ELISA). There have also been reports of IgA autoantibodies directed against the C-terminal portion of the BP180 ectodomain in a PG patient with extensive oral involvement.[14] In addition, sera of PG patients may recognize the BP230 antigen.[13]

Epitope spreading upon exposure of the BP180 molecule to the maternal immune system may account for these additional autoantigens, as is described in other AIBD. None of these studies had sequenced the infant's BP180 gene to see if there was a polymorphism from a paternal allele that may have allowed the infant to recognize the mother's BP180 as foreign. The latter would fit with the history of 50% of pregnancies being affected in large families, as there would be a 50% chance of the fetus inheriting a polymorphism from the father. Such polymorphisms have been found in patients with other AIBD, such as pemphigus foliaceus.[17,18] Upon binding to the target antigen, IgG activates the classical complement pathway, resulting in tissue injury and blister formation. This is evidenced by deposition of C3 along the basement membrane zone during direct immunofluorescence.[9]

PG is associated with the presence of maternal MHC class 2 antigens DR3 and DR4.[9,10,19,20] A study done in the United States on 23 patients with PG showed that 61% of patients express HLA-DR3; 52% express HLA-DR4, and 43% express a combination of HLA-DR3/DR4.[19] This observation seems to be similar across ethnic groups, and has been reported in 8 Mexican patients with PG.[20] In a review of 22 cases of PG in Kuwait, predominance of HLA-DR3 and DQ2 antigens were observed, with no predominance of HLA-DR4.[21] They have also found anti-HLA antibodies to paternal HLA molecules in all cases studied.[22]

## ROLE OF HORMONES

The disease course of PG is related to changes in female hormone levels of estrogen and progesterone. In addition to its association with pregnancy, PG has been found to flare after administration of oral contraceptives and during menstruation.[2,9] Progesterone, a hormone that is elevated in the last few weeks of pregnancy, depresses antibody production, while estrogen enhances antibody production.[23] This could explain why PG usually improves just before delivery, but is usually characterized by an immediate postpartum flare, as levels of progesterone go back down.

## CLINICAL FEATURES

PG or herpes gestationis as initially described by Dr John Milton in 1872, was present in a 45-year-old woman who had nine pregnancies. She developed a severe annular erythema-like vesicular dermatosis leading to blistering during her first, fifth, eighth, and ninth pregnancies, with resolution of the eruption soon after delivery. He described the phenomenon of skipped pregnancies, which is often seen in PG.[1] Pruritus is the main feature of this disease. The patient initially presents with pruritic urticarial papules and annular plaques, followed by vesicles, and finally, large tense bullae (Fig. 1A). The time interval from onset of urticarial plaques to bullae formation ranges from a few days to around 4 weeks. The most common site of the eruption is the periumbilical area (see Fig. 1B) in about 90% of patients, later spreading to the rest of the abdomen, thighs (see Fig. 1C), palms, and soles. Fig. 1 shows grouped tense bullae overlying erythematous urticarial plaques in a patient with PG. Oral involvement is rare, but has been reported.[13] PG is reported to occur more frequently in multigravid women, and can invariably recur in their subsequent pregnancies, often with an earlier presentation if recurrent. Most cases present in the second or third trimester of pregnancy, with a period of remission during the last 6 weeks of pregnancy, followed by a flare immediately after delivery. The average duration postpartum was reported to be 4 weeks for the bullous eruption, and 60 weeks for the urticarial lesions. In some cases, disease activity lasted for up to 12 years

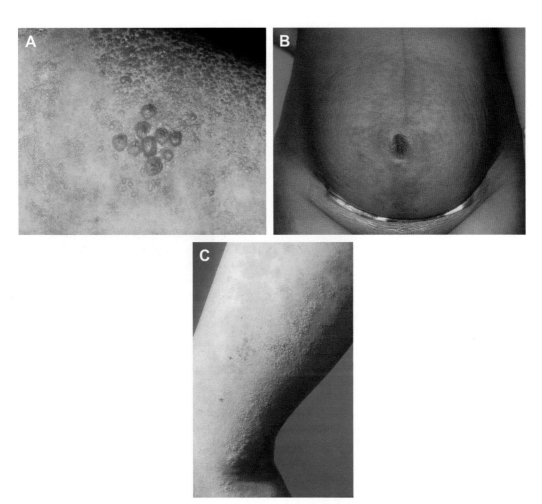

**Fig. 1.** (*A–C*) Grouped, tense bullae on an erythematous, urticarial base on the periumbilical area and leg of a patient with pemphigoid gestationis.

postpartum.[2,3,5] The disease is often severe enough that it requires potent topical or high-dose systemic corticosteroids (ie, 0.5–1 mg/kg/d of prednisone).[2–5,9] Intravenous immunoglobulin (IVIG) and rituximab postpartum have been used off-label to control disease flares.[24,25]

## ASSOCIATED AUTOIMMUNE DISEASES

There has been an increased frequency of Graves' disease being found in association with PG. This can be partially explained by the presence of HLA-DR3 and DR4, as these antigens have been independently associated with other autoimmune diseases, including autoimmune thyroiditis and pernicious anemia.[26]

## RISKS TO THE FETUS AND NEWBORN

An early study of 74 patients with PG showed that although there was an increased risk for prematurity and small-for-gestational-age babies, there was no increase in spontaneous abortions or stillbirths, nor was there an adverse association with the use of systemic steroids.[27] A more recent study of 61 patients has shown that early onset of the disease (ie, during the first or second trimester) and the presence of blisters are associated with adverse pregnancy outcomes, including preterm birth and low birth weight babies. The authors also concluded that the use of systemic corticosteroids does not affect pregnancy outcomes, and is an ideal treatment.[28] There have also been reports of the neonate born to a mother with PG also affected, but the incidence is rare and has been estimated at 1 case per 100,000 affected mothers.[29] Newborns affected with the disease have mild and transient blistering, resolving untreated over days to weeks, without any observed long-term sequelae.[2] A well-documented case in a 33-year-old mother and her affected newborn showed that the same level of pathogenic antibodies was transferred from the mother to the fetus, but that the vesiculo-bullous lesions in the neonate resolved without treatment long before the antibody disappeared.[29]

## DIAGNOSIS

In addition to the clinical presentation, diagnosis is confirmed by histology and direct immunofluorescence (DIF). If required, indirect immunofluorescence (IIF), ELISA, and immunoblotting may be performed. An HLA profile may also be taken to determine the presence of HLA-DR3, DR4, or a combination of both.

### Histology

The classic histologic picture is that of eosinophilic spongiosis, progressing to a subepidermal blister with eosinophils in the blister fluid, and dermal edema with a mixed perivascular infiltrate of eosinophils and lymphocytes.[2,3,9,30] **Fig. 2** shows the typical histopathology of PG.

### Immunofluorescence

The typical pattern on DIF is linear deposition of C3 plus or minus IgG along the basement membrane zone (BMZ). C3 is reported in 100% of cases, while IgG is seen in 25% to 50% of cases. Typically, these linear deposits of C3 plus or minus IgG would bind to the epidermal side of salt-split skin.[4,9,30] On IIF, circulating IgG antibodies would target the BMZ. **Fig. 3** shows the DIF of perilesional skin of a patient with PG showing linear deposition of C3 along the BMZ.

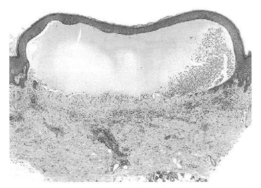

**Fig. 2.** H&E showing a subepidermal blister with predominance of eosinophils. (*From* Ambros-Rudolph CM, Müllegger RR, Vaughan-Jones SA, et al. The specific dermatoses of pregnancy revisited and reclassified: results of a retrospective two-center study on 505 pregnant patients. J Am Acad Dermatol 2006;54:401; with permission.)

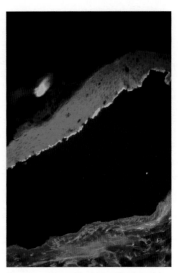

**Fig. 3.** Salt-split skin showing linear immunoglobulin-G binding to the roof of the blister.

### ELISA

ELISA would typically reveal circulating IgG antibodies against collagen XVII (BP180), in particular against the NC16A domain of BP180.[31] Antibodies against some adjacent epitopes have also been reported.[12] A commercially available BP180-NC16A domain ELISA kit was introduced in 2004, and has been useful in studies of the pemphigoid group of diseases. In a recent paper, ELISA was compared with IIF in a large group of patients with bullous pemphigoid (BP) and PG. Sensitivity was 93%, and specificity was 96% (*P*<.001) for ELISA versus a sensitivity of 74% and a similar specificity of 96% (*P*<.001) for IIF testing.[31]

### Immunoblotting

Circulating IgG antibodies to 180 kDa and/or 230 kDa protein bands are seen during immunoblotting (IB).[9] IB has been found useful for sera that are negative by IIF, as it may reveal circulating antibodies to other antigens (ie, BP230).[32]

## SUMMARY

PG is a rare, AIBD of pregnancy and the peripartum period. It is characterized clinically by severe pruritus, annular urticarial plaques underlying a vesiculobullous eruption usually starting in the third trimester of pregnancy. Autoantibodies, commonly IgG, are directed against the NC16A domain of the BP180 antigen found in both the skin and placenta. Histologic features and immunofluorescence findings are similar to that of bullous pemphigoid. ELISA and IB techniques may be used to confirm the target antigen(s) if required.

## REFERENCES

1. Black MM. The Neil Smith memorial lecture: John Laws Milton. The founder of St John's Hospital for Diseases of the Skin. Clin Exp Dermatol 2003;28:89–91.

2. Shornick JK. Herpes gestationis. J Am Acad Dermatol 1987;17:539–56.

3. Holmes RC, Black MM. The specific dermatoses of pregnancy. J Am Acad Dermatol 1983;8:405–12.

4. Ambros-Rudolph CM, Müllegger RR, Vaughan-Jones SA, et al. The specific dermatoses of pregnancy revisited and reclassified: results of a retrospective two-center study on 505 pregnant patients. J Am Acad Dermatol 2006;54:395–404.

5. Jenkins RE, Hern S, Black MM. Clinical features and management of 87 patients with pemphigoid gestationis. Clin Exp Dermatol 1999;24:255–9.

6. Shornick JK, Bangert JL, Freeman RG, et al. Herpes gestationis: clinical and histologic features of twenty-eight cases. J Am Acad Dermatol 1983;8:214–24.

7. Bedocs PM, Kumar V, Mahon MJ. Pemphigoid gestationis: a rare case and review. Arch Gynecol Obstet 2009;279:235–8.

8. Castro LA, Lundell RB, Krause PK, et al. Clinical experience in pemphigoid gestationis: report of 10 cases. J Am Acad Dermatol 2006;55:823–8.

9. Semkova K, Black M. Pemphigoid gestationis: current insights into pathogenesis and treatment. Eur J Obstet Gynecol Reprod Biol 2009;145:138–44.

10. Yip L, McCluskey J, Sinclair R. Immunological aspects of pregnancy. Clin Dermatol 2006;24:84–7.

11. Chi CC, Wang SH, Prenter A, et al. Basement membrane zone and dermal extracellular matrix of the vulva, vagina and amnion: an immunohistochemical study with comparison with non-reproductive epithelium. Australas J Dermatol 2010;51:243–7.

12. Huilaja L, Hurskainen T, Autio-Harmainen H, et al. Pemphigoid gestationis autoantigen, transmembrane collagen XVII, promotes the migration of cytotrophoblastic cells of placenta and is a structural component of fetal membranes. Matrix Biol 2008;27:190–200.

13. Di Zenzo G, Calabresi V, Grosso F, et al. The intracellular and extracellular domains of BP180 antigen comprise novel epitopes targeted by pemphigoid gestationis autoantibodies. J Invest Dermatol 2007;127:864–73.

14. Shimanovich I, Skrobek C, Rose C, et al. Pemphigoid gestationis with preominant involvement of oral mucous membranes and IgA autoantibodies targeting the C-terminus of BP180. J Am Acad Dermatol 2002;47:780–4.

15. Patton T, Plunkett RW, Beutner EH, et al. IgG4 as the predominant IgG subclass in pemphigoides gestationis. J Cutan Pathol 2006;33:299–302.

16. Noe MH, Messingham KA, Brandt DS, et al. Pregnant women have increased incidence of IgE antibodies reactive with the skin and placental antigen BP180 (type XVII collagen). J Reprod Immunol 2010;85:198–204.

17. Martel P, Gilbert D, Drouot L, et al. A polymorphic variant of the gene coding desmoglein 1, the target autoantigen of pemphigus foliaceus, is associated with the disease. Genes Immun 2001;2:41–3.

18. Martel P, Gilbert D, Busson M, et al. Epistasis between DSG1 and HLA class II genes in pemphigus foliaceus. Genes Immun 2002;3:205–10.

19. García-González E, Castro-Llamas J, karchmer S, et al. Class II major histocompatibility complex typing across the ethnic barrier in pemphigoid gestationis. A study in Mexicans. Int J Dermatol 1999;38:46–51.

20. Shornick JK, Stastny P, Gilliam JN. High frequency of histocompatibility antigens HLA-DR3 and DR4 in herpes gestationis. J Clin Invest 1981;68:553–5.

21. Nanda A, Al-saeed K, Dvorak R, et al. Clinicopathological features and HLA tissue typing in pemphigoid gestationis patients in Kuwait. Clin Exp Dermatol 2003;28:301–6.

22. Shornick JK, Jenkins RE, Briggs DC, et al. Anti-HLA antibodies in pemphigoid gestationis (herpes gestationis). Br J Dermatol 1993;129:257–9.

23. Da Silva JAP. Sex hormones and glucocorticoids: Interactions with the immune system. Ann N Y Acad Sci 1999;876:102–18.

24. Kreuter A, Harati A, Breuckmann F, et al. Intravenous immune globulin in the treatment of persistent pemphigoid gestationis. J Am Acad Dermatol 2004;51:1027–8.

25. Cianchini G, Masini C, Lupi F, et al. Severe persistent pemphigoid gestationis: long-term remission with rituximab. Br J Dermatol 2007;157:388–9.

26. Shornick JK, Black MM. Secondary autoimmune diseases in herpes gestationis (pemphigoid gestationis). J Am Acad Dermatol 1992;26:563–6.

27. Shornick JK, Black MM. Fetal risks in herpes gestationis. J Am Acad Dermatol 1992;26:63–8.

28. Chi CC, Wang SH, Charles-Holmes R, et al. Pemphigoid gestationis: early onset and blister formation are associated with adverse pregnancy outcomes. Br J Dermatol 2009;160:1222–8.

29. Aoyama Y, Asai K, Hioki K, et al. Herpes gestationis in a mother and newborn. Arch Dermatol 2007;143:1168–72.

30. Cobo MF, Santi CG, Maruta CW, et al. Pemphigoid gestationis: clinical and laboratory evaluation. Clinics 2009;64:1043–7.

31. Barnadas MA, Rubiales V, González J, et al. Enzyme-linked immunosorbent assay (ELISA) and indirect immunofluorescence testing in a bullous pemphigoid and pemphigoid gestationis. Int J Dermatol 2008;47:1245–9.

32. Ghohestani R, Kanitakis J, Nicolas JF, et al. Comparative sensitivity of indirect immunofluorescence to immunoblot assay for the detection of circulating antibodies to bullous pemphigoid antigens 1 and 2. Br J Dermatol 1996;135:74–9.

# Linear IgA Disease: Clinical Presentation, Diagnosis, and Pathogenesis

Vanessa A. Venning, BMBCh, DM, FRCP

## KEYWORDS

- Linear IgA disease • LAD
- Chronic bullous dermatosis of childhood • CBDC

## DEFINITION

Linear IgA disease (LAD) is a chronic, acquired, autoimmune blistering disease. It is characterized by subepidermal blistering and linear deposition of immunoglobulin A (IgA) basement membrane antibodies. The disease affects both children and adults and, although there are some differences in their clinical presentations, there is considerable overlap with shared immunopathology and immunogenetics.[1]

## DEMOGRAPHICS AND GENETIC BACKGROUND

LAD is one of the rarer subepidermal blistering diseases, with an incidence of only 0.5 per $10^6$ in western Europe. It is commoner in other parts of the world, including China, southeast Asia, and Africa, where there is a higher frequency of childhood disease.[2–4] Although LAD can come on at any age, there are 2 peaks of onset, 1 in early childhood and the other after the age of 60 years. Most children present as toddlers or preschool children, although a few have presented as neonates or in later childhood and in their teens.[1,5] Although it can affect young adults, there is a second peak of onset after the age of 60 years. The sex incidence is about equal, or there may be a slight excess of female patients.

There is a strong association between LAD and the extended autoimmune haplotype HLA-B8, HLA-CW7, HLA-DR3 in British and black South African patients, and possession of this haplotype is associated with an early disease onset. This extended haplotype is in linkage disequilibrium with an activating allele of tumor necrosis factor (TNF), and this association exists in patients with LAD and seems to worsen prognosis and prolong the disease.[6]

## CLINICAL FEATURES

Children with LAD show differences in clinical presentation compared with adults, reflected in the common usage of the term chronic bullous disease of childhood, although the immunopathology of the childhood and adult diseases are the same.

### Chronic Bullous Disease of Childhood

The typical presentation is a small child with an acute episode of blistering with variable symptoms of mild pruritus to severe burning. The first attack is usually more severe than later relapses. The face and perineal area are commonly affected with lesions around the mouth and eyes, including the eyelids or on the lower abdomen vulva, thighs, and buttocks (**Fig. 1**). Blistering on the genitalia may be mistaken for sexual abuse. The lesions may spread to the abdomen and limbs, including the hands and feet. Lesions comprise urticated plaques that frequently assume annular or polycyclic patterns, with blistering around the edge producing the so-celled string-of-pearls sign (**Fig. 2**). Blisters may become large or even hemorrhagic.

Department of Dermatology, Churchill Hospital, Old Road, Oxford OX3 7LJ, UK
*E-mail address:* vanessa.venning@orh.nhs.uk

Dermatol Clin 29 (2011) 453–458
doi:10.1016/j.det.2011.03.013
0733-8635/11/$ – see front matter © 2011 Elsevier Inc. All rights reserved.

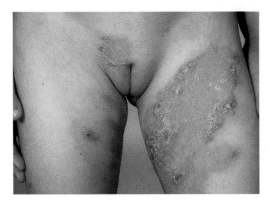

**Fig. 1.** LAD in childhood: blistering around the margins of annular and polycyclic lesions.

Mucosal lesions are common, with oral ulcers and erosions, nasal stuffiness or bleeding, and conjunctivitis.[1]

### Differential diagnosis

In young children, bullous impetigo may resemble the initial lesions. Genetic epidermolysis bullosa is often present at birth and is also differentiated from LAD by the family history. Bullous papular urticaria rarely affects the face or genital region

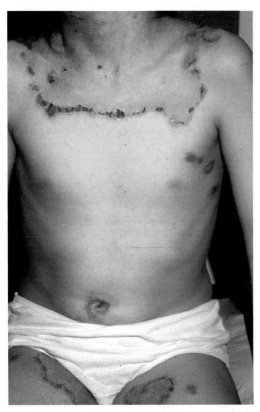

**Fig. 2.** LAD in childhood: blistering around the margins of annular and polycyclic lesions.

and is usually of short duration. Childhood bullous pemphigoid may resemble LAD.

### LAD in Adults

The disease usually starts abruptly but may be insidious, with variable pruritus or a burning sensation. The trunk is almost always involved but lesions on the face, scalp, and limbs, including the hands and feet, are also common. The lesions comprise urticated plaques and papules with vesicles and blisters arising either from normal skin or from the urticated areas (**Fig. 3**). The distinctive annular and string-of-pearls grouping of blisters around the edge are less common than in children. Some cases of LAD, in particular drug-related cases, have resembled other disorders, including erythema multiforme, toxic epidermal necrolysis, and morbilliform rash without blisters.[7,8]

Mucosal involvement is common with oral ulcers and erosions. Hoarseness may indicate pharyngeal involvement. There is often nasal stuffiness and crusting, and eyes are often sore or gritty. Involvement of the genitals and also the vagina can occur.

### Differential diagnosis

The adult disease is frequently confused with bullous pemphigoid in most cases, and less often

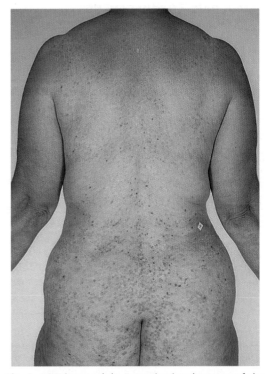

**Fig. 3.** LAD in an adult: extensive involvement of the torso with papulovesicular rash.

with atypical erythema multiforme, nodular prurigo with excoriations, and dermatitis herpetiformis. Histology is helpful and direct immunofluorescence (IMF) is essential for diagnosis.

## LAD: TRIGGERS AND DISEASE ASSOCIATIONS
### Drugs

Most cases start spontaneously but drug-induced LAD is well recognized. Vancomycin is the drug most frequently implicated, diclofenac and other nonsteroidal antiinflammatory drugs being less commonly reported, as well as single cases with a large range of other drugs.[7,9–12]

### Skin Trauma

Skin injury including burns have been associated with triggering disease onset.[1,13,14]

### Malignant Disease

Adults with LAD have an increased incidence of lymphoproliferative disorders that develop even after remission of the skin disease.[14–16] There are several case reports of other malignancies, of which bladder and renal cancer are commonest.[17–19]

### Gastrointestinal Disease

LAD has been associated with both ulcerative colitis and Crohn disease in small numbers of patients.[20,21] Patients with LAD were originally believed to have dermatitis herpetiformis. It is now clear that these 2 IgA-mediated diseases are distinct. LAD shows no association with gluten-sensitive enteropathy and does not respond to dietary gluten exclusion.[22–24]

## CLINICAL COURSE AND PROGNOSIS

Most patients respond well to treatment with dapsone or other sulfone drugs, antiinflammatory antibiotics, and topical steroids,[1] This will be covered in more detail in the article by Ng and Venning in the next issue. After an initial acute attack, the disease may wax and wane slightly, with subsequent flares usually being less severe than the first. In most patients, the disease remits during the course of a few years (3–6 years) and treatment can be discontinued.[1,25] Most children remit before puberty, although it occasionally persists into adult life.[26] In general LAD does not cause scarring. A small number children and adults have exceptionally severe mucosal disease that progresses to cicatrizing conjunctivitis and even blindness.[27–29] This rare subgroup is best regarded as having mucous membrane pemphigoid in accordance with the 2002 International Consensus on Mucous Membrane Pemphigoid: Definition and Diagnostic Criteria.[27]

## DIAGNOSIS

The diagnosis of LAD may be supported by histopathology but is only confirmed by IMF studies.

### Histopathology

The histologic features are not diagnostic for the condition. The blisters are subepidermal but the cellular infiltrate is variable. Some cases show eosinophil predominance suggestive of bullous pemphigoid. In others, the appearances are more in keeping with dermatitis herpetiformis with neutrophils predominating and even dermal papillary microabscesses. Others show subepidermal blisters with entirely nonspecific features.

### IMF

IMF studies are essential for diagnosis. Direct IMF should be performed on clinically uninvolved skin. The back is a suitable site and is a good practical choice for biopsy in a child. Forearm skin gives lower pickup rates of positive results.[28]

On direct IMF, there is linear deposition of IgA along the basement membrane zone and, in some cases, other immunoreactants, immunoglobulin G (IgG), immunoglobulin M, or C3 are also seen.[1] In rare cases, a granular linear pattern of IgA at the basement membrane zone is seen.[29]

Indirect IMF for IgA basement membrane zone antibodies is more often positive in children (about 75%) than adults (about 30%).[1] The titers are usually low, on the order of 1:5 or 1:10, but occasionally much higher. The use as substrate of normal human skin split through the lamina lucida by incubation in saline increases the sensitivity and gives additional information as to the site of the target antigen. Most sera are roof binding, a few are floor binding, and a smaller number show a mixed pattern. Blister fluid is a suitable alternative to serum for indirect IMF testing and may be easier to obtain in a child.[30]

The presence of IgG autoantibodies on direct or indirect IMF causes problems with disease definition, occurs in both children and adults, and has been called mixed immunobullous disease. In most cases, the patients have had a clinical picture compatible with LAD and a good response to dapsone or sulfonamides. The exact position of dual responders is unclear but, for practical purposes, the patients are best managed as LAD.[31–33]

### Immunoblotting

Immunoblotting of linear IgA sera may pick up a variety of target antigens, in keeping with the multiple localizations found using IMF with split skin. Using an epidermal extract for immunoblotting, the positivity rate for IgA is higher than with IMF and is positive in about 83% of adult sera and 64% of children. IgG antibodies may also be detected in more than 50% of adults and children.[34]

### PATHOGENESIS

There is indirect evidence for the pathogenicity of the IgA antibodies. In an in vitro model, IgA binding caused splitting of skin in culture and binding of neutrophils to the basement membrane zone.[35] An animal model has demonstrated that linear IgA bullous disease sera passively transferred to severe combined immunodeficient mice with human skin grafts are capable of promoting neutrophil infiltration and basement membrane vesiculation.[36]

Using split skin as a substrate for IMF, most sera bind to the epidermal side of the split, implying an antigen associated with hemidesmosomes or the upper lamina lucida; a minority bind to the dermal aspect of the artificial blister suggesting a lower lamina lucida or dermal antigen, and a few sera have a combined pattern. In keeping with the IMF findings, immunoelectron microscopy (IEM) studies have shown that the immunoreactants and target antigens are either associated with the hemidesmosomes, within the lamina lucida, in the subbasal lamina zone, or in a mirror-image pattern on each side of the lamina densa.[37,38]

### TARGET ANTIGENS

In keeping with both the IMF and IEM findings, the IgA antibody response in LAD in children and adults is heterogeneous, being directed at several different target antigens within the adhesion complex, and most sera have more than 1 target antigen.

The major target antigen is BP180/collagen XVII, a key structural component of the dermoepidermal adhesion complex (**Fig. 4**). It has an intracellular globular domain where its NH2 terminal interacts with the NH2 terminal of BPAg1 (BP230) and other hemidesmosomal components.[39] The long, extracellular, collagenous domain of collagen XVII traverses the lamina lucida in the region of the anchoring filaments and its COOH terminal embeds into the lamina densa. Part of the extracellular portion of the collagen XVII molecule is

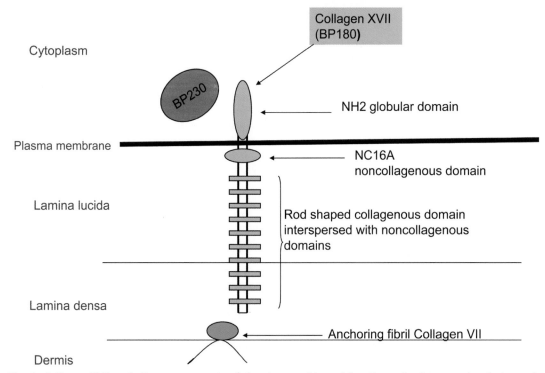

**Fig. 4.** Collagen XVII and other components of the dermoepidermal junction adhesion complex that may be target antigens in LAD. The NC16A domain may be a target epitope and is also the site through which enzymatic cleavage takes place to produce the shed ectodomain and neoantigens.

physiologically shed and is also further degraded by proteolytic action to produce extracellular fragments, molecular weight 120 kDa and 97 kDa respectively. Ectodomain shedding seems to generate neoepitopes in collagen XVII, possibly by conformational changes in the molecule.

Most sera in LAD (in both adults and children) target part or all of the collagen XVII molecule, and T cell responses to it have also been shown.[40] Epitope mapping of the sera has produced variable results[34,41–43] but it seems that sera preferentially react with the shed ectodomain of collagen XVII or its fragment and less with its full-length form. The juxtamembranous NC16A domain collagen XVII, an important immunodominant epitope in both bullous and mucous membrane pemphigoid, is also a target for IgA antibodies in LAD, frequently in conjunction with other antigenic targets.

The intracellular BP230, originally described as the major antigen in bullous pemphigoid,[34] is also targeted by IgA antibodies, more commonly in adult than childhood LAD sera. A unique antigen, LAD285, has a molecular weight of 285 kDa and has been found in patients whose sera have both dermal and epidermal binding on IMF testing using split skin. Collagen VII, a component of the anchoring fibril, is a rare antigen. Unlike classic epidermolysis bullosa acquisita, in which there is anti–collagen VII IgG, LAD is almost never associated with a mechanobullous scarring phenotype. There are also other unidentified dermal antigens.[41]

The detection of multiple antigens by IgA suggests that there is a primary disease-provoking epitope with spread of the immune response to other epitopes on the same or adjacent molecules. Multiple target antigens occur more commonly in adults than in children, possibly reflecting more prolonged antigenic stimulation.[34] In contrast with the heterogeneity of the IgA antibody response, binding of IgG autoantibodies to multiple antigens is rare and the role of the IgG response in the development and spread of the immune response in LAD is unknown.

## REFERENCES

1. Wojnarowska F, Marsden RA, Bhogal B, et al. Chronic bullous disease of childhood, childhood cicatricial pemphigoid, and linear IgA disease of adults. A comparative study demonstrating clinical and immunopathologic overlap. J Am Acad Dermatol 1988;19:792–805.

2. Adam BA. Bullous diseases in Malaysia: epidemiology and natural history. Int J Dermatol 1992;31:42–5.

3. Aboobaker J, Wojnarowska FT, Bhogal B, et al. Chronic bullous dermatosis of childhood–clinical and immunological features seen in African patients. Clin Exp Dermatol 1991;16:160–4.

4. Jin P, Shao C, Ye G. Chronic bullous dermatoses in China. Int J Dermatol 1993;32:89–92.

5. Kishida Y, Kameyama J, Nei M, et al. Linear IgA bullous dermatosis of neonatal onset: case report and review of the literature. Acta Paediatr 2004;93:850–2.

6. Collier PM, Wojnarowska F, Welsh K, et al. Adult linear IgA disease and chronic bullous disease of childhood: the association with human lymphocyte antigens Cw7, B8, DR3 and tumour necrosis factor influences disease expression. Br J Dermatol 1999;141:867–75.

7. Dellavalle RP, Burch JM, Tayal S, et al. Vancomycin-associated linear IgA bullous dermatosis mimicking toxic epidermal necrolysis. J Am Acad Dermatol 2003;48:S56–7.

8. Billet SE, Kortuem KR, Gibson LE, et al. A morbilliform variant of vancomycin-induced linear IgA bullous dermatosis. Arch Dermatol 2008;144:774–8.

9. Collier PM, Wojnarowska F. Drug-induced linear immunoglobulin A disease. Clin Dermatol 1993;11:529–33.

10. Palmer RA, Ogg G, Allen J, et al. Vancomycin-induced linear IgA disease with autoantibodies to BP180 and LAD285. Br J Dermatol 2001;145:816–20.

11. Camilleri M, Pace JL. Linear IgA bullous dermatosis induced by piroxicam. J Eur Acad Dermatol Venereol 1998;10:70–2.

12. Bouldin MB, Clowers-Webb HE, Davis JL, et al. Naproxen-associated linear IgA bullous dermatosis: case report and review. Mayo Clin Proc 2000;75:967–70.

13. Girao L, Fiadeiro T, Rodrigues JC. Burn-induced linear IgA dermatosis. J Eur Acad Dermatol Venereol 2000;14:507–10.

14. Godfrey K, Wojnarowska F, Leonard J. Linear IgA disease of adults: association with lymphoproliferative malignancy and possible role of other triggering factors. Br J Dermatol 1990;123:447–52.

15. Jacyk WK, Nagel GJ, van der Hoven AE. Linear IgA dermatosis and Hodgkin's lymphoma–report of a case in an African and review of the literature. J Dermatol 1990;17:633–7.

16. Usmani N, Baxter KF, Child JA, et al. Linear IgA disease in association with chronic lymphocytic leukaemia. Br J Dermatol 2004;151:710–1.

17. McEvoy MT, Connolly SM. Linear IgA dermatosis: association with malignancy. J Am Acad Dermatol 1990;22:59–63.

18. van der Waal RI, van de Scheur MR, Pas HH, et al. Linear IgA bullous dermatosis in a patient with renal cell carcinoma. Br J Dermatol 2001;144:870–3.

19. Rodenas JM, Herranz MT, Tercedor J, et al. Linear IgA disease in a patient with bladder carcinoma. Br J Dermatol 1997;136:257–9.

20. Paige DG, Leonard JN, Wojnarowska F, et al. Linear IgA disease and ulcerative colitis. Br J Dermatol 1997;136:779–82.

21. Birnie AJ, Perkins W. A case of linear IgA disease occurring in a patient with colonic Crohn's disease. Br J Dermatol 2005;153:1050–2.

22. Sachs JA, Leonard J, Awad J, et al. A comparative serological and molecular study of linear IgA disease and dermatitis herpetiformis. Br J Dermatol 1988;118:759–64.

23. Leonard JN, Griffiths CE, Powles AV, et al. Experience with a gluten free diet in the treatment of linear IgA disease. Acta Derm Venereol 1987;67:145–8.

24. Leonard JN, Haffenden GP, Unsworth DJ, et al. Evidence that the IgA in patients with linear IgA disease is qualitatively different from that of patients with dermatitis herpetiformis. Br J Dermatol 1984; 110:315–21.

25. Marsden RA, McKee PH, Bhogal B, et al. A study of benign chronic bullous dermatosis of childhood and comparison with dermatitis herpetiformis and bullous pemphigoid occurring in childhood. Clin Exp Dermatol 1980;5:159–76.

26. Burge S, Wojnarowska F, Marsden A. Chronic bullous dermatosis of childhood persisting into adulthood. Pediatr Dermatol 1988;5:246–9.

27. Chan LS, Ahmed AR, Anhalt GJ, et al. The First International Consensus on Mucous Membrane Pemphigoid: definition, diagnostic criteria, pathogenic factors, medical treatment, and prognostic indicators. Arch Dermatol 2002;138:370–9.

28. Collier PM, Wojnarowska F, Millard PR. Variation in the deposition of the antibodies at different anatomical sites in linear IgA disease of adults and chronic bullous disease of childhood. Br J Dermatol 1992; 127:482–4.

29. Leonard JN, Haffenden GP, Ring NP, et al. Linear IgA disease in adults. Br J Dermatol 1982;107: 301–16.

30. Zhou S, Wakelin SH, Allen J, et al. Blister fluid for the diagnosis of subepidermal immunobullous diseases: a comparative study of basement membrane zone autoantibodies detected in blister fluid and serum. Br J Dermatol 1998;139:27–32.

31. Powell J, Kirtschig G, Allen J, et al. Mixed immunobullous disease of childhood: a good response to antimicrobials. Br J Dermatol 2001;144:769–74.

32. Sheridan AT, Kirtschig G, Wojnarowska F. Mixed immunobullous disease: is this linear IgA disease? Australas J Dermatol 2000;41:219–21.

33. Viglizzo G, Cozzani E, Nozza P, et al. A case of linear IgA disease in a child with IgA and IgG circulating antibodies directed to BPAg2. Int J Dermatol 2007; 46:1302–4.

34. Allen J, Wojnarowska F. Linear IgA disease: the IgA and IgG response to the epidermal antigens demonstrates that intermolecular epitope spreading is associated with IgA rather than IgG antibodies, and is more common in adults. Br J Dermatol 2003;149:977–85.

35. Hendrix JD, Mangum KL, Zone JJ, et al. Cutaneous IgA deposits in bullous diseases function as ligands to mediate adherence of activated neutrophils. J Invest Dermatol 1990;94:667–72.

36. Zone JJ, Egan CA, Taylor TB, et al. IgA autoimmune disorders: development of a passive transfer mouse model. J Investig Dermatol Symp Proc 2004;9:47–51.

37. Bhogal B, Wojnarowska F, Marsden RA, et al. Linear IgA bullous dermatosis of adults and children: an immunoelectron microscopic study. Br J Dermatol 1987;117:289–96.

38. Prost C, De Leca AC, Combemale P, et al. Diagnosis of adult linear IgA dermatosis by immunoelectronmicroscopy in 16 patients with linear IgA deposits. J Invest Dermatol 1989;92:39–45.

39. Hopkinson SB, Baker SE, Jones JC. Molecular genetic studies of a human epidermal autoantigen (the 180-kD bullous pemphigoid antigen/BP180): identification of functionally important sequences within the BP180 molecule and evidence for an interaction between BP180 and alpha 6 integrin. J Cell Biol 1995;130:117–25.

40. Lin MS, Fu CL, Olague-Marchan M, et al. Autoimmune responses in patients with linear IgA bullous dermatosis: both autoantibodies and T lymphocytes recognize the NC16A domain of the BP180 molecule. Clin Immunol 2002;102:310–9.

41. Allen J, Wojnarowska F. Linear IgA disease: the IgA and IgG response to dermal antigens demonstrates a chiefly IgA response to LAD285 and a dermal 180-kDa protein. Br J Dermatol 2003;149:1055–8.

42. Nishie W, Lamer S, Schlosser A, et al. Ectodomain shedding generates neoepitopes on collagen XVII, the major autoantigen for bullous pemphigoid. J Immunol 2010;185:4938–47.

43. Zillikens D, Herzele K, Georgi M, et al. Autoantibodies in a subgroup of patients with linear IgA disease react with the NC16A domain of BP1801. J Invest Dermatol 1999;113:947–53.

# Clinical Features, Diagnosis, and Pathogenesis of Chronic Bullous Disease of Childhood

Emily M. Mintz, MD, Kimberly D. Morel, MD*

## KEYWORDS

- Chronic bullous disease of childhood • Bullous
- Linear IgA • IgA

Chronic bullous disease of childhood (CBDC) is a nonfamilial, autoimmune blistering disease that occurs in prepubertal children and is characterized by linear IgA staining of the basement membrane zone (BMZ) on direct immunofluorescence. The condition has been recognized since the late nineteenth century, when it was initially thought to be a variant of dermatitis herpetiformis (DH).[1] CBDC was recognized as clinically distinct from DH by Kim and Winkelmann[2] in 1961 and ultimately differentiated as a unique disorder in 1970 by Jordon and colleagues[3] who proposed the term benign chronic bullous dermatosis of childhood. In 1988, CBDC was recognized as the childhood counterpart of the adult linear IgA disease.[4,5] The historical confusion regarding the distinction of CBDC is reflected in the nomenclature. The terms bullous DH, juvenile DH, bullous pemphigoid of childhood, and linear IgA dermatosis of childhood have been used to describe the entity now known as CBDC.[6]

## DISEASE PRESENTATION

CBDC is the most common acquired autoimmune blistering disorder of childhood, and it occurs without preference to race or gender. CBDC is often initially diagnosed as bullous impetigo and may even temporarily improve with the brief course of antibiotics prescribed by the primary provider. It is when the eruption recurs or persists that the initial diagnosis of bullous impetigo is questioned. Disease onset usually occurs at the age of 6 months to 10 years with a mean age of 4.5 years.[5] However, disease onset has been reported as early as within 24 to 48 hours after birth[7,8] and up to the age of 12 years.[9] Children present with the abrupt onset of tense, clear, or hemorrhagic vesicles and bullae on normal or erythematous skin. New lesions often arise around resolving lesions, and these arciform or annular bullae surrounding a central crust have been described as a string of pearls, cluster of jewels, or rosette pattern (**Fig. 1**). The eruption occurs on the face, trunk, and extremities. There is a predilection for the lower trunk, genital area, and medial thighs; disease onset in the perineum has been mistaken for sexual abuse.[10] On the face, lesions tend to occur in a perioral pattern. Younger children more often have the classic distribution of facial and perineal lesions, whereas older children are more likely to present with a generalized eruption (**Fig. 2**).[5] Mucous membranes may be involved, and the severity ranges from mild oral ulcers to severe oral and conjunctival disease.[11] Clinical symptoms are variable, ranging from asymptomatic to severe pruritus, sometimes with a burning sensation. The disease generally remits

The authors have no funding support to disclose.

Department of Dermatology, Columbia University, 161 Fort Washington Avenue, 12th Floor, New York, NY 10032, USA

* Corresponding author.

*E-mail address:* km208@columbia.edu

Dermatol Clin 29 (2011) 459–462

doi:10.1016/j.det.2011.03.022

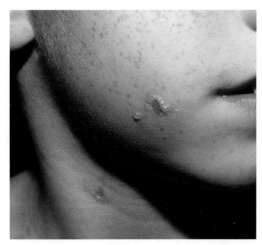

Fig. 1. Tense bulla arranged in a string of pearls distribution. (*Courtesy of* Dr Maria Garzon, Columbia University, New York, NY.)

spontaneously several months to 4 years after onset, leaving dyspigmentation but not scars. A subset of patients manifest clinically as those with CBDC but show a mixed pattern of IgA and IgG antibodies on immunofluorescence testing; this entity has been termed mixed immunobullous disease of childhood and is similar to CBDC in terms of target antigens, disease presentation and course, and response to treatment.[12]

## DIAGNOSIS

CBDC is diagnosed by hematoxylin-eosin–stained biopsy and immunofluorescence testing. Histology is characterized by a subepidermal blister with a primarily neutrophilic infiltrate in the papillary dermis, although mononuclear cells and occasional eosinophils are also seen (**Fig. 3**). Immunofluorescence testing of perilesional skin is the gold standard for diagnosis and shows linear IgA staining along the BMZ (**Fig. 4**). For unclear

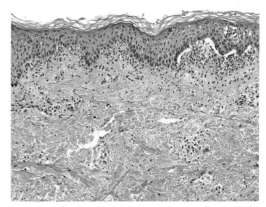

Fig. 3. Biopsy result showing a subepidermal split with a predominantly neutrophilic infiltrate in the papillary dermis (hematoxylin-eosin stain, original magnification ×20). (*Courtesy of* Dr Sameera Husain, Columbia University, New York, NY.)

reasons, the volar forearm seems to be an inferior site for biopsy because immunofluorescence testing may give a negative result.[13] Circulating autoantibodies are of the IgA1 subclass[14] and can be found in more than 90% of patients.[15] Autoantibodies bind the epidermal side of salt-split skin in most patients; however, antibody binding to the dermal side of salt-split skin or to both the epidermal and dermal sides occurs in some.[16] The heterogeneous indirect immunofluorescence pattern is explained by the variety of antigenic epitopes, as described later. The lesions are sterile unless they have become secondarily colonized or superinfected with bacteria.

In addition to the common initial clinical suspicion for bullous impetigo, the differential diagnosis of CBDC includes epidermolysis bullosa acquisita and other autoimmune bullous disorders.

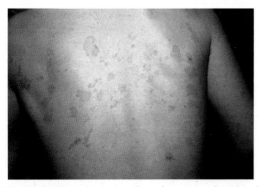

Fig. 2. Erythematous annular plaques and crusted erosions. (*Courtesy of* Dr Maria Garzon, Columbia University, New York, NY.)

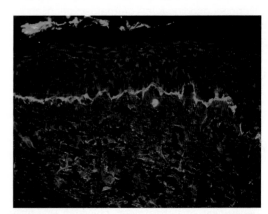

Fig. 4. Direct immunofluorescence demonstrating linear deposition of IgA along the BMZ. (*Courtesy of* Dr John J. Zone, Immunodermatology Laboratory, Department of Dermatology, University of Utah Health Care, Salt Lake City, UT.)

## DISEASE PATHOGENESIS

CBDC is associated with autoimmune haplotypes HLA-B8, Cw7, and DR3, suggesting an underlying genetic susceptibility to this acquired disorder.[17] The disease is often idiopathic but may be triggered by infections, drugs, vaccinations, ultraviolet radiation, or malignancy.[11,18] Presumably, such events somehow cause a normal component of the BMZ to become antigenic, but the sequence of events triggering this change is unknown. The production of an IgA autoantibody suggests either that a cross-reacting antigen enters via the mucosa or that an IgA diathesis exists in affected patients.[4] Autoantibodies are most often directed against proteolytic fragments of collagen XVII. Collagen XVII, also known as the 180-kDa bullous pemphigoid antigen (BP180), is a hemidesmosomal transmembrane protein characterized by a globular cytosolic amino-terminal domain and a rodlike, flexible extracellular carboxy-terminal domain, which is shed physiologically.[19] The 120-kDa shed ectodomain of collagen XVII has been recognized as a key autoantigen in adult linear IgA disease (and subsequently CBDC) and was termed LAD-1, the linear IgA disease antigen.[20] This 120-kDa protein is further processed into a 97-kDa protein, which is another principal autoantigen in CBDC.[21,22] The full-length collagen XVII protein (BP180) is also targeted by IgA in CBDC, but less efficiently than the 120-kDa and 97-kDa protein fragments. The better reactivity of CBDC sera to the shed ectodomain rather than to the full-length molecule suggests that novel epitopes are exposed during physiologic shedding of the ectodomain.[19] These novel epitopes may be more easily targeted by IgA antibodies. Autoimmune CD4+ T cells have also been shown to respond to BP180 antigens.[23] Less-commonly identified antigens for circulating IgA autoantibodies include BP230,[24] collagen VII,[25,26] and antigens of molecular weights 145 kDa,[27] 200 kDa,[28] 255 kDa,[29] 285 kda,[30] and 290 kDa,[31] among others. Consistent with indirect immunofluorescence results, immunoelectron microscopy has demonstrated antibody labeling of heterogeneous components of the BMZ, including the hemidesmosomes, lamina lucida, lamina densa, and sublamina densa. Autoantibodies binding to the hemidesmosomes or lamina lucida (epidermal side of salt-split skin) recognize BP180 (and its 120-kDa and 97-kDa breakdown products) as well as the 200-kDa and 230-kDa antigens. Antibodies binding to the lamina densa recognize the 180-kDa or 285-kDa proteins, and antibodies binding to the sublamina densa/ anchoring fibrils recognize collagen VII.[28,32]

Hence, CBDC is characterized by heterogeneous autoantibodies targeting a variety of antigens localized to various components of the BMZ.

## PROGNOSIS

CBDC is generally considered to have a good prognosis, with spontaneous resolution within months to years, usually by puberty. However, persistence beyond puberty has been described. It should be noted that even in those with short-lived disease, CBDC may carry significant morbidity. Neonatal CBDC has been associated with severe mucosal involvement and respiratory failure.[7,33] Permanent sequelae, including blindness[7] and dysphagia,[8] have been described. Treatment is aimed at controlling disease while avoiding side effects. Management options will be reviewed in an upcoming issue of *Dermatologic Clinics*.

## ACKNOWLEDGMENTS

The authors would like to thank Dr Maria Garzon for providing the clinical figures, Dr Sameera Husain for preparing the photograph of the H&E, and Dr John J. Zone for providing the photograph of the direct immunofluorescence testing.

## REFERENCES

1. Grant PW. Juvenile dermatitis herpetiformis. Trans St Johns Hosp Dermatol Soc 1968;54(2):128–36.
2. Kim R, Winkelmann RK. Dermatitis herpetiformis in children. Relationship to bullous pemphigoid. Arch Dermatol 1961;83:895–902.
3. Jordon RE, Bean SF, Triftshauser CT, et al. Childhood bullous dermatitis herpetiformis. Negative immunofluorescent tests. Arch Dermatol 1970;101(6):629–34.
4. Wojnarowska F. Chronic bullous disease of childhood. Semin Dermatol 1988;7(1):58–65.
5. Wojnarowska F, Marsden RA, Bhogal B, et al. Chronic bullous disease of childhood, childhood cicatricial pemphigoid, and linear IgA disease of adults. A comparative study demonstrating clinical and immunopathologic overlap. J Am Acad Dermatol 1988;19(5 Pt 1):792–805.
6. Sweren RJ, Burnett JW. Benign chronic bullous dermatosis of childhood: a review. Cutis 1982; 29(4):350–2, 356–7.
7. Hruza LL, Mallory SB, Fitzgibbons J, et al. Linear IgA bullous dermatosis in a neonate. Pediatr Dermatol 1993;10(2):171–6.
8. Kishida Y, Kameyama J, Nei M, et al. Linear IgA bullous dermatosis of neonatal onset: case report and review of the literature. Acta Paediatr 2004; 93(6):850–2.

9. Rogers M, Bartlett B, Walder B, et al. Chronic bullous disease of childhood–aspects of management. Australas J Dermatol 1982;23(2):62–9.

10. Coleman H, Shrubb VA. Chronic bullous disease of childhood- another cause for potential misdiagnosis of sexual abuse? Br J Gen Pract 1997;47(421):507–8.

11. Patricio P, Ferreira C, Gomes MM, et al. Autoimmune bullous dermatoses: a review. Ann N Y Acad Sci 2009;1173:203–10.

12. Powell J, Kirtschig G, Allen J, et al. Mixed immuno-bullous disease of childhood: a good response to antimicrobials. Br J Dermatol 2001;144(4):769–74.

13. Collier PM, Wojnarowska F, Millard PR. Variation in the deposition of the antibodies at different anatomical sites in linear IgA disease of adults and chronic bullous disease of childhood. Br J Dermatol 1992;127(5):482–4.

14. Wojnarowska F, Bhogal BS, Black MM. Chronic bullous disease of childhood and linear IgA disease of adults are IgA1-mediated diseases. Br J Dermatol 1994;131(2):201–4.

15. Willsteed E, Bhogal BS, Black MM, et al. Use of 1M NaCl split skin in the indirect immunofluorescence of the linear IgA bullous dermatoses. J Cutan Pathol 1990;17(3):144–8.

16. Wojnarowska F, Collier PM, Allen J, et al. The localization of the target antigens and antibodies in linear IgA disease is heterogeneous, and dependent on the methods used. Br J Dermatol 1995;132(5):750–7.

17. Collier PM, Wojnarowska F, Welsh K, et al. Adult linear IgA disease and chronic bullous disease of childhood: the association with human lymphocyte antigens Cw7, B8, DR3 and tumour necrosis factor influences disease expression. Br J Dermatol 1999;141(5):867–75.

18. Salmhofer W, Soyer HP, Wolf P, et al. UV light-induced linear IgA dermatosis. J Am Acad Dermatol 2004;50(1):109–15.

19. Schumann H, Baetge J, Tasanen K, et al. The shed ectodomain of collagen XVII/BP180 is targeted by autoantibodies in different blistering skin diseases. Am J Pathol 2000;156(2):685–95.

20. Marinkovich MP, Taylor TB, Keene DR, et al. LAD-1, the linear IgA bullous dermatosis autoantigen, is a novel 120-kDa anchoring filament protein synthesized by epidermal cells. J Invest Dermatol 1996;106(4):734–8.

21. Zone JJ, Taylor TB, Kadunce DP, et al. Identification of the cutaneous basement membrane zone antigen and isolation of antibody in linear immunoglobulin A bullous dermatosis. J Clin Invest 1990;85(3):812–20.

22. Zone JJ, Taylor TB, Kadunce DP, et al. IgA antibodies in chronic bullous disease of childhood react with 97 kDa basement membrane zone protein. J Invest Dermatol 1996;106(6):1277–80.

23. Lin MS, Fu CL, Olague-Marchan M, et al. Autoimmune responses in patients with linear IgA bullous dermatosis: both autoantibodies and T lymphocytes recognize the NC16A domain of the BP180 molecule. Clin Immunol 2002;102(3):310–9.

24. Ghohestani RF, Nicolas JF, Kanitakis J, et al. Linear IgA bullous dermatosis with IgA antibodies exclusively directed against the 180- or 230-kDa epidermal antigens. J Invest Dermatol 1997;108(6):854–8.

25. Hashimoto T, Ishiko A, Shimizu H, et al. A case of linear IgA bullous dermatosis with IgA anti-type VII collagen autoantibodies. Br J Dermatol 1996;134(2):336–9.

26. Allen J, Zhou S, Wakelin SH, et al. Linear IgA disease: a report of two dermal binding sera which recognize a pepsin-sensitive epitope (?NC-1 domain) of collagen type VII. Br J Dermatol 1997;137(4):526–33.

27. Yamane Y, Sato H, Higashi K, et al. Linear immunoglobulin A (IgA) bullous dermatosis of childhood: identification of the target antigens and study of the cellular sources. Br J Dermatol 1996;135(5):785–90.

28. Zhou S, Ferguson DJ, Allen J, et al. The localization of target antigens and autoantibodies in linear IgA disease is variable: correlation of immunogold electron microscopy and immunoblotting. Br J Dermatol 1998;139(4):591–7.

29. Dmochowski M, Hashimoto T, Bhogal BS, et al. Immunoblotting studies of linear IgA disease. J Dermatol Sci 1993;6(3):194–200.

30. Wojnarowska F, Whitehead P, Leigh IM, et al. Identification of the target antigen in chronic bullous disease of childhood and linear IgA disease of adults. Br J Dermatol 1991;124(2):157–62.

31. Zambruno G, Manca V, Kanitakis J, et al. Linear IgA bullous dermatosis with autoantibodies to a 290 kd antigen of anchoring fibrils. J Am Acad Dermatol 1994;31(5 Pt 2):884–8.

32. Ishiko A, Shimizu H, Masunaga T, et al. 97-kDa linear IgA bullous dermatosis (LAD) antigen localizes to the lamina lucida of the epidermal basement membrane. J Invest Dermatol 1996;106(4):739–43.

33. Salud CM, Nicolas ME. Chronic bullous disease of childhood and pneumonia in a neonate with VATERL association and hypoplastic paranasal sinuses. J Am Acad Dermatol 2010;62(5):895–6.

# An Exception Within the Group of Autoimmune Blistering Diseases: Dermatitis Herpetiformis, the Gluten-Sensitive Dermopathy

Sarolta Kárpáti, MD, PhD, DrSc[a,b,*]

## KEYWORDS

- Dermatitis herpetiformis • Gluten sensitivity
- IgA precipitate • Transglutaminase autoimmunity

Dermatitis herpetiformis (DH) is special among the classic autoimmune blistering skin diseases when considering its dermatologic symptoms, associated diseases, and pathomechanisms. The granular IgA precipitates present at the tips of the papillary dermis of the patients, an observation made by van der Meer in 1969 in Groningen,[1] proved to be pathognomonic for the disease. Contrary to other autoimmune blistering diseases, whereby tissue-bound and serum autoantibodies bind the same target molecule in the skin, no circulating IgA has been detected in DH sera reacting with normal tissue components of the sub-basal membrane zone or any other connective tissue particles within the healthy papillary dermis. The antigenicity of skin-bound IgA remained unknown for 3 decades, until 2002, when epidermal transglutaminase (TG3) was identified by the author's research group as its main antigen, an enzyme never detected in that area of the normal skin.[2] It has also been confirmed that DH patients have serum IgA autoantibodies to TG3. This article focuses on the clinical data concerning DH, rather than its detailed pathomechanism.

## SKIN SYMPTOMS AND DISEASE MANAGEMENT

DH can start at any age; rarely, it can be present in toddlers or in the very elderly, but the mean onset is generally in young adulthood or middle age. It is a chronic, very pruritic skin disease, characterized by 1- to 3-mm large papules, seropapules, vesicles, crusted erosions, and excoriations (Fig. 1). Rarely, larger blisters can also develop. The lesions heal with hypopigmentation or hyperpigmentation. In young patients, urticarial plaques might be the predominant skin symptoms (Fig. 2). The severe pruritus and scratching can result in extended lichenification (Fig. 3). In the majority of cases DH is a polymorphic skin disease, and only rarely presents as a bullous

[a] Department of Dermatology, Venereology and Dermato-Oncology, Semmelweis University, Mária utca 41, Budapest 1085, Hungary
[b] Hungarian Academy of Sciences, Molecular Research Group, Mária utca 41, Budapest 1085, Hungary
* Corresponding author. Hungarian Academy of Sciences, Molecular Research Group, Mária utca 41, Budapest 1085, Hungary.
E-mail address: skarpati@t-online.hu

Dermatol Clin 29 (2011) 463–468
doi:10.1016/j.det.2011.03.019
0733-8635/11/$ – see front matter © 2011 Published by Elsevier Inc.

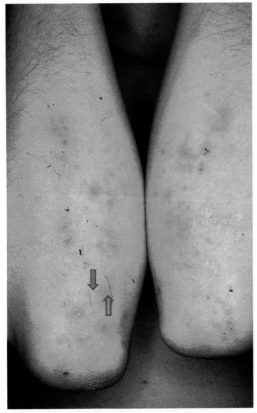

**Fig. 1.** Grouped polymorphic eruption above the elbows in dermatitis herpetiformis. Red arrow indicates the best site for a lesional biopsy for routine histology, and the blue arrow the best site for a perilesional biopsy for direct immunofluorescence.

dermatosis.[3–5] Specific symptoms, not always present, are purpura on the fingers and toes, which alone may focus attention on the diagnosis (Fig. 4).

DH has a typical distribution of the skin symptoms; these are, in order of frequency (strongly supported by the author's personal observations): 1, elbows and knees; 2, buttock; 3, shoulders, middle

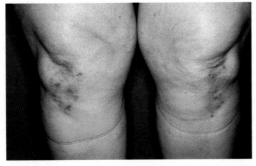

**Fig. 2.** Note the symmetric crusted erosions above the knees.

line of the back, and scapula; 4, scalp; 5 (rarely), purpura on the fingers and toes (see **Figs 1–4**).[3,4]

Although severe DH is almost a continuous disease with some fluctuation in the severity and itch, it might also present as a relatively mild lichenification, with alternating remissions and relapses: a few patients have skin disease only for a few days between long symptom-free periods. The symptom-free periods may only be in the warmer months when it is sunny. By contrast, in some DH patients sweating may induce disease progression in hot weather. There are patients who, without a gluten-free diet or other medication, remain free of skin symptoms for at least 6 months, in so-called spontaneous remission.[6] One must bear in mind that the underlying celiac disease (CD) and the possibility for further secondary disease development will persist. Spontaneous remissions are rare, but might develop and may last for years, life-long, or just for a short time. Pruritus can precede the skin symptoms and rarely also challenge the otherwise symptom-free time of the patients.

Untreated DH can be a life-long disease with variable severity. Associated uncontrolled diabetes, autoimmune diseases, underlying tumors, and iodine challenges might induce permanent very severe skin symptoms. During pregnancy the disease may improve, but in some cases it is worse. The reason for iodine sensitivity of DH patients is unknown, but is common. A possible relationship with thyroid diseases also remains unraveled. The sensitivity can be proved by patch testing, but iodine-containing drugs also flare up the disease. One of the author's young patients underwent a thyrotoxic crisis together with a severe DH flare-up after one short visit to a salt cave suggested for her as a "natural therapy."

## DIAGNOSIS CONFIRMATION

Diagnosis should be made by histologic and direct immunofluorescence (IF) analysis of the skin. The former sample should be taken from the lesional skin, the latter from perilesional, close to symptom-free tissue. On urticaria like lesions the presence of IgA, C3, and eventually IgM and IgG vasculitis is commonly associated with granular IgA and C3 staining of the dermis.[7] In the serum the presence of circulating IgA endomysial antibodies (EMA) or tissue transglutaminase (TG2) autoantibodies should be checked by indirect IF and by enzyme-linked immunosorbent assay (ELISA), respectively. The sensitivity and specificity of these tests are very high for CD, between or above 90% to 95%, whereas for DH it is less: about 75% to 90%. Serum samples from autoimmune

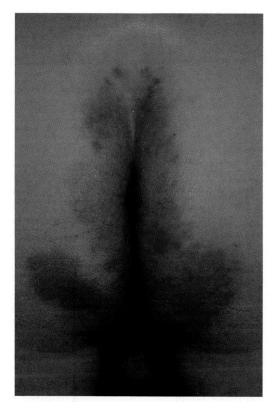

**Fig. 3.** Skin along the gluteal cleft is commonly involved in dermatitis herpetiformis: eczema-like chronic, livid erythema and mild lichenification without vesicles and crusts.

diseases as well as sera from normal individuals treated by heat or pH shift might show nonspecific TG2 reactivity.[8,9] The TG3 antibodies (ELISA) are also gluten dependent and slowly disappear under gluten-free diet (GFD), but later than the EMA or TG2. TG3 antibodies are more commonly present in DH than in CD patients, and in DH patients they have higher avidity and affinity.[2,10,11] An upper gastroduodenoscopy and a small bowel histology is strongly advised to visualize and document the

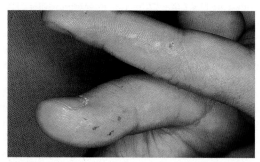

**Fig. 4.** Purpura on the fingers in dermatitis herpetiformis, a rare but specific sign.

upper part of the gastroinstestine and to analyze the initial jejunal histology, due to its strong association with CD.[3,4]

### Enteropathy and Malabsorption

The majority (75%–90%) of DH patients have an associated small bowel disease, a latent or silent CD. It persists and without treatment leads to malabsorption, which may induce secondary diseases: microcytic or macrocytic anemia due to iron, folate, or B12 deficiency, caries, alopecia due to zinc deficiency (see also dental problems), and early or very severe osteoporosis. Weight loss but also weight gain is possible, with unfavorable body mass index (BMI). Most patients have no typical gastrointestinal symptoms, but symptoms may include any of the following: diarrhea, constipation, bloating, abdominal discomfort or pain, and secondary lactose intolerance. Similarly to other gluten-sensitive enteropathy (GSE) patients, in DH patients with severe insulin-dependent diabetes, because of malabsorption the diabetes will be controlled only under a combined, strict GFD and diabetic diet. In childhood short stature, delayed development and puberty, or a high BMI might indicate the underlying GSE. Dental enamel defects, and mineralization disturbances of permanent and decidual teeth may be evident. Half of DH patients have celiac-type permanent-tooth enamel defects, milder than those described for severe celiac disease, and secondary severe caries or early tooth loss is also more common.[3–6,12,13] Although the skin can go into spontaneous remission,[3–6] the underlying CD and the possibility for further secondary disease development persist.

### OTHER ASSOCIATED DISEASES
#### Autoimmune Diseases

Due to the high frequency of associated autoimmune diseases, the author recommends screening and following the patients for autoimmune thyroiditis, type 1 diabetes (anti-islet AB), lupus erythematosus, Sjögren syndrome, vitiligo, primary biliary cirrhosis, pernicious anemia, and alopecia areata.[14] Screening the family for DH, CD, and autoimmune diseases is suggested.

### Neurologic Associations

Gluten sensitivity presenting with ataxia (gluten ataxia) is approximately one-quarter of the sporadic idiopathic cerebellar ataxia, the single most common cause of the disease.[15]

Rarely, gluten-induced axonal and demyelinating neuropathy, and myopathies have also been identified. In the central nervous system epilepsy, myoclonus, dementia, and multifocal leukoencephalopathy were detected in patients with GSE.[16]

## Tumors

Long-lasting GSE is significantly more commonly associated with jejunal adenocarcinomas and lymphomas. Enteropathy-associated T-cell lymphomas encompass about 1% of the non-Hodgkin lymphomas, and these usually have a very poor prognosis. Other lymphomas, such as B or cutaneous lymphomas, have also been described. The relative risk of any lymphoma in untreated CD and DH is significantly enhanced, while a risk reduction is well documented under strict GFD.[17–19]

## Other Disease Associations

Iodine sensitivity (cause is unknown), selective immunoglobulin A deficiency (more common also in CD), Down syndrome, and Turner syndrome have been reported.[3,4]

## GENETIC BACKGROUND AND FAMILY SCREENING

There is no difference between CD and DH patients: HLA could be a nonspecific diagnostic marker for both diseases. Ninety-five percent of DH patients are HLA DQ2 positive with DQA1* 0501/DQB1*0201; DQA1*0501/DQB1*0202; DRB1*03/DRB1*05/07 alleles, while 5% of them are HLA-DQ8 positive and carry the DQA1*0301/DQB1*0302, DRB1*4 alleles.[6,20] Asiatic races lack this HLA pattern, therefore DH and CD are rare and in these patients because this association cannot be detected. There are a few patients reported from Japan with only epidermal but not with tissue TG autoantibodies.[21]

GSE is more common among the family members of DH patients. Therefore it is strongly suggested to screen the first-degree and second-degree relatives for the presence of tissue TG antibodies (or EMA) to identify latent or silent forms of gluten sensitivity.[20]

## TREATMENT

A strict, long-lasting (according to current knowledge life-long) GFD is the most advisable treatment for DH patients, which is healthy and seems to prevent the development of lymphomas and diseases associated with gluten-induced enteropathy and malabsoportion.[3–5] The GFD should be maintained in DH patients who become free from skin symptoms while on the diet. Also, patients with spontaneous regression need to take the diet because the GSE persists. The skin symptoms rarely disappear even under a strict GFD within a few weeks, and commonly persist for months or for a year. Gastroenterological and dietician consultations are necessary.

A secondary lactose intolerance might accompany the GSE, and in these cases a temporary lactose-gluten–free diet combination is advised.

In severe or insulin-resistant diabetic patients, only the combination of low-carbohydrate diet and GFD seems to be effective, because severe diabetes can be only stabilized if the enteropathy is reversed and the absorption is normalized. Low iodine intake like iodine-free salt, avoidance of fruit of meer (eg, shellfish), and GFD might be necessary for DH cases with iodine sensitivity. A dose of 50 to 150 mg dapsone per day could be a quick help for severe skin symptoms, because all DH patients react well to this medication. Dapsone, however, has no effect on the underlying GSE, nor on the secondary malabsorption and the enhanced risk of lymphomas. Dapsone may induce peripheral neuropathy and in glucose-6-phosphate–deficient patients, hemolysis. Rarely, it may be toxic to the bone marrow or might induce drug hypersensitivity syndrome. A high-dose vitamin C supplementation is suggested with dapsone to reduce methemoglobinemia.[12] In the first months of dapsone treatment blood counts, including reticulocyte counts, and bilirubin and liver enzyme values should be repeatedly determined. For more detailed information on dapsone, see the article elsewhere in this issue. Sunshine or ultraviolet A are beneficial for the skin symptoms and may keep mild cases in good condition, but cannot be considered as a sole treatment (personal observation by the author). In GFD refractory cases, patients should be screened for underlying diseases, particularly for tumors.[13]

## DISEASE PATHOGENESIS: CLINICAL RELEVANCE

When and how the tolerance to alimentary gluten is lost in DH patients is not known exactly. The presence of IgA antibodies against gliadin and TG2 in the circulation prove the activity of enteropathy or a too short or improper diet adherence, therefore they should be regularly monitored. The major difference between CD and DH is the presence of skin symptoms, and the IgA precipitates in the papillary skin that may persist for years even in symptom-free patients. Furthermore, only in DH skin a pathologic epidermal TG3 is also deposited, colocalizing there with the granular IgA staining.[2,22,23] TG3-IgA immune complexes can be also detected in the small vessels of the papillary dermis.[7] These data show that DH can be considered as a gluten-induced immune-complex disease of the skin developing in some patients suffering from milder CD. The presence of cutaneous immune complexes also explains the purpura on the fingers and toes. The gluten-induced skin and small bowel pathology develops only in genetically determined individuals who carry specific HLADQ8 or DQ2 haplotypes (see earlier discussion).

Although an interesting animal model of a gluten-sensitive skin disease was presented in HLA-DQ8 transgenic NOD mice, and this animal model demonstrated well the role of HLA molecules in gluten-induced immunologic reactions, a DH similar TG3 autoimmunity could not be reproduced.[24] It is likely that there are additional genetic or environmental factors that might contribute to gluten-dependent TG autoimmunity.[25,26]

## MANAGEMENT OF DH

Management of DH will be discussed in more detail in the next issue, but a summary guideline is given in **Table 1**.

## REFERENCES

1. van der Meer JB. Granular deposits of immunoglobulins in the skin of patients with dermatitis herpetiformis. An immunofluorescent study. Br J Dermatol 1969;81(7):493–503.
2. Sárdy M, Kárpáti S, Merkl B, et al. Epidermal transglutaminase (TGase 3) is the autoantigen of dermatitis herpetiformis. J Exp Med 2002;195(6):747–57.
3. Collin P, Reunala T. Recognition and management of the cutaneous manifestations of celiac disease: a guide for dermatologists. Am J Clin Dermatol 2003;4(1):13–20.
4. Kárpáti S. Dermatitis herpetiformis: close to unravelling a disease. J Dermatol Sci 2004;34(2):83–90.
5. Junkins-Hopkins JM. Dermatitis herpetiformis: pearls and pitfalls in diagnosis and management. J Am Acad Dermatol 2010;63(3):526–8.
6. Paek SY, Steinberg SM, Katz SI. Remission in dermatitis herpetiformis: a cohort study. Arch Dermatol 2011;147(3):301–5.
7. Preisz K, Sárdy M, Horváth A, et al. Immunoglobulin, complement and epidermal transglutaminase deposition in the cutaneous vessels in dermatitis herpetiformis. J Eur Acad Dermatol Venereol 2005;19(1):74–9.
8. Zöller-Utz IM, Esslinger B, Schulze-Krebs A, et al. Natural hidden autoantibodies to tissue transglutaminase cross-react with fibrinogen. J Clin Immunol 2010;30(2):204–12.
9. Sárdy M, Csikós M, Geisen C, et al. Tissue transglutaminase ELISA positivity in autoimmune disease independent of gluten-sensitive disease. Clin Chim Acta 2007;376(1–2):126–35.
10. Marietta EV, Camilleri MJ, Castro LA, et al. Transglutaminase autoantibodies in dermatitis herpetiformis and celiac sprue. J Invest Dermatol 2008;128(2):332–5.
11. Dahlbom I, Korponay-Szabó IR, Kovács JB, et al. Prediction of clinical and mucosal severity of coeliac disease and dermatitis herpetiformis by quantification of IgA/IgG serum antibodies to tissue transglutaminase. J Pediatr Gastroenterol Nutr 2010;50(2):140–6.
12. Dunne J, Caron A, Menu P, et al. Ascorbate removes key precursors to oxidative damage by cell-free

**Table 1**
**Dermatitis herpetiformis is a multidisciplinary disease: a guideline summary for patient care**

| | |
|---|---|
| Skin | Skin histology (lesional) and direct IF for papillary IgA (perilesional) |
| Serum | Detect IgA to TG2 (ELISA) or endomysium (EMA, indirect IF), and TG3 (ELISA). Total serum IgA level |
| Gut | Gastroenterology consult: endoscopy/small bowel biopsy for H&E and IgA |
| Family | Screen the first- and second-degree relatives for gluten-sensitive diseases by IgA-TG2 antibody test (ELISA) |
| Associations | Autoimmune diseases, osteoporosis, enemal deficiencies, and neurologic symptoms. Correct the symptoms of malabsorption |
| Diet | Dietician consult; healthy, strict GFD; control the patients following the titer of serum IgA to TG2 or EMA. SLOW improvement! (months). Relapses indicate diet failure or tumor |
| Follow-up | Regular checkup for associated diseases. Be aware of the rare possibility of lymphoma development in patients under gluten-containing diet |

*Abbreviations:* ELISA, enzyme-linked immunosorbent assay; EMA, endomysial antibodies; GFD, gluten-free diet; H&E, hematoxylin and eosin; IF, immunofluorescence; TG, transglutaminase.

haemoglobin in vitro and in vivo. Biochem J 2006; 399(3):513–24.

13. Rubio-Tapia A, Murray JA. Classification and management of refractory coeliac disease. Gut 2010;59(4):547–57.

14. Neuhausen SL, Steele L, Ryan S, et al. Co-occurrence of celiac disease and other autoimmune diseases in celiacs and their first-degree relatives. J Autoimmun 2008;31(2):160–5.

15. Stamnaes J, Dorum S, Fleckenstein B, et al. Gluten T cell epitope targeting by TG3 and TG6; implications for dermatitis herpetiformis and gluten ataxia. Amino Acids 2010;39(5):1183–91.

16. Wills AJ, Turner B, Lock RJ, et al. Dermatitis herpetiformis and neurological dysfunction. J Neurol Neurosurg Psychiatry 2002;72(2):259–61.

17. Collin P, Pukkala E, Reunala T. Malignancy and survival in dermatitis herpetiformis: a comparison with coeliac disease. Gut 1996;38(4):528–30.

18. Viljamaa M, Kaukinen K, Pukkala E, et al. Malignancies and mortality in patients with coeliac disease and dermatitis herpetiformis: 30-year population-based study. Dig Liver Dis 2006;38(6):374–80.

19. Holmes GK, Prior P, Lane MR, et al. Malignancy in coeliac disease—effect of a gluten free diet. Gut 1989;30(3):333–8.

20. Karell K, Korponay-Szabo I, Szalai Z, et al. Genetic dissection between coeliac disease and dermatitis herpetiformis in sib pairs. Ann Hum Genet 2002; 66(Pt 5–6):387.

21. Asano Y, Makino T, Ishida W, et al. Detection of antibodies against epidermal transglutaminase but not tissue transglutaminase in Japanese patients with Dermatitis herpetiformis. Br J Dermatol 2010. DOI:10.1111/j.1365-2133.2010.

22. Dieterich W, Laag E, Bruckner-Tuderman L, et al. Antibodies to tissue transglutaminase as serologic markers in patients with dermatitis herpetiformis. J Invest Dermatol 1999;113(1):133–6.

23. Jaskowski TD, Hamblin T, Wilson AR. IgA anti-epidermal transglutaminase antibodies in dermatitis herpetiformis and pediatric celiac disease. J Invest Dermatol 2009;129(11):2728–30.

24. Marietta E, Black K, Camilleri M, et al. A new model for dermatitis herpetiformis that uses HLA-DQ8 transgenic NOD mice. J Clin Invest 2004;114(8):1090–7.

25. Koskinen LL, Korponay-Szabo IR, Viiri K, et al. Myosin IXB gene region and gluten intolerance: linkage to coeliac disease and a putative dermatitis herpetiformis association. J Med Genet 2008;45(4): 222–7.

26. Blazsek A, Sillo P, Ishii N, et al. Searching for foreign antigens as possible triggering factors of autoimmunity: torque Teno virus DNA prevalence is elevated in sera of patients with bullous pemphigoid. Exp Dermatol 2008;17(5):446–54.

# Pathophysiology of Dermatitis Herpetiformis: A Model for Cutaneous Manifestations of Gastrointestinal Inflammation

Adela Rambi G. Cardones, MD, Russell P. Hall III, MD*

## KEYWORDS

- Dermatitis herpetiformis • Gastrointestinal inflammation
- Cutaneous autoimmune disease

Louis Duhring[1] proposed using the term dermatitis herpetiformis (DH) in 1884 to describe a cutaneous disease that was characterized by violent pruritus. Almost 1 century later, Cormane reported another key feature of this disease: the deposition of immunoglobulins at the dermoepidermal junction.[2] Shortly afterwards, it was described that 85% to 90% of patients with DH had granular and the rest linear, IgA deposits.[3,4] The third key feature was first described in 1966: these patients had an associated gastrointestinal disease, more specifically, a gluten-sensitive enteropathy (GSE).[5–7] Not only was it shown that this disease was GSE, but that dietary control was sufficient in abrogating the cutaneous symptoms of DH.[7,8] The association of GSE with DH was further correlated with the pattern of cutaneous IgA deposits by Lawley and colleagues,[9] who found that patients with clinical DH and an associated GSE had granular IgA deposits only in the skin. This finding defined the significance of DH as a model for an autoimmune disease that linked gastrointestinal mucosal immunity with cutaneous disease. Since that time, much has been done to describe the clinical and immunopathologic features of DH. Although the exact mechanism by which cutaneous lesions appear is still unclear, much has been uncovered in the pathophysiology of the disease.

## CLINICAL PRESENTATION

The classic cutaneous manifestations of DH, true to Duhring's original description, are markedly pruritic, symmetrically distributed papulovesicles that usually affect the extensor surfaces: scalp, especially the posterior hairline, elbows, knees, back, and buttocks.[1,10] Certainly variations exist, and frankly bullous, pustular, or eczematous lesions can sometimes be found. Patients can have only multiple erosions or small ulcerations, with or without crust, as a result of the severe pruritus. Rarely, atypical morphologies and locations, such as purpuric macules on the palms or tips of fingers,[11–13] can be found as presenting features, especially in children. The mucous membranes are only rarely, if ever, involved, but have certainly been reported as an initial manifestation of the disease.[14,15] The patients typically report a tingling or burning sensation 12 to 24 hours before the appearance of clinically evident lesions, which persists until the vesicle is broken and a crust is formed. DH typically presents in

Department of Dermatology, Duke University, DUMC 3135, Durham, NC 27710, USA
* Corresponding author. Room 4044, Purple Zone, Duke South, Durham NC, 27710-0001.
*E-mail address:* hall0009@mc.duke.edu

Dermatol Clin 29 (2011) 469–477
doi:10.1016/j.det.2011.03.005
0733-8635/11/$ – see front matter © 2011 Published by Elsevier Inc.

the second or third decade of life, with some investigators reporting a mean age of onset in the 40s, but it can certainly appear at any age.[16–19] The condition is chronic, but waxes and wanes with no clear triggering factors. This disease tends to be chronic, although around 12% of these patients can go into spontaneous remission.[20] Those who were 39 years or older at the age of onset and those who had already had longer duration of disease were more likely to experience remission. It is more prevalent among Anglo-Saxons and Scandinavians, with the estimated frequency between 10 and 39 per 100,000.[21,22] This frequency seems to be similar among Whites in the United States.[23] It is less common among other ethnic groups, such as African Americans and Asians, presumably because of differences in the frequency of HLA antigens associated with DH.[24–26] Furthermore, clinical variations may exist among different ethnicities. An increased incidence of fibrillar pattern of IgA deposits in the skin of patients with a clinical presentation consistent with DH has been reported in a Japanese cohort.[26] In addition, these Japanese patients seem to have a decreased frequency of GSE. It is not clear if this situation is because of a true difference in the pathogenesis of the disease, decreased exposure to gluten in the Japanese patients, or a less aggressive diagnostic approach to the potential gut disease. Although DH in the past has not been considered to be a familial disease, recent studies have indicated an indicated prevalence of both DH and isolated GSE in families. The incidence of familial occurrence (ie, a first-degree relative with DH) has been reported at 2.3% to 4.4%.[19,27,28] In a series from Finland, as many as 6.1% of patients with DH have first-degree relatives with celiac disease.[27]

## HISTOLOGY AND IMMUNOPATHOLOGY

Histology of skin in DH is characterized by a subepidermal blister with a predominantly neutrophilic infiltrate in the dermal papillary tips,[18] although a mixed or even predominantly lymphocytic dermal infiltrate may also be found.[19,29] Direct immunofluorescence reveals granular deposition of IgA at the dermoepidermal junction in both involved and uninvolved skin as well as the oral mucosa.[30–32] However, IgA deposition is not evenly distributed in the skin of patients with DH.[33] Deposition is most intense in noninflamed perilesional skin, and is decreased in skin that has never been involved. Erythematous or lesional skin in patients with DH may not show IgA deposition, perhaps as a result of neutrophil destruction of the IgA. Therefore, the ideal site

for a skin biopsy in DH is uninvolved, perilesional skin. Patients with isolated GSE without DH do not have cutaneous IgA deposition,[34] showing that this phenomenon is related to DH itself, and not the underlying GSE.

Complement deposition, specifically C3,[31,33,35,36] can be found along with IgA in the skin of patients with DH. There is evidence that IgA activates complement in DH via the alternative pathway.[35,37]

A fibrillar pattern of IgA deposition in a subset of patients with DH has also been described.[38–40] Although these patients typically have other clinical features consistent with DH, it has been suggested that these patients may have a higher incidence of atypical features, such as a urticarial or psoriasiform clinical presentation, the absence of GSE, or HLA-B8/DR3/DQ2 haplotype.[39] Some of these patients have been reported to lack circulating antibodies against tissue transglutaminase and endomysium.[40] Whether or not these patients represent a true distinct subset or variant of DH or another disease entity altogether remains to be seen.[41]

## ASSOCIATED CONDITIONS

Patients with DH have an associated GSE. In contrast to patients with GSE alone, most patients with DH have little or no gastrointestinal symptoms, in spite of the almost invariable presence of demonstrable pathologic changes in the gastrointestinal tract when there is active cutaneous disease. Even when cutaneous disease is controlled with dapsone or sulfapyridine, the mucosal changes are persistent. Twenty percent to 30% of patients with DH have mild steatorrhea, and even fewer complain of bloating, diarrhea, and malabsorption. The gross and histologic changes of the small bowel in DH are identical, although less severe, to that found in isolated GSE or celiac disease. There is often patchy involvement, with changes confined to the small bowel, typically the jejenum. There is flattening of the intestinal villi, elongation of intestinal crypts, and flattening of the intestinal epithelial cells. A mononuclear infiltrate of plasma cells and lymphocytes is found in the lamina propria and intraepithelially. These changes persist even when cutaneous symptoms are controlled with dapsone and sulfapyridine but normalize with dietary therapy or strict avoidance of gluten.

Aside from GSE, several diseases are associated with DH. It has been reported that up to 41% of patients with DH have hypochlorhydria or achlorhydria, and most of these patients have gastric atrophy.[42] As many as 38% of patients with DH have been found to have thyroid microsomal antibodies, and patients with DH have a higher incidence of thyroid abnormalities, including hypothyroidism, thyroid nodules, and thyroid cancer.[43,44] Other autoimmune diseases have been reported to be associated with DH as well: systemic lupus erythematosus, dermatomyositis, myasthenia gravis, Sjögren syndrome, and rheumatoid arthritis.[45] IgA nephropathy has also been described in patients with DH, and mesangial changes and IgA deposition can be found even in the absence of overt renal symptoms.[46]

Patients with DH have been reported to have an increased risk of gastric lymphoma 2.3 times higher than the normal population, with the incidence as high as 6.4%.[47] However, others have reported a lower rate. Hervonen and colleagues[48] reported that only 1% of a series of 1104 patients with DH developed gastrointestinal lymphoma 2 to 31 years after the onset of DH and these patients were less likely to have adhered to adhere to a gluten-free diet. More recent reports have found no increased incidence of malignancy or mortality among patients with DH and matched controls.[49,50]

## IMMUNOGENETICS

DH has striking HLA associations, specifically with class I antigens HLA-B8[51–53] and HLA-A1[54] and the class II antigens HLA-DR3 and HLA-DQw2.[54–56] Initial studies showed that 58% of patients with DH had HLA-B8, as opposed to 20% to 30% of normal controls. This same genetic marker was found to be present in 88% of patients with GSE as opposed to 22% of controls.[51–53,57] Furthermore, patients with GSE also have an increased frequency of HLA-A1, HLA-DR3 and HLA-DQw2, genetically linking DH and GSE. An even stronger association was found with HLA-DR3 and HLA-DQw2 because 95% and 100%, respectively, of patients with DH with confirmed granular IgA papillary dermal deposition expressed these markers.[55]

## IMMUNOPATHOGENESIS

Although it is clear that gastrointestinal inflammation is integral in the pathophysiology of DH, the exact mechanism of antibody production as well as the cascade by which gastrointestinal inflammation translates into cutaneous disease is not known. Our laboratory has been interested in how the inflammatory response to gluten in patients with DH results in an itchy blistering skin disease with rare gastrointestinal symptoms, whereas patients with isolated GSE have no skin disease with significant gastrointestinal symptoms.

Patients with DH can control the appearance of cutaneous lesions by restricting themselves to a gluten-free diet. Moreover, eliminating gluten intake leads to a decrease and eventual clearance of IgA deposits in the skin.[58,59] Although the presence of IgA in the skin is well documented, we set out to determine if the IgA in the skin could be of gut origin. Evaluation of the IgA subclass present in DH skin revealed that the cutaneous IgA deposits were IgA1 and that joining chain could not be detected.[60] Because IgA1 is the predominant subclass of serum IgA whereas IgA2 is the predominant subclass in mucosal secretions this finding suggested that the IgA was not of mucosal origin. Patients with circulating IgA antibodies against reticulin and endomysium also had these antibodies in their intestinal secretions.[61] These studies showed that the presence of IgA autoantibodies in the serum is concordant with the presence of IgA antibodies in intestinal secretions. Furthermore, whereas normal gut secretions contained more IgA2, gut secretions from patients with DH were predominantly IgA1, showing that the IgA immune response in the gut was predominantly IgA1. Characterization of the serum and gastrointestinal IgA antibodies directed against dietary proteins revealed that both serum and intestinal antibodies had similar isoelectric spectrotypes and IgA subclass composition and that was distinct from the pattern seen with total serum IgA.[62] These studies showed that IgA1 antibodies in the serum can be of gut origin, linking closely the IgA immune response in the gut to the IgA deposits in DH skin. Although attempts to elute IgA from DH skin have not been successful, recent studies by Sardy and colleagues[63] and Donaldson and colleagues[64] have shown that the IgA in DH skin seems to bind to epidermal transglutaminase (eTG) in the dermis.

These studies, together with the clinical studies, have shown that the mucosal immune response to gluten can lead to IgA antibodies of mucosal origin, which can persist in circulation, and that a specific group of these antibodies, IgA antitransglutamase 3 (anti-TG3) (eTG), deposit in the skin. The mechanism of that binding remains unknown. However, these studies do not explain how the IgA deposits may relate to the development of skin lesions, nor do they explain the clinically different presentations of DH and isolated GSE.

eTG or TG3 has been identified as the target autoantigen in DH.[63,64] It is strongly expressed in the upper epidermis but may also be found in renal basement membrane. Patients with DH have detectable eTG in the papillary dermis, overlapping with the same sites that have IgA deposition. It was not found in sites where IgA was not found. It has been hypothesized that eTG is released from keratinocytes and drops to the basement membrane in response to trauma, and is subsequently bound by circulating IgA. Another hypothesis is that preformed circulating complexes of IgA and eTG deposit in the papillary dermis.[63] Evidence of the presence of these circulating complexes is shown by the precipitation of these complexes in vessel walls of patients with DH.[65] It has also been hypothesized that these dermal deposits are somehow the end product of a reaction against TG3 in kidneys. IgA nephropathy has been associated with DH, and mesangial deposits were detected in as many as 45% of patients with DH without any overt clinical signs of nephropathy.[46,66] Although IgA deposition in the kidney was not related to epidermal deposits or degree of gut involvement, this was associated with a high frequency of circulating IgA against gliadin and reticulin.[46] In 1 series of patients with DH, Jaskowski and colleagues[67] reported that serum eTG IgA compared with eTG IgA and IgG was more sensitive in detecting GSE; however, sensitivity of IgA anti-eTG was only 71%. Furthermore, dietary intake seems to correlate with eTG IgA; that is, avoidance of gluten resulted in the gradual decrease of antibody levels.

Despite the difference in the clinical presentations of patients with DH and those with isolated GSE, patients with DH and isolated GSE share many common features. In addition to sensitivity to gluten, patients with DH and those with isolated GSE share the same strong HLA association: HLA-A1, B8, DR3, DQ2.[68,69] Patients with DH and isolated GSE also both have circulating IgA anti-tissue and eTG antibodies and have the same typical histologic features of villous atrophy of the small intestine. In contrast most patients with DH do not complain of the bloating, abdominal cramps, and diarrhea that typically affect patients with isolated GSE. Only around 20% of patients with DH experience steatorrhea, and even fewer (<10%) have bloating, diarrhea, and malabsorption. In addition, patients with isolated GSE do not have cutaneous IgA deposits or skin blisters. These differences in clinical features may be because of a difference in the intestinal cytokine response to dietary gluten. Real-time polymerase chain reaction analysis of small bowel biopsies of patients with DH showed a greater expression of interleukin 4 (IL-4) mRNA and less expression of interferon γ (IFN-γ) compared with patients with isolated GSE.[70] In both DH and GSE, small bowel biopsy often shows a mononuclear infiltrate of plasma cells and lymphocytes if found in the lamina propria and intraepithelially. T-cell lines derived from small bowel mucosa of patients with DH were predominantly CD4+/IL-4+, and less frequently CD4+/IFN-γ+. In contrast,

T-cell lines from isolated patients with GSE were predominantly CD8+ with a similar frequency of IL-4+ and IFN-γ+ cells.[71] In vitro culture of these T-cell lines with phorbol myristate acetate and ionomycin revealed that the T-cell lines produced IL-4 whereas isolated GSE T-cell lines produced both IL-4 and IFN-γ. These studies suggest that the increased expression of IL-4 mRNA in the gut of patients with DH when compared with patients with isolated GSE may modulate the inflammatory response and play a role in the lack of symptoms in patients with DH. T-cell receptor $V_\beta$ expression also seems to be more restricted among patients with DH who continue to ingest gluten when compared with patients with isolated GSE on a gluten-containing diet.[72] Therefore, differences in the symptoms exhibited by patients with DH and isolated GSE may be the result of a difference in the local immune response and cytokine production.

Although these studies showed that patients with DH have an ongoing chronic mucosal immune response that results in mucosal IgA in the serum with deposition of IgA in the skin, the factors that lead to the development of the skin lesions were not clearly understood. Neutrophils play a central role in pathogenesis of the skin lesions seen in patients with DH. Histopathologic evaluation of involved skin shows neutrophil deposits in the papillary dermis. The development of skin lesions is also exquisitely responsive to dapsone, a drug known to inhibit neutrophil function, without changing the small bowel mucosal immune response. Patients with DH have a predominantly asymptomatic, chronic mucosal immune response in the gut, and control of the mucosal immune response through dietary gluten restriction can control the skin disease; it was certainly possible that the ongoing gut small bowel mucosa inflammation could partially prime both the skin and the circulating neutrophil with resultant skin blister formation. Evaluation of serum cytokine levels revealed that patients with DH with inactive skin disease secondary to use of dapsone but on a gluten-containing diet had increased levels of cytokines, including IL-8 and tumor necrosis factor α (TNF-α). We then compared the serum IL-8 and IgA anti-tissue transglutaminase levels in patients with DH before beginning a gluten-free diet and after an average of 24.5 months (range 0.5–40 months) of a gluten-free diet.[73] Patients who were placed on a gluten-free diet had a significant decrease in their serum IL-8 and IgA anti-tissue transglutaminase levels (**Fig. 1**). In contrast, those who were kept on a gluten-containing diet had persistently increased serum IL-8 and IgA anti-tissue transglutaminase levels even if their cutaneous disease was well

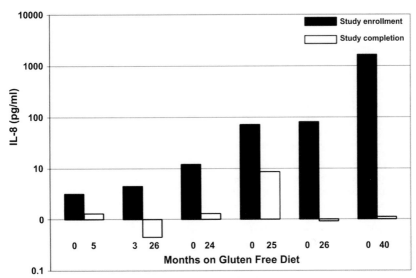

**Fig. 1.** Serum IL-8 levels in patients with DH on regular and gluten-free diets. Serum IL-8 is significantly reduced in patients with DH after maintaining a gluten-free diet (*open bars*) when compared with levels while on a gluten-containing normal diet (*solid bars*) (*P* = .0156, Wilcoxon signed rank test). (*From* Hall RP 3rd, Benbenisty KM, Mickle C, et al. Serum IL-8 in patients with dermatitis herpetiformis is produced in response to dietary gluten. J Invest Dermatol 2007;127:2159; with permission.)

controlled on dapsone or sulfapyridine. IL-8 mRNA message in small bowel biopsies of those on a gluten-containing diet was increased, whereas those patients on a gluten-free diet had IL-8 mRNA levels similar to normal controls. Thus, studies showed that the persistent mucosal immune response to gluten in the gut of patients with DH resulted in a chronic increase of proinflammatory cytokines in the circulation.

Neutrophils from patients with DH with active disease have an increased expression of CD11b when compared with those from patients with quiescent disease or normal controls. In addition, neutrophils from patients with DH with active disease had similar numbers of Fc IgA receptors but were able to bind more IgA compared with those from normal controls.[74] This finding suggests that in patients with DH, the circulating neutrophils are partially primed to allow for increased adherence to endothelial cells and potentially responding to the cutaneous IgA deposits.

Although increased expression of CD11b is important in neutrophils exiting the circulation, the circulating neutrophil must also be able to firmly adhere to the cutaneous endothelium. Cytokines released from ongoing gastrointestinal inflammation may also be responsible for the activation of cutaneous endothelial cells. E-selectin is a type 1 protein that mediates stable arrest and adhesion of neutrophils on endothelial cells.[75,76] Normal inner arm skin in patients with DH on gluten-containing diets but without active skin

lesions have an increased level of mRNA expression for E-selectin, when compared with E-selectin expression in the inner arm skin from normal individuals (**Fig. 2**).[77]

These studies show that in patients with DH on gluten-containing diets there is a chronic mucosal immune response that results in increases in circulating cytokines, including IL-8, a chemokine that is important in neutrophil function. This cytokine production is directly related to the mucosal immune response and is associated with increased expression of neutrophil CD11b and increased function of neutrophil Fc IgA receptors. This mucosal immune response is also associated with priming of the skin for an inflammatory response through a markedly increased expression of endothelial cell expression of E-selectin. However, the question remains why skin lesions are predominantly associated with the elbows, knees, buttocks, and other extensor areas. This regional localization may be caused by the constant minor trauma to extensor areas of the skin, and this trauma could result in local cytokine production in the skin, leading to chemotaxis of the partially primed neutrophils out of the blood vessels and into the skin at these sites of trauma. Minor trauma to the inner arm skin results in a striking increase in IL-8 and E-selectin mRNA and production of E-selectin protein in cutaneous endothelium.[78] This evidence supports the hypothesis that local trauma to the skin can establish the conditions necessary for neutrophils with an activated Fc IgA receptor to move into skin,

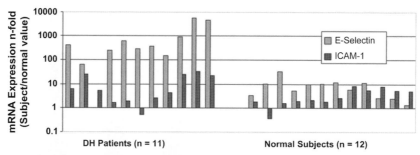

**Fig. 2.** Expression of E-selectin mRNA is increased in normal-appearing skin of patients with DH compared with normal individuals. mRNA expression represents fold expression of an individual compared with a constant single normal individual value. Expression of E-selectin mRNA in the skin of patients with DH is significantly increased compared with that seen in normal individuals ($P = .0001$, Mann-Whitney $U$ test). No significant difference is seen in intercellular adhesion molecule 1 mRNA expression. (*From* Hall RP 3rd, Takeuchi F, Benbenisty KM, et al. Cutaneous endothelial cell activation in normal skin of patients with dermatitis herpetiformis associated with increased serum levels of IL-8, sE-Selectin and TNF-$\alpha$. J Invest Dermatol 2006;126:1332; with permission.)

localize to the dermal epidermal junction where the IgA deposits are found, and result in the development of blisters in the skin.

## SUMMARY

DH is an autoimmune blistering skin disease in which antigen presentation in the gastrointestinal mucosa results in cutaneous IgA deposition and a distinct, neutrophil-driven cutaneous lesions. These studies taken in total provide us with a potential explanation of the pathophysiology of DH. The development of skin lesions in patients with DH is intimately linked to an active and chronic gastrointestinal mucosal inflammation as a result of persistent gluten challenge, resulting in a local immune response, with a production of mucosal IgA antibodies. This mucosal IgA reaches the circulation and a portion of it (potentially IgA anti-eTG) bind to skin. Because this IgA accumulates in the skin, the gastrointestinal mucosal immune response results in increased levels of circulating cytokines such as TNF-$\alpha$ and IL-8, which may partially prime neutrophils as well as activate cutaneous endothelial cells. Minor trauma to the skin increases local cytokine production, leading to egress of neutrophils and migration to the IgA at the dermal epidermal junction and the skin lesions of DH. This model is consistent with the clinical observation that skin disease can be prevented by use of dapsone, which affects neutrophil function but allows for ongoing gluten ingestion, or by a gluten-free diet, which inhibits the gut inflammation and controls the disease by stopping the inflammatory response in the gut. Our findings suggest that the qualitatively different immune response to gluten in the intestinal mucosa of patients with DH (increased IL-4 and decreased IFN-$\gamma$) results in minimal clinical

symptoms, thus allowing the continued ingestion of gluten and the eventual development of the skin disease DH.

Although all of the elements of this hypothesis have not been firmly established they remain testable. Evaluation of patients for the induction of skin lesions by controlled trauma while on a gluten-containing diet would confirm the final pathway. In addition, further characterization of the mucosal immune response to gluten including antigen specificities and more defined cytokine patterns in patients with DH compared with isolated GSE is needed. This model suggests that chronic inflammation of an epithelial surface (lung, intestine, or skin), exposed to the external environment, whether by dietary or other environmental antigen, may have systemic effects through chronic cytokine expression or modulation of effector cells, which could play a critical role in disease processes in other organs. This model may provide a new way to understand the pathogenesis of other skin diseases associated with gastrointestinal inflammation such as pyoderma gangenosum or erythema nodosum, or explain association of seronegative inflammatory arthritis with inflammatory bowel disease.

## REFERENCES

1. Duhring LA. Landmark article, Aug 30, 1884: dermatitis herpetiformis. By Louis A. Duhring. JAMA 1983; 250(2):212–6.
2. Cormane RH. Immunofluorescence studies of the skin in lupus erythematosus and other diseases. Pathologica Eur 1967;2:170.
3. van der Meer JB. Granular deposits of immunoglobulins in the skin of patients with dermatitis herpetiformis. An immunofluorescent study. Br J Dermatol 1969;81(7):493–503.

4. Chorzelski TP, Beutner EH, Jablonska S, et al. Immu-nofluorescence studies in the diagnosis of dermatitis herpetiformis and its differentiation from bullous pemphigoid. J Invest Dermatol 1971;56(5):373–80.

5. Marks J, Shuster S, Watson AJ. Small-bowel changes in dermatitis herpetiformis. Lancet 1966; 2(7476):1280–2.

6. Shuster S, Watson AJ, Marks J. Coeliac syndrome in dermatitis herpetiformis. Lancet 1968;1(7552): 1101–6.

7. Fry L, McMinn RM, Cowan JD, et al. Effect of gluten-free diet on dermatological, intestinal, and haemato-logical manifestations of dermatitis herpetiformis. Lancet 1968;1(7542):557–61.

8. Fry L, McMinn RM, Cowan JD, et al. Gluten-free diet and reintroduction of gluten in dermatitis herpetifor-mis. Arch Dermatol 1969;100(2):129–35.

9. Lawley TJ, Strober W, Yaoita H, et al. Small intestinal biopsies and HLA types in dermatitis herpetiformis patients with granular and linear IgA skin deposits. J Invest Dermatol 1980;74(1):9–12.

10. Katz SI. Dermatitis herpetiformis. Clinical, histologic, therapeutic and laboratory clues. Int J Dermatol 1978;17(7):529–35.

11. Flann S, Degiovanni C, Derrick EK, et al. Two cases of palmar petechiae as a presentation of dermatitis herpetiformis. Clin Exp Dermatol 2010;35(2):206–8.

12. Hofmann SC, Nashan D, Bruckner-Tuderman L. Petechiae on the fingertips as presenting symptom of dermatitis herpetiformis Duhring. J Eur Acad Der-matol Venereol 2009;23(6):732–3.

13. McGovern TW, Bennion SD. Palmar purpura: an atypical presentation of childhood dermatitis herpe-tiformis. Pediatr Dermatol 1994;11(4):319–22.

14. Economopoulou P, Laskaris G. Dermatitis herpetifor-mis: oral lesions as an early manifestation. Oral Surg Oral Med Oral Pathol 1986;62(1):77–80.

15. Fraser NG, Kerr NW, Donald D. Oral lesions in dermatitis herpetiformis. Br J Dermatol 1973;89(5): 439–50.

16. Gawkrodger DJ, Blackwell JN, Gilmour HM, et al. Dermatitis herpetiformis: diagnosis, diet and demography. Gut 1984;25(2):151–7.

17. Buckley DB, English J, Molloy W, et al. Dermatitis herpetiformis: a review of 119 cases. Clin Exp Der-matol 1983;8(5):477–87.

18. Rose C, Brocker EB, Zillikens D. Clinical, histological and immunopathological findings in 32 patients with dermatitis herpetiformis Duhring. J Dtsch Dermatol Ges 2010;8(4):265–70, 265–71.

19. Alonso-Llamazares J, Gibson LE, Rogers RS 3rd. Clinical, pathologic, and immunopathologic features of dermatitis herpetiformis: review of the Mayo Clinic experience. Int J Dermatol 2007;46(9):910–9.

20. Paek SY, Steinberg SM, Katz SI. Remission in dermatitis herpetiformis: a cohort study. Arch Dermatol 2011;147(3):301–5.

21. Moi H. Incidence and prevalence of dermatitis her-petiformis in a country in central Sweden, with comments on the course of the disease and IgA deposits as diagnostic criterion. Acta Derm Venereol 1984;64(2):144–50.

22. Reunala T, Lokki J. Dermatitis herpetiformis in Finland. Acta Derm Venereol 1978;58(6):505–10.

23. Smith JB, Tulloch JE, Meyer LJ, et al. The incidence and prevalence of dermatitis herpetiformis in Utah. Arch Dermatol 1992;128(12):1608–10.

24. Hall RP, Clark RE, Ward FE. Dermatitis herpetiformis in two American blacks: HLA type and clinical char-acteristics. J Am Acad Dermatol 1990;22(3):436–9.

25. Hashimoto K, Miki Y, Nishioka K, et al. HLA antigens in dermatitis herpetiformis among Japanese. J Dermatol 1980;7(4):289–91.

26. Shibahara M, Nanko H, Shimizu M, et al. Dermatitis herpetiformis in Japan: an update. Dermatology 2002;204(1):37–42.

27. Reunala T. Incidence of familial dermatitis herpetifor-mis. Br J Dermatol 1996;134(3):394–8.

28. Meyer LJ, Zone JJ. Familial incidence of dermatitis herpetiformis. J Am Acad Dermatol 1987;17(4): 643–7.

29. Warren SJ, Cockerell CJ. Characterization of a subgroup of patients with dermatitis herpetiformis with nonclassical histologic features. Am J Dermato-pathol 2002;24(4):305–8.

30. Seah PP, Fry L, Stewart JS, et al. Immunoglobulins in the skin in dermatitis herpetiformis and coeliac disease. Lancet 1972;1(7751):611–4.

31. Haffenden G, Wojnarowska F, Fry L. Comparison of immunoglobulin and complement deposition in multiple biopsies from the uninvolved skin in dermatitis herpetiformis. Br J Dermatol 1979; 101(1):39–45.

32. Nisengard RJ, Chorzelski T, Maciejowska E, et al. Dermatitis herpetiformis: IgA deposits in gingiva, buccal mucosa, and skin. Oral Surg Oral Med Oral Pathol 1982;54(1):22–5.

33. Zone JJ, Meyer LJ, Petersen MJ. Deposition of gran-ular IgA relative to clinical lesions in dermatitis her-petiformis. Arch Dermatol 1996;132(8):912–8.

34. Karlsson IJ, Dahl MG, Marks JM. Absence of cuta-neous IgA in coeliac disease without dermatitis her-petiformis. Br J Dermatol 1978;99(6):621–5.

35. Provost TT, Tomasi TB Jr. Evidence for the activation of complement via the alternate pathway in skin diseases. II. Dermatitis herpetiformis. Clin Immunol Immunopathol 1974;3(2):178–86.

36. Katz SI, Hertz KC, Crawford PS, et al. Effect of sulfones on complement deposition in dermatitis herpetiformis and on complement-mediated guinea-pig reactions. J Invest Dermatol 1976;67(6): 688–90.

37. Seah PP, Fry L, Mazaheri MR, et al. Alternate-pathway complement fixation by IgA in the skin

in dermatitis herpetiformis. Lancet 1973;2(7822): 175–7.

38. Kawana S, Segawa A. Confocal laser scanning microscopic and immunoelectron microscopic studies of the anatomical distribution of fibrillar IgA deposits in dermatitis herpetiformis. Arch Dermatol 1993;129(4):456–9.

39. Shimizu K, Hashimoto T, Fukuda T, et al. A Japanese case of the fibrillar type of dermatitis herpetiformis. Dermatology 1995;191(2):88–92.

40. Ko CJ, Colegio OR, Moss JE, et al. Fibrillar IgA deposition in dermatitis herpetiformis–an underreported pattern with potential clinical significance. J Cutan Pathol 2010;37(4):475–7.

41. Clements SE, Stefanato CM, Bhogal B, et al. Atypical dermatitis herpetiformis with fibrillar IgA deposition. Br J Dermatol 2007;157:17.

42. Gillberg R, Kastrup W, Mobacken H, et al. Gastric morphology and function in dermatitis herpetiformis and in coeliac disease. Scand J Gastroenterol 1985; 20(2):133–40.

43. Gaspari AA, Huang CM, Davey RJ, et al. Prevalence of thyroid abnormalities in patients with dermatitis herpetiformis and in control subjects with HLA-B8/-DR3. Am J Med 1990;88(2):145–50.

44. Cunningham MJ, Zone JJ. Thyroid abnormalities in dermatitis herpetiformis. Prevalence of clinical thyroid disease and thyroid autoantibodies. Ann Intern Med 1985;102(2):194–6.

45. Reunala T, Collin P. Diseases associated with dermatitis herpetiformis. Br J Dermatol 1997; 136(3):315–8.

46. Reunala T, Helin H, Pasternack A, et al. Renal involvement and circulating immune complexes in dermatitis herpetiformis. J Am Acad Dermatol 1983;9(2):219–23.

47. Leonard JN, Tucker WF, Fry JS, et al. Increased incidence of malignancy in dermatitis herpetiformis. Br Med J (Clin Res Ed) 1983;286(6358):16–8.

48. Hervonen K, Vornanen M, Kautiainen H, et al. Lymphoma in patients with dermatitis herpetiformis and their first-degree relatives. Br J Dermatol 2005; 152(1):82–6.

49. Lewis NR, Logan RF, Hubbard RB, et al. No increase in risk of fracture, malignancy or mortality in dermatitis herpetiformis: a cohort study. Aliment Pharmacol Ther 2008;27(11):1140–7.

50. Viljamaa M, Kaukinen K, Pukkala E, et al. Malignancies and mortality in patients with coeliac disease and dermatitis herpetiformis: 30-year population-based study. Dig Liver Dis 2006;38(6):374–80.

51. Katz SI, Hertz KC, Rogentine N, et al. HLA-B8 and dermatitis herpetiformis in patients with IgA deposits in skin. Arch Dermatol 1977;113(2):155–6.

52. White AG, Barnetson RS, Da Costa JA, et al. The incidence of HL-A antigens in dermatitis herpetiformis. Br J Dermatol 1973;89(2):133–6.

53. Katz SI, Falchuk ZM, Dahl MV, et al. HL-A8: a genetic link between dermatitis herpetiformis and gluten-sensitive enteropathy. J Clin Invest 1972;51(11): 2977–80.

54. Sachs JA, Awad J, McCloskey D, et al. Different HLA associated gene combinations contribute to susceptibility for coeliac disease and dermatitis herpetiformis. Gut 1986;27(5):515–20.

55. Hall RP, Sanders ME, Duquesnoy RJ, et al. Alterations in HLA-DP and HLA-DQ antigen frequency in patients with dermatitis herpetiformis. J Invest Dermatol 1989;93(4):501–5.

56. Karpati S, Kosnai I, Verkasalo M, et al. HLA antigens, jejunal morphology and associated diseases in children with dermatitis herpetiformis. Acta Paediatr Scand 1986;75(2):297–301.

57. Falchuk ZM, Rogentine GN, Strober W. Predominance of histocompatibility antigen HL-A8 in patients with gluten-sensitive enteropathy. J Clin Invest 1972;51(6):1602–5.

58. Fry L, Leonard JN, Swain F, et al. Long term follow-up of dermatitis herpetiformis with and without dietary gluten withdrawal. Br J Dermatol 1982;107(6): 631–40.

59. Leonard J, Haffenden G, Tucker W, et al. Gluten challenge in dermatitis herpetiformis. N Engl J Med 1983;308(14):816–9.

60. Hall RP, Lawley TJ, Heck JA, et al. IgA-containing circulating immune complexes in dermatitis herpetiformis, Henoch-Schonlein purpura, systemic lupus erythematosus and other diseases. Clin Exp Immunol 1980;40(3):431–7.

61. McCord ML, Hall RP 3rd. IgA antibodies against reticulin and endomysium in the serum and gastrointestinal secretions of patients with dermatitis herpetiformis. Dermatology 1994;189(Suppl 1): 60–3.

62. Hall RP 3rd, McKenzie KD. Comparison of the intestinal and serum antibody response in patients with dermatitis herpetiformis. Clin Immunol Immunopathol 1992;62(1 Pt 1):33–41.

63. Sardy M, Karpati S, Merkl B, et al. Epidermal transglutaminase (TGase 3) is the autoantigen of dermatitis herpetiformis. J Exp Med 2002;195(6): 747–57.

64. Donaldson MR, Zone JJ, Schmidt LA, et al. Epidermal transglutaminase deposits in perilesional and uninvolved skin in patients with dermatitis herpetiformis. J Invest Dermatol 2007;127(5): 1268–71.

65. Preisz K, Sardy M, Horvath A, et al. Immunoglobulin, complement and epidermal transglutaminase deposition in the cutaneous vessels in dermatitis herpetiformis. J Eur Acad Dermatol Venereol 2005;19(1): 74–9.

66. Helin H, Mustonen J, Reunala T, et al. IgA nephropathy associated with celiac disease and dermatitis

herpetiformis. Arch Pathol Lab Med 1983;107(6): 324–7.

67. Jaskowski TD, Hamblin T, Wilson AR, et al. IgA anti-epidermal transglutaminase antibodies in dermatitis herpetiformis and pediatric celiac disease. J Invest Dermatol 2009;129(11):2728–30.

68. Otley CC, Wenstrup RJ, Hall RP. DNA sequence analysis and restriction fragment length polymorphism (RFLP) typing of the HLA-DQw2 alleles associated with dermatitis herpetiformis. J Invest Dermatol 1991;97(2):318–22.

69. Fronek Z, Cheung MM, Hanbury AM, et al. Molecular analysis of HLA DP and DQ genes associated with dermatitis herpetiformis. J Invest Dermatol 1991; 97(5):799–802.

70. Smith AD, Bagheri B, Streilein RD, et al. Expression of interleukin-4 and interferon-gamma in the small bowel of patients with dermatitis herpetiformis and isolated gluten-sensitive enteropathy. Dig Dis Sci 1999;44(10):2124–32.

71. Hall RP 3rd, Smith AD, Streilein RD. Increased production of IL-4 by gut T-cell lines from patients with dermatitis herpetiformis compared to patients with isolated gluten-sensitive enteropathy. Dig Dis Sci 2000;45(10):2036–43.

72. Hall RP 3rd, Owen S, Smith A, et al. TCR Vbeta expression in the small bowel of patients with dermatitis herpetiformis and gluten sensitive enteropathy. Limited expression in dermatitis herpetiformis and treated asymptomatic gluten sensitive enteropathy. Exp Dermatol 2000;9(4):275–82.

73. Hall RP 3rd, Benbenisty KM, Mickle C, et al. Serum IL-8 in patients with dermatitis herpetiformis is produced in response to dietary gluten. J Invest Dermatol 2007;127(9):2158–65.

74. Smith AD, Streilein RD, Hall RP 3rd. Neutrophil CD11b, L-selectin and Fc IgA receptors in patients with dermatitis herpetiformis. Br J Dermatol 2002; 147(6):1109–17.

75. Bevilacqua MP, Stengelin S, Gimbrone MA Jr, et al. Endothelial leukocyte adhesion molecule 1: an inducible receptor for neutrophils related to complement regulatory proteins and lectins. Science 1989; 243(4895):1160–5.

76. Milstone DS, Fukumura D, Padgett RC, et al. Mice lacking E-selectin show normal numbers of rolling leukocytes but reduced leukocyte stable arrest on cytokine-activated microvascular endothelium. Microcirculation 1998;5(2–3):153–71.

77. Hall RP 3rd, Takeuchi F, Benbenisty KM, et al. Cutaneous endothelial cell activation in normal skin of patients with dermatitis herpetiformis associated with increased serum levels of IL-8, sE-Selectin, and TNF-alpha. J Invest Dermatol 2006;126(6):1331–7.

78. Takeuchi F, Sterilein RD, Hall RP 3rd. Increased E-selectin, IL-8 and IL-10 gene expression in human skin after minimal trauma. Exp Dermatol 2003;12(6): 777–83.

# Pathogenesis of Mucous Membrane Pemphigoid

A. Shadi Kourosh, MD*, Kim B. Yancey, MD

## KEYWORDS

- Mucous membrane • Pemphigoid • Autoimmune
- Pathogenesis

Mucous membrane pemphigoid (MMP) is the designation for a class of rare autoimmune blistering disorders in which autoantibodies directed against structural proteins of the epidermal basement membrane cause erosive lesions followed by scarring of the skin and mucous membranes. It is for their shared cicatrizing clinical phenotype that disorders of immunologic heterogeneity and of predilection for different sites of the body have been classified together using the designation MMP.

As an orphan disease with an approximate incidence of 1 person per million annually, and with early presenting symptoms that can be subtle and nonspecific, the signs of MMP often go unrecognized until the resulting erosions and scarring are established.[1] As a chronic and progressive disorder with sequelae that are irreversible and often debilitating, early diagnosis is critical because the limited therapeutic options available have the greatest potential to affect the course of the disease before scarring develops. Thus, the challenge for clinicians lies in recognizing an uncommon disorder underlying seemingly common complaints, and to establish timely diagnosis and appropriate interventions.

## CLINICAL FEATURES

MMP was first differentiated from other bullous disorders based on its predominance on mucous membranes, tendency for scarring, and resistance to treatment.[2,3] Multiple mucosal sites may be simultaneously affected, and occasionally the skin, particularly on the head and upper body. Although scarring is its clinical hallmark, this may not always be obvious, particularly in sites such as the oral mucosa. Clinical manifestations and the form and gravity of possible complications, such as blindness and life-threatening airway obstruction, depend on the sites involved.[4]

MMP is generally a disease of later life, with mean age of onset between 60 and 80 years. Women seem to be more often affected than men by a factor of 1.5 to 2. No geographic or racial predilection has been found; however, associations with certain human leukocyte antigen (HLA) haplotypes (HLA-DQB1*0301) have been described.[5]

Although the onset of lesions may begin or occur at any mucosal site, the oral mucosa seems to be most commonly affected, followed by the ocular, then the nasal, nasopharyngeal, anogenital, skin, laryngeal, and the esophageal mucosa (Table 1).[6–8]

Lesions in the mouth typically consist of erosions and blisters that may be covered by pseudomembranes. Such lesions often recur at the same sites and/or progress to scarring and focal sites of tissue loss or alternation. Depending on its progress at the time when intraoral disease is recognized, the clinician may find signs of acute disease (eg, inflammation, erosions, desquamative gingivitis) or their sequelae, which can range from a delicate white pattern of reticulated

Disclosures: None.
Conflicts of Interest: None.
Department of Dermatology, University of Texas Southwestern Medical Center in Dallas, 5323 Harry Hines Boulevard, Dallas, TX 75390-9069, USA
* Corresponding author.
E-mail address: askderm@gmail.com

Dermatol Clin 29 (2011) 479–484
doi:10.1016/j.det.2011.03.011

**Table 1**
**Manifestations and diagnosis by mucosal site**

| Site | Symptoms/Signs | History/Examination | Possible Complications |
|------|----------------|---------------------|------------------------|
| Mouth | Painful, erosive/blistering lesions: More common: gingival, buccal mucosa, and palate Less common: tongue, lips, alveolar ridge Desquamative gingivitis Tense blisters on oral mucosa Mucosal erosions Delicate white pattern of reticulated scarring | Question regarding: Pain/sensitivity on eating or brushing teeth Gum, dental pain Bleeding, mucosal lesions On Examination[a]: Erythema or erosions of the gingiva Delicate pattern of reticulate scarring | Adhesions between tongue and floor of mouth and around uvula and tonsils Dental complications: Caries Periodontal ligament damage Loss of bone mass Loss of teeth |
| Eye | Conjunctivitis slowly progressing to scarring Subtle and nonspecific symptoms, usually first in one eye, then both: Foreign body sensation Photophobia Tearing Itching Dryness Blurry vision, decreased visual acuity | Question regarding chronic symptoms such as: Burning, dryness, itching, tearing Photophobia or photosensitivity Persistent foreign body sensation Blurry vision, decreased visual acuity Unilateral or bilateral symptoms On examination[a]: Red/pink eyes, resembling conjunctivitis Malalignment of eyelashes Inward turning eyelashes Tarsal conjunctivitis | Painful, erosive conjunctivitis Conjunctival scarring Shortened fornices Loss of goblet cells Decrease in tear mucus content Unstable tear film Symblepharon Ankyloblepharon Ectropion Trichiasis Corneal irritation Superficial punctate keratinopathy Corneal neovascularization Corneal ulcers Scarring, occlusion, secondary infection of the tear ducts Blindness |
| Nose | Discharge Epistaxis Excessive crust formation Impaired air flow Chronic sinusitis | Question regarding: Chronic sinus symptoms Discharge Epistaxis Pain Congestion | Scarring Tissue loss Loss of air passages |
| Larynx | Hoarseness Chronic sore throat Loss of phonation Frequent throat clearing | Question regarding: Hoarseness, loss of voice, or sore throat Frequent throat clearing Symptoms last more than a few week Exacerbation by GERD | Chronic erosions, edema, scarring leading to: Stenosis of hypopharyngeal region\aspiration Airway compromise |
| Esophagus | Dysphagia Odynophagia Reflux symptoms/GERD Weight loss | Questions regarding: Difficulty eating/ swallowing Pain with swallowing Rapid and/or unintentional weight loss | Esophageal dysfunction and reflux causing: Exacerbation of laryngeal disease Bronchospasm Stricture formation Weight loss Aspiration |
| Anogenital region | Dysuria Constipation Pain on voiding Rectal bleeding Dyspareunia | Question regarding: Pain, difficulty and/or bleeding on voiding Pain during intercourse | Urethral strictures Vaginal and/or anal stenosis Secondary infection |

*Abbreviation:* GERD, gastroesophageal reflux disease.
[a] It is rare to see frank blisters on conjunctival surfaces.

scarring to severe tissue loss, dental complications (eg, caries, periodontal ligament damage, and loss of bone mass and teeth), or adhesions fusing the buccal mucosa and alveolar processes, the uvula and tonsillar fossa, or the tongue with the floor of the mouth.[4,9]

Ocular disease, also sometimes the only site of involvement, follows a course of conjunctival inflammation and erosions that scar and may cause symblepharon, ankyloblepharon, entropion, trichiasis, corneal damage, and neovascularization. Ocular MMP can result in blindness. The clinician should not expect to see vesicles or frank blisters in ocular MMP. Conversely, initial stages of ocular disease are often subtle, with vague symptoms (ie, burning, dryness, photophobia, or foreign body sensation) that could arise from other causes. Disease progression may be slow, taking several years, may initially affect 1 eye, and only gradually involve the other. Detection of early disease may require slit lamp examination and eversion of upper eyelids. Evaluation by an experienced ophthalmologist is critical to differentiate MMP from other ocular problems.[4,9]

Nasopharyngeal involvement can mimic allergic or infectious upper respiratory diseases, with signs of discharge, epistaxis, airway congestion, sore throat, hoarseness, and loss of phonation. MMP must be differentiated from these other disorders before acute symptoms and erosions progress to scarring, tissue loss, airway compromise, and tracheostomy.[10] It has been theorized that disease-related esophageal dysfunction and gastroesophageal reflux might trigger or exacerbate bronchospasm and/or laryngeal disease. Esophageal involvement can be complicated by stricture formation, dysphagia, odynophagia, weight loss, and/or aspiration. Anogenital involvement, although rare, when present causes significant pain and morbidity because blisters, erosions, and scarring can cause fusion of the labial tissues, urethral strictures, vaginal stenosis, and anal narrowing.[4,9]

Skin lesions in a patient with MMP tend to be few in number and commonly affect the head, neck, and upper trunk in the form of tense vesicles and erosions. These lesions tend to heal with atrophic scars and milia.

## DIFFERENTIAL DIAGNOSIS

The differential diagnosis of MMP includes other immunobullous diseases, erythema multiforme, lupus erythematosus, lichen planus, and lichenoid drug eruptions. Cicatrizing ocular disease may represent the sequela of a prior bout of Stevens-Johnson syndrome, occurring a few months to as much as 30 years previously. Drug-induced cicatrizing or inflammatory conjunctivitis, also known as ocular pseudopemphigoid, can arise from long-term use of certain ophthalmologic preparations (antiviral and glaucoma medications) or biologic drugs (epidermal growth factor receptor tyrosine kinase inhibitors).[4,9]

## LABORATORY FEATURES

As implied by the term pemphigoid, the diseases displaying the phenotype of MMP share the histologic feature of subepidermal blistering. Blisters are typically characterized by a lymphohistiocytic infiltrates admixed with some granulocytes and plasma cells in early lesions. Older lesions typically display scant infiltrates, fibroblast proliferation, and sites of lamellar fibrosis in the upper dermis.[11]

Direct immunofluorescence microscopy of normal-appearing perilesional mucosa (or skin) from patients with MMP typically shows linear deposits of immunoglobulin G (IgG), immunoglobulin A (IgA), or C3 in epithelial basement membranes, in contrast with pemphigus vulgaris, in which IgG deposits occur on the plasma membranes of epithelial cells, and oral lichen planus, in which fibrinogen rather than immunoreactants is typically seen in epithelial basement membranes.

Further differentiation of the disorders classified as MMP requires identification of the specific autoantigens targeted by patient autoantibodies. Subtypes of MMP and their corresponding autoantibody:autoantigen pair include:

- Antiepiligrin MMP: autoantibodies to laminin-332
- Ocular MMP: autoantibodies to integrin subunit $\beta_4$
- Oral MMP: autoantibodies to the NC16 and C-terminal regions of BPAG2 (seen in oral MMP as well as other forms of MMP [eg, ocular, nasal, hypopharyngeal]), or autoantibodies to integrin subunit $\alpha_6$
- Mucosal-predominant epidermolysis bullosa acquisita: autoantibodies to the NC1 domain of collagen VII.

The pattern and distribution of immunoreactants identified in indirect immunofluorescence microscopy studies of 1 M NaCl split skin differ among MMP subtypes. More specifically, autoantibodies targeting BPAG2 (BP 180), $\alpha_6$ integrin, or $\beta_4$ integrin bind the epidermal side of 1 M NaCl split skin, whereas autoantibodies versus laminin-332 or collagen VII bind the dermal side of this test substrate.

## PATHOGENESIS

Current evidence suggests that MMP develops as a consequence of the loss of immunologic tolerance to structural proteins in epidermal basement membrane. This loss of tolerance culminates in the development of circulating autoantibodies that bind epidermal basement membrane, elicit inflammation, and weaken adhesion of the overlying epidermis. As noted earlier, a variety of different autoantigens are recognized by circulating autoantibodies from patients with MMP. This article provides a brief summary of what is known about the pathogenic activity of these autoantibodies.

Passive transfer studies in newborn mice have shown that experimental antibodies directed against the murine homologue of the NC16A domain of human BPAG2 bind epidermal basement membrane; fix complement; elicit mast cell degranulation; and create neutrophil-rich, subepidermal blisters that resemble those seen in patients with bullous pemphigoid and some forms of MMP.[12] In this model, neutrophil-derived MMP-9 inactivates $\alpha$1-proteinase inhibitor, allowing unrestrained activity of neutrophil elastase to weaken basal keratinocyte adhesion to epidermal basement membrane and result in subepidermal blister formation.[13] These experimental observations have served as proof of concept that IgG versus NC16A can cause blister formation in vivo. Recently, Nishie and colleagues[14] extended these observations by showing that passive transfer of IgG from patients with bullous pemphigoid to BPAG2 humanized mice creates inflammatory subepidermal blisters like those seen in patients with pemphigoid. Nishie and colleagues[14] could block the binding of pemphigoid IgG to the epidermal basement membrane of these humanized mice (and hence neutralize their ability to induce subepidermal blisters) through the coadministration of decoy peptides corresponding with the NC16A domain of human BPAG2. Although no studies have yet shown that experimental or patient IgG versus the carboxyl terminal domain of BPAG2 are pathogenic in vivo, conventional thinking posits that such autoantibodies (which have been identified in sera from patients with MMP) are pathogenic (ie, blister inducing).

Passive transfer studies in newborn and adult mice have shown that experimental antibodies directed against laminin-332 bind epidermal basement membrane and produce noninflammatory subepidermal blisters of skin and mucous membranes like those seen in patients with MMP.[15] Such antibodies produce subepidermal blisters in mice that lack complement, mast cells, or T lymphocytes—findings indicating that anti–laminin-332 IgG can cause subepidermal blisters through noninflammatory mechanisms. Additional evidence in support of this hypothesis was developed in studies showing that Fab fragments of anti–laminin-332 antibodies could blister mouse skin in vivo.[16] These experimental findings are consistent with the subsequent demonstration that intradermal injection of IgG from patients with antiepiligrin MMP cause completely noninflammatory subepidermal blisters in human skin grafts on immunodeficient mice.[17] Although these studies support the conclusion that anti–laminin-332 IgG is pathogenic in vivo, the exact manner (eg, steric hindrance, cell signaling, protease activation) by which such autoantibodies produce subepidermal blisters is currently unknown.

Although the pathogenic activity of experimental or patient IgG versus integrin subunits $\alpha_6$ or $\beta_4$ have not been shown in passive transfer studies to date, experimental and patient IgGs directed against these integrin subunits have been shown to induce basement membrane separation in skin organ culture models.[18,19] Findings in these studies suggest that antibody-induced epidermal dysadhesion in these models is dependent on binding and inactivation of specific epitopes within these integrin subunits—observations that are of potential pathophysiologic significance to patients with MMP.

As noted earlier, rare patients with epidermolysis bullosa acquisita have disease that is either mucosal predominant or exclusively mucosal at some point in its evolution. Understanding of disease pathophysiology in these and other patients with epidermolysis bullosa acquisita has recently been advanced by the demonstration that passive transfer of experimental or patient IgG versus the NCI domain of type VII collagen to adult mice causes neutrophil-rich subepidermal blisters like those seen in patients with inflammatory epidermolysis bullosa.[20–22] The factors that account for the development of mucosal-predominant or dermolytic (ie, noninflammatory) forms of epidermolysis bullosa acquisita remain to be defined.

## COMPLICATIONS AND PROGNOSIS

MMP is typically a chronic and progressive disease. Its course is usually one of irreversible scarring and the associated loss of function, potentially to the point of blindness, airway compromise, or esophageal strictures.[4,11] Its ultimate effect on longevity and quality of life depends on the sites involved and their likelihood of scarring. Its outcome depends on timely intervention, because scarring in MMP can only be prevented, not reversed.

Disease affecting only the oral mucosa and/or the skin is considered lower risk, because such involvement is often more amenable to treatment. In contrast, ocular, genital, nasopharyngeal, esophageal, and laryngeal involvement is typically associated with a less favorable prognosis. Early intervention is critical for these patients, although, in some cases, the cicatrizing process progresses despite appropriate treatment. These trends should guide physicians in counseling patients and choosing timely and site-appropriate therapeutic regimens.[4,9,23,24]

There is some evidence that the types and titers of patients' autoantibodies can affect prognosis. For example, titers of IgG autoantibodies versus epidermal basement membrane at initial presentation roughly correlate with disease activity and eventual severity. Moreover, the presence of both IgG and IgA anti–basement membrane autoantibodies has been associated with more severe and persistent disease.[25,26] The subtype of MMP in question can also affect prognosis in that patients with antiepiligrin (laminin-332) autoantibodies seem to have an increased relative risk of cancer, an association linked to an unfavorable outcome in many patients with MMP who are so affected.[27–29]

## SUMMARY

MMP is the clinical phenotype of a group of autoimmune blistering diseases characterized by autoantibodies directed against different structural proteins in epidermal basement membranes. The clinical course and prognosis of MMP are affected by the specific autoantigen targeted, the titer and bioactivity profile of corresponding autoantibodies, and the specific mucosal sites of disease activity. Irreversible scarring and loss of function must be prevented by early diagnosis and appropriate interventions.

## REFERENCES

1. Bernard P, Vaillant L, Labeille B, et al. Incidence and distribution of subepidermal autoimmune bullous skin diseases in three French regions. Bullous Diseases French Study Group. Arch Dermatol 1995;131:48–52.
2. Lever W. Pemphigus. Medicine (Baltimore) 1953;32: 1–123.
3. Stanley JR, Amagai M. Autoimmune bullous diseases: historical perspectives. J Invest Dermatol 2008;128:E16–8.
4. Chan LS, Ahmed AR, Anhalt GJ, et al. The first international consensus on mucous membrane pemphigoid: definition, diagnostic criteria, pathogenic factors, medical treatment, and prognostic indicators. Arch Dermatol 2002;138:370–9.
5. Chan LS, Hammerberg C, Cooper KD. Significantly increased occurrence of HLA-DQB1*0301 allele in patients with ocular cicatricial pemphigoid. J Invest Dermatol 1997;108:129–32.
6. Hardy KM, Perry HO, Pingree GC, et al. Benign mucous membrane pemphigoid. Arch Dermatol 1971;104:467–75.
7. Hanson RD, Olsen KD, Rogers RS 3rd. Upper aerodigestive tract manifestations of cicatricial pemphigoid. Ann Otol Rhinol Laryngol 1988;97:493–9.
8. Chan LS, Yancey KB, Hammerberg C, et al. Immune-mediated subepithelial blistering diseases of mucous membranes. Pure ocular cicatricial pemphigoid is a unique clinical and immunopathological entity distinct from bullous pemphigoid and other subsets identified by antigenic specificity of autoantibodies. Arch Dermatol 1993;129:448–55.
9. Yancey KB. Cicatricial pemphigoid. In: Wolff K, Goldsmith LA, Katz SI, et al, editors. Dermatology in general medicine. 7th edition. New York: McGraw-Hill Inc; 2008. p. 481–5.
10. Lazor JB, Varvares MA, Montgomery WW, et al. Management of airway obstruction in cicatricial pemphigoid. Laryngoscope 1996;106:1014–7.
11. Yancey KB, Egan CA. Pemphigoid: clinical, histologic, immunopathologic, and therapeutic considerations. JAMA 2000;284:350–6.
12. Liu Z, Diaz LA, Troy JL, et al. A passive transfer model of the organ-specific autoimmune disease, bullous pemphigoid, using antibodies generated against the hemidesmosomal antigen, BP180. J Clin Invest 1993;92:2480–8.
13. Liu Z, Zhou X, Shapiro SD, et al. The serpin alpha1-proteinase inhibitor is a critical substrate for gelatinase B/MMP-9 in vivo. Cell 2000;102:647–55.
14. Nishie W, Sawamura D, Goto M, et al. Humanization of autoantigen. Nat Med 2007;13:378–83.
15. Lazarova Z, Yee C, Darling T, et al. Passive transfer of anti-laminin 5 antibodies induces subepidermal blisters in neonatal mice. J Clin Invest 1996;98:1509–18.
16. Lazarova Z, Hsu R, Briggaman RA, et al. Fab fragments directed against laminin 5 induce subepidermal blisters in neonatal mice. Clin Immunol 2000;95:26–32.
17. Lazarova Z, Hsu R, Yee C, et al. Human anti-laminin 5 autoantibodies induce subepidermal blisters in an experimental human skin graft model. J Invest Dermatol 2000;114:178–84.
18. Rashid KA, Stern JN, Ahmed AR. Identification of an epitope within human integrin alpha 6 subunit for the binding of autoantibody and its role in basement membrane separation in oral pemphigoid. J Immunol 2006;176:1968–77.
19. Chan RY, Bhol K, Tesavibul N, et al. The role of antibody to human beta4 integrin in conjunctival

basement membrane separation: possible in vitro model for ocular cicatricial pemphigoid. Invest Ophthalmol Vis Sci 1999;40:2283–90.

20. Sitaru C, Mihai S, Otto C, et al. Induction of dermal-epidermal separation in mice by passive transfer of antibodies specific to type VII collagen. J Clin Invest 2005;115:870–8.

21. Woodley DT, Chang C, Saadat P, et al. Evidence that anti-type VII collagen antibodies are pathogenic and responsible for the clinical, histological, and immunological features of epidermolysis bullosa acquisita. J Invest Dermatol 2005;124:958–64.

22. Woodley DT, Ram R, Doostan A, et al. Induction of epidermolysis bullosa acquisita in mice by passive transfer of autoantibodies from patients. J Invest Dermatol 2006;126:1323–30.

23. Tauber J, Sainz de la Maza M, Foster CS. Systemic chemotherapy for ocular cicatricial pemphigoid. Cornea 1991;10:185–95.

24. Mondino BJ, Brown SI. Immunosuppressive therapy in ocular cicatricial pemphigoid. Am J Ophthalmol 1983;96:453–9.

25. Setterfield J, Shirlaw PJ, Kerr-Muir M, et al. Mucous membrane pemphigoid: a dual circulating antibody response with IgG and IgA signifies a more severe and persistent disease. Br J Dermatol 1998;138:602–10.

26. Setterfield J, Shirlaw PJ, Bhogal BS, et al. Cicatricial pemphigoid: serial titres of circulating IgG and IgA antibasement membrane antibodies correlate with disease activity. Br J Dermatol 1999;140:645–50.

27. Domloge-Hultsch N, Gammon WR, Briggaman RA, et al. Epiligrin, the major human keratinocyte integrin ligand, is a target in both an acquired autoimmune and an inherited subepidermal blistering skin disease. J Clin Invest 1992;90:1628–33.

28. Domloge-Hultsch N, Anhalt GJ, Gammon WR, et al. Antiepiligrin cicatricial pemphigoid. A subepithelial bullous disorder. Arch Dermatol 1994;130:1521–9.

29. Egan CA, Lazarova Z, Darling TN, et al. Anti-epiligrin cicatricial pemphigoid and relative risk for cancer. Lancet 2001;357:1850–1.

# Diagnosis and Clinical Features of Epidermolysis Bullosa Acquisita

Frédéric Caux, MD, PhD

## KEYWORDS

- Epidermolysis bullosa acquisita • Blistering disease
- Collagen VII • Autoimmunity • Anchoring fibrils • Diagnosis

Epidermolysis bullosa acquisita (EBA) is a rare autoimmune subepidermal bullous disease involving the skin and the mucous membranes. It is characterized by the deposition of autoantibodies directed to the anchoring fibrils of the basement membrane zone of stratified squamous epithelia. These autoantibodies recognize type VII collagen, which is the major component of anchoring fibrils. The incidence of EBA is estimated to be between 0.2 and 0.5 new cases per million inhabitants per year.[1,2] Several clinical presentations have been reported; classical EBA includes skin fragility, blisters over the trauma-prone surfaces, and milium cysts. Making a definitive diagnosis of EBA may be difficult because specialized tests only available in certain laboratories are necessary to confirm the clinical suspicion. This orphan disease is often misdiagnosed, explaining an important delay in its diagnosis and the difficulty of performing therapeutic trials.

## PATHOGENESIS
### Type VII Collagen

Type VII collagen is a homotrimer composed of 3 identical α chains. Each chain includes a 145-kDa central helical region characterized by the repeated Gly-X-Y amino acid sequence; this region is flanked by a large 145-kDa amino-terminal noncollagenous (NC1) domain and a small 34-kDa carboxyl-terminal noncollagenous (NC2) domain. Type VII collagen molecules form dimers through their NC2 domains and are stabilized by

disulfide bridges. Then these antiparallel dimers aggregate laterally to form the anchoring fibrils. The NC1 globular domains are located at the end of these fibrils and interact with other extracellular matrix proteins, such as laminin 332, type IV collagen, type I collagen, and fibronectin.[3] These domains probably stabilize the basement membrane zone to the underlying dermis. Autoantibodies of patients with EBA preferentially recognize epitopes located in the NC1 domain[4–6] but epitopes in the NC2 domain and the helical region also are reported.[7] Binding of autoantibodies to type VII collagen induces a reduction in the number of anchoring fibrils and consequently a skin fragility and a cleavage between epidermis and dermis.

### Pathogenicity of Autoantibodies

Because EBA is often associated with low titers of autoantibodies directed to the basement membrane zone, the pathogenicity of these autoantibodies has been difficult to demonstrate for a long time. Cases of spontaneous EBA have been described in dogs, such as great Danes,[8] but this animal model did not permit a better understanding of the pathogenesis of this disease. Pathogenicity of autoantibodies that target type VII collagen was proved when two research teams demonstrated that (1) iterative passive transfer of antibodies directed to murine type VII collagen induces subepidermal blisters in mice,[9] (2) repeated injections of autoantibodies from EBA

Department of Dermatology & Reference Center on Autoimmune Bullous Diseases, University Paris 13, Avicenne Hospital, AP-HP, 125 rue de Stalingrad, 93000 Bobigny, France
E-mail address: frederic.caux@avc.aphp.fr

Dermatol Clin 29 (2011) 485–491
doi:10.1016/j.det.2011.03.017

patients in hairless mice produce a phenotype reminiscent of EBA,[10] and (3) immunization of mice with recombinant murine type VII collagen results in a subepidermal phenotype closely resembling human EBA.[11] The development of an active experimental model permitted dissection of the molecular events after the binding of auto-antibodies to the basement membrane zone and the demonstration that dermoepidermal cleavage is dependant on the capacity of antibodies to activate the alternative pathway of complement.[12]

## CLINICAL MANIFESTATIONS

The mean age of onset is approximately 50 years, although some cases in the elderly, in childhood, and even in neonates through passive transfer of maternal autoantibodies have been described.[13] EBA has been encountered in all ethnic groups but its incidence seems increased in patients of sub-Saharan African descent, in particular African Americans; this genetic predisposition may be

related to a particular HLA phenotype (HLA DRB1*1503) as it has recently been demonstrated in experimental EBA.[14] There are 4 main clinical variants of EBA: classical, inflammatory, cicatricial pemphigoid–like, and Brunsting-Perry pemphigoid–like forms, all of which have an IgG as well as an IgA-EBA form.

### Classical Form

The classical form is characterized by skin fragility and tense blisters occurring on noninflamed skin (**Fig. 1**A). Lesions develop over the trauma-prone surfaces, such as the extensor aspect of the limbs (elbows, knees, dorsal aspect of the hands, toes, and ankles). They heal with atrophic scarring and/or milium cysts (see **Fig. 1**B). Scarring alopecia and nail dystrophy even leading to acquired anonychia may be seen in the more severe evolution of the disease. Mucous membrane involvement is rare and involves the mouth, if present. This classical presentation is

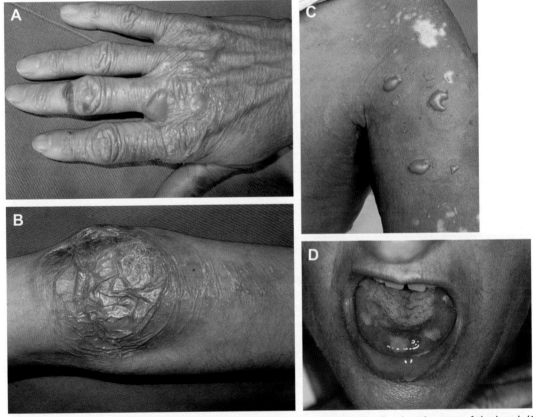

**Fig. 1.** Clinical features of EBA: (*A*) tense blister, crusts, and atrophic scars over the dorsal aspect of the hand; (*B*) cigarette paper–like scar and milium cysts on an elbow in a classical form of EBA; (*C*) tense blisters surrounded by urticarial plaques on the arm and trunk in an inflammatory form of EBA; (*D*) and flaccid blisters and erosions on the edges of the tongue in a cicatricial pemphigoid–like form of EBA.

reminiscent of dystrophic bullous epidermolysis of childhood when it is severe and of porphyria cutanea tarda (PCT) in adults when it is mild.

### Inflammatory Form

The presentation of the inflammatory form looks like bullous pemphigoid with widespread tense blisters surrounded by urticarial plaques (see **Fig. 1**C) involving the trunk, the folds, and the extremities of limbs. Itching may be associated and large erythematous areas and urticarial plaques without blisters may be seen.

### Cicatricial Pemphigoid–Like Form

The mucous membranes form of EBA is reminiscent of cicatricial pemphigoid with lesions on the mucosal surfaces of the mouth, conjunctiva, nose, larynx, esophagus, genitals, and anus. The buccal lesions are fibrinous erosions occurring on a noninflammatory basis and preferentially develop on the lips and tongue, allowing a clinical difference with classical cicatricial pemphigoid (see **Fig. 1**D). Alternatively, the ophthalmologic lesions of EBA are similar to those encountered in cicatricial pemphigoid. Ocular involvement includes conjunctival inflammation and fibrosis with an initial conjunctival shrinkage leading to synechia between palpebral and bulbar conjunctivae and finally ankyloblepharon. These ocular lesions may result in blindness. Ear, nose, and throat involvement presents with crusted rhinitis, nasal synechiae, pharyngeal erythema, or laryngeal erosions or stenosis.[15] Strictures of the first third of the esophagus may also occur, leading to dysphagia and risk of false passage.[16]

### Brunsting-Perry Pemphigoid–Like Form

Some EBA patients with a phenotype of Brunsting-Perry pemphigoid have been reported. Patients presented with vesicles and blisters located only over the head, the neck, and the upper aspect of the trunk. In contrary to the classical cicatricial pemphigoid, they have no mucous membranes involvement. Cutaneous lesions heal with atrophic scarring.

### IgA-EBA

Most patients with IgA-mediated EBA develop their first symptoms after their third decade but disease may start at childhood. Skin symptoms vary from erythematous urticarial plaques to vesicles, bullae, erythema multiforme–like lesions, and skin erosions. Almost all patients complain about an intense itch before or during the skin eruption.[17] Atrophic scars and milium cysts are

rare. Involvement of mucous membranes, mainly the oral mucosa, is seen in 30% of the cases. Severe, therapy-resistant ocular scarring leading to blindness has rarely been described.[18,19]

## POSITIVE DIAGNOSIS

Routine tests, such as skin standard pathology and direct immunofluorescence (IF), allow the diagnosis of autoimmune subepidermal blistering disease but do not specify a diagnosis of EBA with certainty. Specialized tests available in only certain laboratories are necessary to confirm EBA.

### Standard Pathology

Routine skin biopsy shows a subepidermal blister with an intact epidermis and a dermal inflammatory infiltrate. The classical form of EBA usually presents with a scarce infiltrate of neutrophils, whereas the inflammatory form of EBA is associated with a rich infiltrate of lymphocytes, neutrophils, and eosinophils (**Fig. 2**A).

### Direct Immunofluorescence

Patients with EBA have linear deposits of IgG along the basement membrane zone of the skin or mucous membranes detected by direct IF (see **Fig. 2**B). Additional deposits of C3, IgM, and IgA may more rarely been present on the same location.

### Indirect Immunofluorescence

Indirect IF is performed on human skin, or rat or monkey esophagus, and demonstrates antibodies recognizing the basement membrane zone in EBA. It is often negative, however, and titers are low if positive. Indirect IF detected antibodies in 37% of the patients in a series of 39 EBA patients[20]; it is more frequently positive in the inflammatory form than in the classical form of the disease. Indirect IF may also be done after splitting the skin using 1M NaCl.[21] This method permits increasing the level of positivity of indirect IF and helps distinguish between the different types of subepidermal autoimmune blistering diseases. Autoantibodies of EBA patients decorate the dermal side of the salt-split skin whereas bullous pemphigoid sera label the epidermal side of the separated skin. The detection of antibodies recognizing the dermal side of the separation, excluding the diagnosis of bullous pemphigoid, however, does not make the diagnosis of EBA certain because dermal staining is also observed in patients with anti-p200 pemphigoid whose sera recognize the γ1 chain of laminin[22] or in patients with a subset of

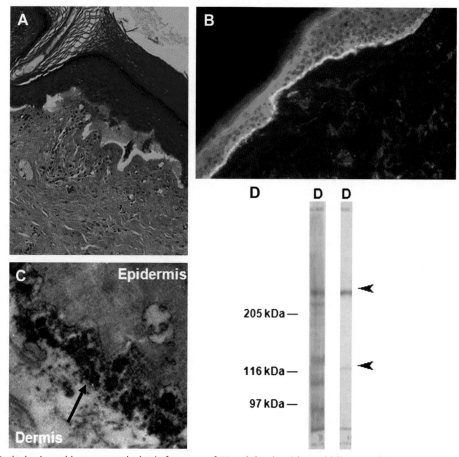

**Fig. 2.** Pathologic and immunopathologic features of EBA: (*A*) subepidermal blister and scarce dermal inflammatory infiltrate; (*B*) linear deposits of IgG along the basement membrane zone by direct IF; (*C*) intense immune
deposits located under the lamina densa (*arrow*) demonstrated by direct immunoelectron microscopy; and (*D*)
presence of antibodies binding dermal proteins of 290-kDa weight and 145-kDa weight (*arrowheads*) comigrat-
ing with the monoclonal antibody LH7.2 recognizing type VII collagen (lane LH7.2) in the serum of an EBA
patient (lane P) by immunoblotting using dermal extracts. Migration of molecular weight markers is shown on
the left. ([*B*]*Courtesy of* C. Prost, MD, PhD.)

cicatricial pemphigoid who have antibodies
directed to laminin 332, formerly laminin 5.

## Immunoblotting

Antibodies in EBA recognize the target antigen,
type VII collagen, by immunoblotting. Two bands
of 290-kDa weight and/or 145-kDa weight comi-
grating with type VII collagen detected by the
monoclonal antibody LH7.2 are observed using
dermal extract (see **Fig. 2**D). Immunoblotting
may be performed using tissue extracts (dermal
extract, epidermal sheets, and amniotic
membrane), cellular extracts (WISH cells), or recombinant proteins coding for a segment of type
VII collagen. Quantities of type VII collagen may
vary in the different extracts explaining the
discrepancies observed in the sensitivity of

detection of autoantibodies. Sensitivity of immunoblotting is approximately 60% using dermal
extract[20,23] but increases to 80% if several recombinant proteins covering 4 immunodominant
epitopes of NC1 domain are used.[4] Approximately
20% of EBA sera recognize the NC2 domain of
type VII collagen.[24,25]

### ELISA
ELISA is a method that is an alternative to immunoblotting to detect autoantibodies directed to type
VII collagen and is easier to perform. ELISA using
the NC1 domain is sensitive, with a detection level
close to 100%, but it is not highly specific because
it may be positive in patients with Crohn disease or
ulcerative colitis without cutaneous manifestations
of EBA.[26] Autoantibodies to NC2 recombinant
protein are detected in 20% of patients by ELISA

as observed by immunoblotting.[25] Autoantibody detection in EBA increases to 66% by ELISA if several recombinant proteins covering the NC1 domain are combined.[27] An ELISA using a recombinant homotrimer of type VII collagen tested in 44 EBA patients had a sensitivity of 70% and a specificity of 95% in the authors' experience.[28]

### Direct Immunoelectron Microscopy

Direct immunoelectron microscopy permits localization of which precise structure of basement membrane zone the autoantibodies of the patients are binding in vivo. It is the gold standard for the diagnosis of EBA, allowing asserting a diagnosis with good sensitivity, showing intense immune deposits under the lamina densa on the anchoring fibrils (see **Fig. 2**C). Immunoreactivity may sometimes be observed on the lower part of the lamina densa or in the sublamina densa, which is distinct from the deposits encountered on the lamina lucida and/or the lamina densa observed in antilaminin 5 cicatricial pemphigoid[29] or in anti-p200 pemphigoid.[22]

## DIFFERENTIAL DIAGNOSIS

The classical form of EBA may mimic PCT. Skin fragility, tense blisters healing with scars, and milium cysts are present in PCT. Lesions are located on photodistributed areas, such as the hands and face, in PCT whereas they also involve covered areas (feet, elbows, and knees) in EBA. Standard cutaneous pathology is identical in both conditions but direct IF demonstrates a dull staining on the basement membrane zone of the skin and also the vessels. Diagnosis of porphyria is confirmed by elevations in blood, urine, and fecal porphyrins, allowing an accurate classification (PCT, coproporphyria, or variegate porphyria). Other differential diagnoses are discussed more rarely, such as the recessive form of dystrophic epidermolysis bullosa, pseudoporphyria, and bullous amyloidosis.

The cicatricial pemphigoid–like form and the inflammatory form of EBA are reminiscent of cicatricial pemphigoid and bullous pemphigoid. Direct IF shows a similar staining in bullous pemphigoid, cicatricial pemphigoid, and EBA but if mucous membranes involvement is present, additional investigations in specialized centers are needed. These specialized tests allow distinguishing EBA from classical cicatricial pemphigoid (antibodies directed to BP180/type XVII collagen by immunoblotting or ELISA and immune deposits localized on the lamina densa by direct immunoelectron microscopy) or antilaminin 5 cicatricial pemphigoid (antibodies recognizing one of the 3 chains of laminin 5 by immunoblotting or ELISA and immune deposits present on the lower part of the lamina lucida by direct immunoelectron microscopy). These additional investigations are also necessary if a patient has clinical features of an inflammatory autoimmune subepidermal blistering disease but the clinical criteria of bullous pemphigoid are not fulfilled. Moreover, the diagnosis of bullous pemphigoid may be established clinically with a positive predictive value of 95% if 3 of 4 criteria are present: age over 70 years, absence of involvement of the head and neck, absence of atrophic scarring, and absence of mucosal involvement.[30] If 2 of these 4 clinical criteria are present, specialized tests are mandatory because diagnosis of bullous pemphigoid is improbable.

IgA-EBA is one of the several diseases included in the heterogeneous group of linear IgA dermatosis characterized by exclusive linear IgA deposition along the basement membrane zone. In IgA-EBA, IgA immune deposits are present on the anchoring fibrils by direct immunoelectron microscopy and circulating IgA autoantibodies bind to the floor of the salt-split skin and recognize type VII collagen by immunoblotting.

## ASSOCIATED DISEASES

EBA is associated with inflammatory bowel diseases, in particular Crohn disease.[31] This association has been estimated in 25% of the EBA patients in an US series[26] and in a French series.[20] Crohn disease has to be investigated if an EBA patient develops intestinal clinical manifestations, such as diarrhea, abdominal pain, or malabsorption. Many other diseases have been reported with EBA but these associations seem anecdotal.

EBA may also been associated with systemic lupus erythematosus (SLE). SLE may occur before, simultaneously, or after the onset of EBA, which is related to the development of autoimmunity directed to type VII collagen. Vesiculobullous lupus affects young adults in the second or third decade of life. Tense vesicles and bullae arise on sun-exposed areas but can appear at any cutaneous site. Skin fragility, scars, and milium cysts are usually absent.[32] Cutaneous lesions of discoid lupus, subacute lupus, or SLE are infrequent. Histopathologic analysis of skin biopsy shows a subepidermal blister associated with a neutrophilic infiltrate in the papillary dermis. Direct IF reveals linear immune deposits on the basement membrane zone, which can be associated with granular deposits similar to a lupus band. Direct immunoelectron microscopy demonstrates the same site of immune deposition in EBA but additional immune deposits can be observed beyond the area where anchoring fibrils are usually seen into the deeper portion of the dermis. Patients have circulating antibodies directed to type VII collagen. They usually meet the American Rheumatism Association revised criteria for SLE. Vesiculobullous lupus has a striking therapeutic response to dapsone and has a less chronic evolution than EBA.[33]

## SUMMARY

EBA is one of the more rare forms of subepidermal autoimmune blistering diseases. To distinguish it from the other subepidermal blistering diseases with absolute certainty, patients should have one of the several consistent clinical manifestations along with either autoantibodies to collagen VII by ELISA or immunoblotting or directed against anchoring fibrils on immunoelectron microscopy.

## REFERENCES

1. Bernard P, Vaillant L, Labeille B, et al. Incidence and distribution of subepidermal autoimmune bullous skin diseases in three French regions. French Bullous Study Group. Arch Dermatol 1995;131(1): 48–52.

2. Bertram F, Bröcker EB, Zillikens D, et al. Prospective analysis of the incidence of autoimmune bullous disorders in Lower Franconia, Germany. J Dtsch Dermatol Ges 2009;7(5):434–40.

3. Woodley DT, Remington J, Chen M. Autoimmunity to type VII collagen: epidermolysis bullosa acquisita. Clin Rev Allergy Immunol 2007;33(1–2):78–84.

4. Lapiere JC, Woodley DT, Parente MG, et al. Epitope mapping of type VII collagen. Identification of discrete peptide sequences recognized by sera from patients with acquired epidermolysis bullosa. J Clin Invest 1993;92(4):1831–9.

5. Gammon WR, Murrell DF, Jenison MW, et al. Autoantibodies to type VII collagen recognize epitopes in a fibronectin-like region of the noncollagenous (NC1) domain. J Invest Dermatol 1993;100(5): 618–22.

6. Tanaka T, Furukawa F, Imamura S. Epitope mapping for epidermolysis bullosa acquisita autoantibody by molecularly cloned cDNA for type VII collagen. J Invest Dermatol 1994;102(5):706–9.

7. Ishii N, Yoshida M, Ishida-Yamamoto A, et al. Some epidermolysis bullosa acquisita sera react with epitopes within the triple-helical collagenous domain as indicated by immunoelectron microscopy. Br J Dermatol 2009;160(5):1090–3.

8. Hill PB, Boyer P, Lau P, et al. Epidermolysis bullosa acquisita in a great Dane. J Small Anim Pract 2008;49(2):89–94.

9. Sitaru C, Mihai S, Otto C, et al. Induction of dermal-epidermal separation in mice by passive transfer of antibodies specific to type VII collagen. J Clin Invest 2005;115(4):870–8.

10. Woodley DT, Ram R, Doostan A, et al. Induction of epidermolysis bullosa acquisita in mice by passive transfert of autoantibodies from patients. J Invest Dermatol 2006;126(6):1323–30.

11. Sitaru C, Chiriac MT, Mihai S, et al. Induction of complement-fixing autoantibodies against type VII collagen results in subepidermal blistering in mice. J Immunol 2006;177(5):3461–8.

12. Mihai S, Chiriac MT, Takahashi K, et al. The alternative pathway of complement activation is critical for blister induction in experimental epidermolysis bullosa acquisita. J Immunol 2007;178(10):6514–21.

13. Abrams ML, Smidt A, Benjamin L, et al. Congenital epidermolysis bullosa acquisita. Arch Dermatol 2011; 147(3):337–41.

14. Ludwig R, Recke A, Bieber K, et al. Generation of antibodies of distinct subclasses and specificity is linked to H2s in an active mouse model of epidermolysis bullosa acquisita antigen. J Invest Dermatol 2011;131(1):167–76.

15. Alexandre M, Brette MD, Pascal F, et al. A prospective study of upper aerodigestive tract manifestations of mucous membrane pemphigoid. Medicine 2006; 85(4):239–52.

16. Shipman AR, Agero AL, Cook I, et al. Epidermolysis bullosa acquisita requiring multiple oesophageal dilatations. Clin Exp Dermatol 2008;33(6):787–9.

17. Vodegel RM, de Jog MC, Pas HH, et al. IgA-mediated epidermolysis bullosa acquisita: two cases and review of the literature. J Am Acad Dermatol 2002;47(6):919–25.

18. Caux F, Kirtschig G, Lemarchand-Venencie F, et al. IgA-epidermolysis bullosa acquisita in a child resulting in blindness. Br J Dermatol 1997;137(2): 270–5.

19. Cox NH, Bearn MA, Herold J, et al. Blindness due to the IgA variant of epidermolysis bullosa acquisita, and treatment with osteo-odonto-keratoprosthesis. Br J Dermatol 2007;156(4):775–7.

20. Le Roux-Villet C, Prost-Squarcioni C, Heller M, et al. Epidermolysis bullosa acquisita: a clinical, histological and immunological study of 39 cases. Ann Dermatol Venereol 2002;129. 1S71–1S72.

21. Gammon WR, Briggaman RA, Inman AO 3rd, et al. Differentiating anti-lamina lucida and antisublamina densa anti-BMZ antibodies by indirect immunofluorescence on 1.0 M sodium chloride-separated skin. J Invest Dermatol 1984;82(2):139–44.

22. Dainichi T, Kurono S, Ohyama B, et al. Anti-laminin gamma-1 pemphigoid. Proc Natl Acad Sci U S A 2009;106(8):2800–5.

23. Grootenboer-Mignot S, Descamps V, Picard-Dahan C, et al. Place of human amniotic membrane

immunoblotting in the diagnosis of autoimmune bullous dermatoses. Br J Dermatol 2010;162(4):743–50.

24. Ishii N, Yoshida M, Hisamatsu Y, et al. Epidermolysis bullosa acquisita sera react with distinct epitopes on the NC1 and NC2 domains of type VII collagen: study using immunoblotting of domain-specific recombinant proteins and postembedding immunoelectron microscopy. Br J Dermatol 2004;150(5):843–51.

25. Chen M, Keene DR, Costa FK, et al. The carboxyl terminus of type VII collagen mediates antiparallel dimer formation and constitutes a new antigenic epitope for epidermolysis bullosa acquisita autoantibodies. J Biol Chem 2001;276(24):21649–55.

26. Chen M, O'Toole EA, Sanghavi J, et al. The epidermolysis bullosa acquisita antigen (type VII collagen) is present in human colon and patients with Crohn's disease have autoantibodies to type VII collagen. J Invest Dermatol 2002;118(6):1059–64.

27. Müller R, Dahler C, Möbs C, et al. T and B cells target identical regions of the non-collagenous domain 1 of collagen VII in epidermolysis bullosa acquisita. Clin Immunol 2010;135(1):99–107.

28. Pendaries V, Le Roux C, Vitezica ZG, et al. Valeur diagnostique et pronostique d'un test Elisa sur un homotrimère recombinant de collagène VII dans l'épidermolyse bulleuse acquise et le lupus érythémateux vésiculobulleux. Ann Dermatol Venereol 2008;135S:A68–9.

29. Chan LS, Majmudar AA, Tran HH, et al. Laminin-6 and laminin-5 are recognized by autoantibodies in a subset of cicatricial pemphigoid. J Invest Dermatol 1997;108(6):848–53.

30. Vaillant L, Bernard P, Joly P, et al. Evaluation of clinical criteria for diagnosis of bullous pemphigoid. French Bullous Study Group. Arch Dermatol 1998; 134(9):1075–80.

31. Hundorfean G, Neurath MF, Sitaru C. Autoimmunity against type VII collagen in inflammatory bowel disease. J Cell Mol Med 2010;14(10):2393–403.

32. Gammon WR, Briggaman RA. Epidermolysis bullosa acquisita and bullous systemic lupus erythematosus. Dermatol Clin 1993;11(3):535–47.

33. Vassileva S. Bullous systemic lupus erythematosus. Clin Dermatol 2004;22(2):129–38.

# Pathogenesis of Epidermolysis Bullosa Acquisita

Ralf J. Ludwig, MD*, Detlef Zillikens, MD

**KEYWORDS**

- Skin • Epidermolysis bullosa acquisita • Autoimmunity
- Blister • Animal model

In 1904, the term epidermolysis bullosa acquisita (EBA) was proposed as a descriptive clinical diagnosis for patients with adult onset and features resembling those of hereditary dystrophic epidermolysis bullosa.[1] Almost 70 years later, EBA was distinguished from other bullous diseases based on distinctive clinical and histologic features, implementing the first diagnostic criteria for the disease.[2] Since then, the understanding of the clinical presentation, histopathologic features, and pathogenesis of EBA has significantly increased. Despite these insights, therapy for patients with EBA still relies on general immunosuppression and overall remains unsatisfactory.

## LOSS OF TOLERANCE TO TYPE VII COLLAGEN
### Identification of Type VII Collagen as the Autoantigen in EBA

In 1984, a skin basement membrane component was identified as the target of the autoantibody response in EBA.[3] Subsequently, autoantibody specificity of sera from patients with EBA was mapped to the noncollagenous (NC) 1 domain of type VII collagen (COL7).[4] Fine epitope mapping studies indicated that sera from patients with EBA bind to numerous antigens located within the NC1 domain (**Fig. 1**). More specifically, major antigenic sites recognized by antibodies from patients with EBA clustered on fibronectin type (Fn) III–like domains and the von Willebrand factor domain.[5,6] After successful expression of the cartilage matrix protein (CMP) domain of COL7, this domain was identified to also harbor major antigenic sites.[7] Recent reports have indicated that some patients with EBA also recognize epitopes located within the NC2 domain[8] or the triple-helical collagenous domain[9] of COL7 (see **Fig. 1**). Further fine mapping studies identified octapeptide sequences within the NC1 domain as the major binding sites of anti-COL7 antibodies. However, in contrast to previous work, autoantibody binding was shown to be restricted to certain epitopes within the NC1 domain, which may be due to a relatively small sample size.[10]

The pathogenic relevance of anti-COL7 antibodies has been demonstrated both in vitro and in vivo: in the presence of neutrophils, serum from patients with EBA induces dermal-epidermal separation when incubated with cryosections of human skin. This blister-inducing potential is retained if immunoglobulin G (IgG) from the serum is affinity purified using recombinant NC1. In contrast, the corresponding flow-through fraction fails to induce dermal-epidermal separation.[11] When injected into mice, either human or rabbit anti-COL7 IgG elicits skin lesions, resembling those observed in human patients with EBA.[7,12–14] In these anti-COL7 IgG transfer models of EBA, autoantibodies were directed against different epitopes within the murine NC1 domain, for example, the CMP domain or various Fn III–like domains. In addition, the disease can be induced in mice by immunization with an immunodominant peptide within the murine

Grant support: DFG Excellence Cluster "Inflammation at Interfaces" (DFG EXC 306/1), DFG LU877/5-1, Focus Program "Autoimmunity" of the University of Lübeck.
Financial disclosures and/or conflict of interest: The authors have nothing to disclose.
Department of Dermatology, University of Lübeck, Ratzeburger Allee 160, D-23538 Lübeck, Germany
* Corresponding author.
E-mail address: ralf.ludwig@uk-sh.de

Dermatol Clin 29 (2011) 493–501
doi:10.1016/j.det.2011.03.003

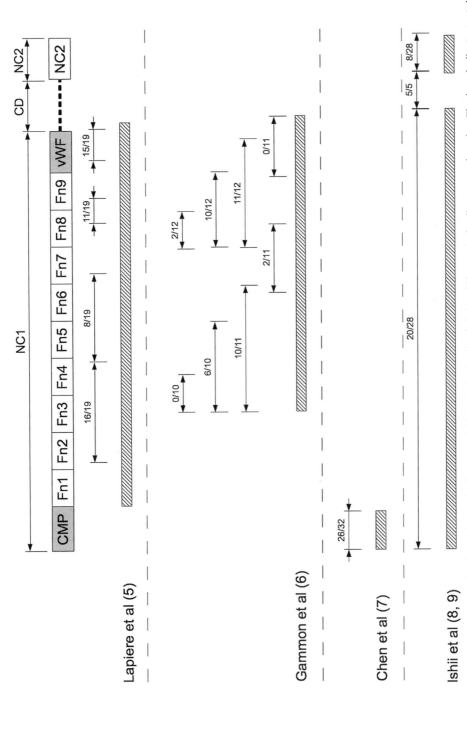

**Fig. 1.** Fine mapping of anti-COL7 antibodies. Schematic diagram of COL7, including both NC and the central collagenous domains. The bars indicate protein sequences included in the respective epitope mapping studies. Numbers in lines correspond to the number of positive sera/total number of samples tested. The study by Dr Chen and colleagues[7] confirmed reactivity of the sera outside the CMP domain from patients, but detailed information has not been provided because of the focus on the CMP domain. In the study by Ishii and colleagues,[8] only EBA sera not reactive to both NC domains were included. (*Data from* Ishii N, Yoshida M, Ishida-Yamamoto A, et al. Some epidermolysis bullosa acquisita sera react with epitopes within the triple-helical collagenous domain as indicated by immunoelectron microscopy. Br J Dermatol 2009;160:1090–93.)

NC1 domain, which includes Fn III–like domains 7 to 9.[15–17] These regions correspond to the similar Fn III–like domains of human COL7 (see **Fig. 1**).

## Susceptibility to EBA is Linked to Major Histocompatibility Complex Genes

The major histocompatibility complex (MHC) or human leukocyte antigen (HLA) region is one of the most extensively studied regions in the genome because of the contribution of multiple variants of this locus to inflammatory diseases, including autoimmune disorders.[18] In contrast to most autoimmune diseases, little is known about the susceptibility genes in EBA. In a small cohort of human patients, an association with HLA-DR2 has been described.[19] Experimental data on immunization-induced EBA in mice[15] support the notion that EBA is associated with MHC genes. In the initial description of this model, immunization with a recombinant fragment of murine COL7 led to clinical disease in 82% of SJL/J mice (H2s), whereas incidence in Balb/c mice (H2d) was significantly lower and outbreed SKH-1 mice were completely protected from EBA induction.[15] Following up on this initial observation, detailed analyses including different inbreed mouse strains showed a clear association of EBA susceptibility with the H2s haplotype. Whereas 75% of mice carrying H2s (SJL/J, C57Bl/10.s) developed clinical EBA lesions, only 5% of inbreed non-H2s mouse strains were prone to EBA. The observation of clinical EBA in C57Bl/10.s mice, but not in genetically identical (with the exception of the MHC locus) C57Bl/10.q mice, underscores the importance of MHC in controlling tolerance to COL7.[17] As murine and human MHC regions share little similarity, direct comparisons of genetic regions within this locus controlling EBA susceptibility cannot be made. However, both observations underscore the importance of the MHC locus in controlling autoimmune diseases such as EBA.

In addition to MHC genes, these experimental studies also indicated that genes outside the MHC locus have a strong influence in the control of tolerance to COL7. More specifically, the otherwise EBA-resistant C57Bl/6 mice become susceptible to EBA development when lacking expression of the inhibitory FcγRIIB receptor.[15] In contrast to SJL/J mice, EBA in C57Bl/10.s mice is mild and mostly transient.[17] Unpublished data from our laboratory, using a family of mice from a large, autoimmune-prone intercross line, has identified non-MHC genes, controlling susceptibility to immunization-induced EBA (unpublished data, 2011).

## T Cells are Required for Induction of Experimental EBA

Induction of autoimmune diseases in experimental animals is generally a T-cell–dependent process.[20,21] However, recent studies in the models of lupus erythematosus have indicated that under certain experimental settings, B cells, independent of T cells, are sufficient for the development of systemic autoimmunity.[22,23] In EBA, T-cell reactivity to COL7 has been reported in individual patients. For example, T-cell reactivity against COL7 paralleled the clinical activity, preceding a delayed response of COL7-specific IgG. Furthermore, by enzyme-linked immunosorbent spot analysis, interleukin (IL)-5–secreting $T_H2$ cells, interferon-γ–secreting $T_H1$ cells, and an IL-10–secreting T-cell subset were detected on ex vivo stimulation of peripheral blood mononuclear cells from patients with EBA.[24] However, the few numbers of patients with EBA investigated does not yet allow further insights into T-cell activation in patients with EBA. The critical contribution of T cells to the pathogenesis of experimental EBA has been demonstrated by recent data obtained from mice immunization-induced EBA,[15] where genetic lack of T cells protected from disease induction. Furthermore, reconstitution of SJL$^{nude}$ mice with lymphocytes from wild-type SJL/J mice restored the susceptibility to immunization-induced EBA.[25]

## Conclusions and Remaining Questions Regarding the Loss of Tolerance

The pathogenic relevance of COL7 as the autoantigen in EBA has been convincingly demonstrated. Data from observational studies in humans with EBA and in model systems of EBA have indicated that the loss of tolerance to COL7 requires T cells and that this process is associated with specific genes (**Fig. 2**). However, several questions need to be addressed for a detailed understanding of the pathogenesis of EBA:

1. Is a distinct autoantibody specificity associated with the different EBA phenotypes?
2. Which cells (if any), in addition to T cells, are involved in the loss of tolerance to COL7?
3. Which individual genes are associated with EBA?

## Autoantibody-induced Tissue Injury in EBA

After mounting an autoantibody response toward COL7, autoantibodies rapidly bind to their targeted antigen in the skin. For example, anti-COL7 IgG deposition is observed at the dermal-epidermal junction within 2 hours after subcutaneous injection at distant sites. Intravenously injected anti-COL7 IgG is detected within

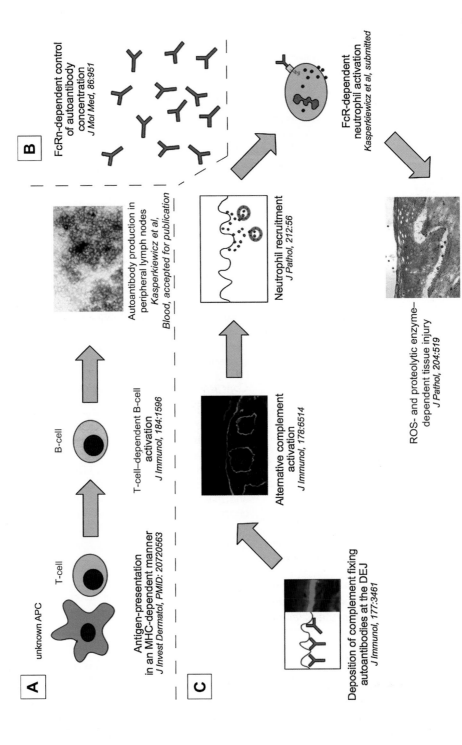

**Fig. 2.** The pathogenesis of EBA is divided into 3 distinct steps: A, loss of tolerance; B, maintenance of the loss of tolerance/autoantibody half-life; and C, tissue injury. The respective events in the pathogenesis have been ordered in a sequence that presumably leads to tissue injury. However, the precise order in which these events take place is currently unknown. DEJ, dermal-epidermal junction.

minutes at the dermal-epidermal junction (Ludwig and Zillikens, unpublished, 2011). After deposition at the dermal-epidermal junction, anti-COL7 autoantibodies can be detected by direct immunofluorescent microscopy for as long as 8 weeks.[16] Anti-COL7 autoantibodies cross the placenta and can be detected in the offspring of the mice with experimental EBA[16] and the neonates of female patients with EBA.[26]

### Autoantibody-induced Tissue Injury Depends on Fc-dependent Mechanisms

Without exception, autoantibody-induced tissue injury in all available experimental models of EBA depends on the Fc fragment of IgG. Incubation of human skin with anti-NC1 polyclonal IgG isolated from patients with EBA or a monoclonal antibody directed to an epitope on the central portion of the NC1 domain (clone LH7.2) leads to dermal-epidermal separation in the presence of neutrophils. Removal of the Fc portion of the autoantibodies by pepsin digestion abolished this pathogenic activity.[11] Correspondingly, mice injected with either human or rabbit anti-COL7 IgG developed clinical lesions when injected with IgG but not when F(ab)$_2$ fragments were used at equimolar doses.[7,12] In addition, chicken immunoglobulin Y (IgY), which is unable to activate murine complement and does not bind to murine Fc receptors,[27] induced neither dermal-epidermal separation ex vivo, nor clinical EBA lesions in mice.[28]

### Distinct Autoantibody Isotypes Mediate Tissue Injury in EBA

However, effector functions of the Fc portion differ among isotypes and subclasses of antibodies. Depending on the subclass, antibodies greatly vary regarding their affinity to inhibiting and activating Fc receptors.[29,30] In patients with EBA, anti-COL7 antibodies of all IgG subclasses can be detected with the following detection frequency: IgG4>IgG1>IgG2>IgG3.[31,32] IgG subclasses of circulating anti-COL7 autoantibodies have not been demonstrated to correlate with the different clinical variants of EBA.[33,34] However, recent work has demonstrated that only IgG1- and IgG3-anti-COL7 autoantibodies are capable to fix complement and induce dermal-epidermal separation ex vivo.[35] This experimental model requires neutrophils for induction of dermal-epidermal separation,[11] thus reflecting the inflammatory variant of EBA. The role of IgG2- and IgG4-anti-COL7 antibodies in the pathogenesis of EBA (especially the noninflammatory manifestation) cannot be excluded.

### Activation of the Alternative Complement Cascade is Required in the Experimental Models of EBA

Injection of rabbit anti-mouse COL7 IgG into mice (passive EBA mouse model) elicits clinical EBA lesions,[12] mimicking the inflammatory variant of the disease. In this model, mice lacking C5 are completely protected from disease induction.[12] In line, chicken IgY did not induce clinical EBA lesions in mice.[28] Further experiments demonstrated a predominant role of the alternative complement pathway, leading to the conversion of C5 to C5a, in lesion formation in this mouse model of EBA. In detail, factor B–deficient mice developed a delayed and significantly less severe blistering disease compared with control mice. Furthermore, local reconstitution of factor B–deficient mice with wild-type neutrophils reestablished disease susceptibility. Mice with defects in the classical- or lectin-complement activation pathways (C1q- or mannose binding lectin–deficient mice, respectively) showed little or no changes in the EBA phenotype compared with the respective wild-type control mice.[36] In summary, this suggests, that complement activation in EBA leads to generation of a chemotactic gradient, which supports recruitment of effector cells into the skin, rather than direct toxic effects. This assumption is supported by the observation that autoantibody-induced tissue injury ex vivo, induced by the incubation of cryosections from human skin with anti-COL7 antibodies and neutrophils, is independent of complement activation.[11]

### Neutrophils are Key Effector Cells in the Pathogenesis of EBA

Complement activation, and presumably also activation of additional resident immune cells (eg, mast cells and dendritic cells), generates a proinflammatory environment in the skin, leading to the recruitment of leukocytes.[37] If neutrophils are depleted by injection of anti–Gr-1 antibody (clone RB6–8C5) during the induction of EBA by repetitive injections of anti-COL7 IgG, mice are completely protected from disease induction,[38] which strongly indicates that neutrophils are the main effector cells for blister formation and tissue injury. However, a contribution of additional cells, especially monocytes, cannot be excluded, because the Gr-1 antibody is also known to deplete monocytes.[39] The observed resistance of CD18-deficient mice, lacking expression of all β2-integrins, required for firm adhesion and subsequent extravasation of leukocytes to the skin,[40] underscores the significant contribution of neutrophils

**Table 1**
**Model systems of EBA**

| Model | Method | Reproduces | References |
|---|---|---|---|
| IC-induced neutrophil activation | - IC fixed on a 96-well plate<br>- Addition of human neutrophils<br>- Measurement of ROS production and lactoferin release | COL7/anti-COL7-IC–induced neutrophil activation | 42<br>(Recke and colleagues, in preparation) |
| Ex vivo dermal-epidermal separation (Cryosection assay) | - Incubation of cryosections of human skin with anti-COL7 autoantibodies (monoclonal autoantibodies, patient serum, total or NC1 affinity-purified IgG from the serum from patients with EBA)<br>- Addition of human polymorphnuclear leukocytes or neutrophils<br>- Determination of the extent of dermal-epidermal separation | Tissue injury of inflammatory EBA | 11,35 |
| Autoantibody transfer ("passive") EBA mouse model | - Isolation of human or rabbit anti-human/mouse COL7 IgG<br>- Repetitive injection of anti-COL7 IgG in mice<br>- Determination of the extent of clinical EBA lesions | Tissue injury of inflammatory EBA | 7,12,13 |
| Immunization-induced ("active") EBA mouse model | - Immunization (1–4 times) of SJL/J, C57Bl/10.s, or female MRL/MpJ mice with an immunodominant peptide within the murine NC1 domain using TiterMax as adjuvant<br>- Analysis of T- and B-cell responses<br>- Determination of the extent of clinical EBA lesions | - Loss of tolerance to COL7<br>- Tissue injury of inflammatory EBA | 15–17 |

*Abbreviation:* IC, a fixed *immune complex* of a human anti-COL7 monoclonal antibody bound to the respective antigen.[35]

(and possibly monocytes) in the pathogenesis of experimental EBA.[38]

## Neutrophil Activation Leads to the Release of Reactive Oxygen Species and Proteolytic Enzymes, Which Induce Blister Formation

Release of reactive oxygen species (ROS) and proteolytic enzymes is a key event in neutrophil activation.[41] Indeed, neutrophils produce ROS and release their granules upon incubation with immune complexes.[42] In addition, after incubation of cryosections of human skin with anti-COL7 antibodies and neutrophils, formazan precipitates are present at the dermal-epidermal junction when nitroblue tetrazolium is present, indicating ROS production. In contrast, neither formazan precipitates nor dermal-epidermal separation was observed when neutrophils from patients with chronic granulomatous disease, in which the ability of phagocytes to produce ROS is lacking, were used.[38] The dependency of autoantibody-induced tissue injury on ROS production is further supported by the observation of a complete protection of Ncf1-deficient mice, which are unable to produce ROS, from experimental EBA.[38]

In addition to ROS release, neutrophil-derived proteases are indispensable for autoantibody-induced tissue injury in experimental models of EBA. In detail, when cryosections of human skin were treated with autoantibodies from patients with EBA and with peripheral blood leukocytes from healthy donors in the presence of a cocktail of broad-spectrum protease inhibitors, including α2-macroglobulin, α1-protease inhibitor, AEBSF, GM6001, E64, and pepstatin A, leukocytes were recruited to the dermal-epidermal junction but failed to induce split formation at the dermal-epidermal junction. When characterizing the proteases involved more specifically, selective inhibition of human leukocyte elastase or gelatinase B/matrix metalloproteinase-9 (MMP-9) was found to result in the suppression of blistering. Therefore, elastase and gelatinase B/MMP-9 mediate dermal-epidermal separation in the ex vivo models of EBA.[43]

## Possible Contribution of Cytokines

There is ample evidence for increased expression of several cytokines in patients with autoimmune blistering skin diseases. However, with few exceptions,[44] there is little experimental evidence that demonstrates a direct contribution of a given cytokine to the pathogenesis of the disease.[45] Regarding EBA, no data on cytokine expression are available. Hence, the contribution of cytokines to the pathogenesis of EBA (and other autoimmune blistering skin diseases) remains an issue of ongoing investigation.

## Conclusions and Remaining Questions Regarding Autoantibody-Induced Tissue Damage

Blister formation in experimental models of EBA clearly depends on the autoantibodies' isotype, complement activation, neutrophils, production of ROS, and release of proteolytic enzymes (see **Fig. 2**). Despite these detailed insights into the pathogenesis of tissue injury in EBA, the exact sequence of events leading to blister formation needs to be defined. Understanding this process in detail may help to identify key molecules in the generation of tissue injury, which, in turn, may be targeted by novel (topical) inflammation-modulating compounds. In addition, several questions regarding the pathogenesis of tissue injury in EBA need to be addressed:

1. What is the contribution of cells other than neutrophils, especially mast cells and monocytes/macrophages, in the pathogenesis of EBA?
2. Are cytokines involved in mediating tissue injury? If yes, which specific cytokines?
3. On the molecular level, which Fc receptors mediate tissue injury?

## GAPS IN THE UNDERSTANDING OF THE PATHOGENESIS OF EBA

In addition to the issues raised above, research on EBA still lacks appropriate model systems for the noninflammatory disease variants and solid epidemiologic data.

### Novel Disease Models are Required

All experimental models of EBA mimic the inflammatory variant of the disease (**Table 1**).[7,12,13,42,46] At present, there is no model available mirroring the noninflammatory variants of EBA. Consequently, most of the above outlined understanding of the pathogenesis of EBA refers only to inflammatory EBA. To fill this gap, development of respective model systems would greatly enhance our overall understanding of EBA.

## REFERENCES

1. Elliott GT. Two cases of epidermolysis bullosa. J Cutan Genitourin Dis 1895;13:10.
2. Roenigk HHJ, Ryan JG, Bergfeld WF. Epidermolysis bullosa acquisita. Report of three cases and review of all published cases. Arch Dermatol 1971;103:1–10.

3. Woodley DT, Briggaman RA, O'Keefe EJ, et al. Identification of the skin basement-membrane autoantigen in epidermolysis bullosa acquisita. N Engl J Med 1984;310:1007–13.

4. Woodley DT, Burgeson RE, Lunstrum G, et al. Epidermolysis bullosa acquisita antigen is the globular carboxyl terminus of type VII procollagen. J Clin Invest 1988;81:683–7.

5. Lapiere JC, Woodley DT, Parente MG, et al. Epitope mapping of type VII collagen. Identification of discrete peptide sequences recognized by sera from patients with acquired epidermolysis bullosa. J Clin Invest 1993;92:1831–9.

6. Gammon WR, Murrell DF, Jenison MW, et al. Autoantibodies to type VII collagen recognize epitopes in a fibronectin-like region of the noncollagenous (NC1) domain. J Invest Dermatol 1993;100:618–22.

7. Chen M, Doostan A, Bandyopadhyay P, et al. The cartilage matrix protein subdomain of type VII collagen is pathogenic for epidermolysis bullosa acquisita. Am J Pathol 2007;170:2009–18.

8. Ishii N, Yoshida M, Hisamatsu Y, et al. Epidermolysis bullosa acquisita sera react with distinct epitopes on the NC1 and NC2 domains of type VII collagen: study using immunoblotting of domain-specific recombinant proteins and postembedding immunoelectron microscopy. Br J Dermatol 2004;150:843–51.

9. Ishii N, Yoshida M, Ishida-Yamamoto A, et al. Some epidermolysis bullosa acquisita sera react with epitopes within the triple-helical collagenous domain as indicated by immunoelectron microscopy. Br J Dermatol 2009;160:1090–3.

10. Jones DA, Hunt SW 3rd, Prisayanh PS, et al. Immunodominant autoepitopes of type VII collagen are short, paired peptide sequences within the fibronectin type III homology region of the noncollagenous (NC1) domain. J Invest Dermatol 1995;104:231–5.

11. Sitaru C, Kromminga A, Hashimoto T, et al. Autoantibodies to type VII collagen mediate Fcgamma-dependent neutrophil activation and induce dermal-epidermal separation in cryosections of human skin. Am J Pathol 2002;161:301–11.

12. Sitaru C, Mihai S, Otto C, et al. Induction of dermal-epidermal separation in mice by passive transfer of antibodies specific to type VII collagen. J Clin Invest 2005;115:870–8.

13. Woodley DT, Chang C, Saadat P, et al. Evidence that anti-type VII collagen antibodies are pathogenic and responsible for the clinical, histological, and immunological features of epidermolysis bullosa acquisita. J Invest Dermatol 2005;124:958–64.

14. Woodley DT, Ram R, Doostan A, et al. Induction of epidermolysis bullosa acquisita in mice by passive transfer of autoantibodies from patients. J Invest Dermatol 2006;126:1323–30.

15. Sitaru C, Chiriac MT, Mihai S, et al. Induction of complement-fixing autoantibodies against type VII collagen results in subepidermal blistering in mice. J Immunol 2006;177:3461–8.

16. Kasperkiewicz M, Hirose M, Recke A, et al. Clearance rates of circulating and tissue-bound autoantibodies to type VII collagen in experimental epidermolysis bullosa acquisita. Br J Dermatol 2010;162:1064–70.

17. Ludwig RJ, Recke A, Bieber K, et al. Generation of antibodies of distinct subclasses and specificity is linked to H2s in an active mouse model of epidermolysis bullosa acquisita. J Invest Dermatol 2011;131(1):167–76.

18. Fernando MM, Stevens CR, Walsh EC, et al. Defining the role of the MHC in autoimmunity: a review and pooled analysis. PLoS Genet 2008;4:e1000024.

19. Gammon WR, Heise ER, Burke WA, et al. Increased frequency of HLA-DR2 in patients with autoantibodies to epidermolysis bullosa acquisita antigen: evidence that the expression of autoimmunity to type VII collagen is HLA class II allele associated. J Invest Dermatol 1988;91:228–32.

20. Connolly K, Roubinian JR, Wofsy D. Development of murine lupus in CD4-depleted NZB/NZW mice. Sustained inhibition of residual CD4+ T cells is required to suppress autoimmunity. J Immunol 1992;149:3083–8.

21. Takahashi H, Amagai M, Nishikawa T, et al. Novel system evaluating in vivo pathogenicity of desmoglein 3-reactive T cell clones using murine pemphigus vulgaris. J Immunol 2008;181:1526–35.

22. Groom J, Mackay F. B cells flying solo. Immunol Cell Biol 2008;86:40–6.

23. Herlands RA, Christensen SR, Sweet RA, et al. T cell-independent and toll-like receptor-dependent antigen-driven activation of autoreactive B cells. Immunity 2008;29:249–60.

24. Muller R, Dahler C, Mobs C, et al. T and B cells target identical regions of the non-collagenous domain 1 of type VII collagen in epidermolysis bullosa acquisita. Clin Immunol 2010;135:99–107.

25. Sitaru AG, Sesarman A, Mihai S, et al. T cells are required for the production of blister-inducing autoantibodies in experimental epidermolysis bullosa acquisita. J Immunol 2010;184:1596–603.

26. Abrams ML, Smidt A, Benjamin L, et al. Congenital epidermolysis bullosa acquisita: vertical transfer of maternal autoantibody from mother to infant. Arch Dermatol 2010.

27. Ambrosius H, Hadge D. Chicken immunoglobulins. Vet Immunol Immunopathol 1987;17:57–67.

28. Sesarman A, Mihai S, Chiriac MT, et al. Binding of avian IgY to type VII collagen does not activate complement and leucocytes fail to induce subepidermal blistering in mice. Br J Dermatol 2008;158:463–71.

29. Nimmerjahn F, Ravetch JV. Divergent immunoglobulin G subclass activity through selective Fc receptor binding. Science 2005;5753:1510–2.

30. Bruhns P, Iannascoli B, England P, et al. Specificity and affinity of human Fcgamma receptors and their polymorphic variants for human IgG subclasses. Blood 2008;16:3716–25.

31. Bernard P, Prost C, Aucouturier P, et al. The subclass distribution of IgG autoantibodies in cicatricial pemphigoid and epidermolysis bullosa acquisita. J Invest Dermatol 1991;97:259–63.

32. Oostingh GJ, Sitaru C, Zillikens D, et al. Subclass distribution of type VII collagen-specific autoantibodies in patients with inflammatory bowel disease. J Dermatol Sci 2005;37:182–4.

33. Cho HJ, Lee IJ, Kim SC. Complement-fixing abilities and IgG subclasses of auto-antibodies in epidermolysis bullosa acquisita. Yonsei Med J 1998;39: 339–44.

34. Gandhi K, Chen M, Aasi S, et al. Autoantibodies to type VII collagen have heterogeneous subclass and light chain compositions and their complement-activating capacities do not correlate with the inflammatory clinical phenotype. J Clin Immunol 2000;20:416–23.

35. Recke A, Sitaru C, Vidarsson G, et al. Pathogenicity of IgG subclass autoantibodies to type VII collagen: induction of dermal-epidermal separation. J Autoimmun 2010;34:435–44.

36. Mihai S, Chiriac MT, Takahashi K, et al. The alternative pathway in complement activation is critical for blister induction in experimental epidermolysis bullosa acquisita. J Immunol 2007;178:6514–21.

37. Schön M, Ludwig RJ. Lymphocyte trafficking to inflames skin—molecular mechanisms and implications for therapeutic target molecules. Expert Opin Ther Targets 2005;9:225–43.

38. Chiriac MT, Roesler J, Sindrilaru A, et al. NADPH oxidase is required for neutrophil-dependent autoantibody-induced tissue damage. J Pathol 2007;212:56–65.

39. Daley JM, Thomay AA, Connolly MD, et al. Use of Ly6G-specific monoclonal antibody to deplete neutrophils in mice. J Leukoc Biol 2008;83:64–70.

40. Radeke HH, Ludwig RJ, Boehncke WH. Experimental approaches to lymphocyte migration in dermatology in vitro and in vivo. Exp Dermatol 2005;14:641–66.

41. van Eeden SF, Klut ME, Walker BA, et al. The use of flow cytometry to measure neutrophil function. J Immunol Methods 1999;232:23–43.

42. Yu X, Holdorf K, Kasper B, et al. FcγRIIA and FcγRIIIB are required for autoantibody-induced tissue damage in experimental human models of bullous pemphigoid. J Invest Dermatol 2010; 130(12):2841–4.

43. Shimanovich I, Mihai S, Oostingh GJ, et al. Granulocyte-derived elastase and gelatinase B are required for dermal-epidermal separation induced by autoantibodies from patients with epidermolysis bullosa acquisita and bullous pemphigoid. J Pathol 2004; 204:519–27.

44. Feliciani C, Toto P, Amerio P, et al. In vitro and in vivo expression of interleukin-1alpha and tumor necrosis factor-alpha mRNA in pemphigus vulgaris: interleukin-1alpha and tumor necrosis factor-alpha are involved in acantholysis. J Invest Derm 2000; 114:71–7.

45. Ludwig RJ, Schmidt E. Cytokines in autoimmune bullous skin diseases. Epiphenomena or contribution to pathogenesis? G Ital Dermatol Venereol 2009;144:339–49.

46. Bieber K, Sun S, Ishii N, et al. Animal models for autoimmune bullous dermatoses. Exp Dermatol 2010;19:2–11.

# Hair Loss in Autoimmune Cutaneous Bullous Disorders

Maryia Miteva, MD[a],
Dédée F. Murrell, MA, BMBCh, FAAD, MD, FACD[b],
Antonella Tosti, MD[a],*

KEYWORDS

• Hair loss • Autoimmune cutaneous bullous disorders
• Alopecia

The expression of the basement membrane zone (BMZ) components in the anagen hair follicles of the human scalp is similar to that of interfollicular epidermis, with expression of plectin, 180-kD bullous pemphigoid antigen (BP180), 230-kD bullous pemphigoid antigen (PB230), a6b4 integrin, laminin 311, laminin 332, and type 4 and type 7 collagen.[1,2] However, expression of the BMZ components varies according to the different follicular portions. In particular, the upper and middle portions of the hair follicle (infundibulum and isthmus), including the bulge region, show expression of all BMZ components with a labeling intensity under immunofluorescence similar to that found in the interfollicular epidermis. In the lower part of the follicle and in the hair bulb, expression of laminin 311 and collagen 4 is continuous, but labeling for other BMZ components shows a gradual decrease with discontinuous expression of a6b4 integrin and laminin 332, particularly outside the hair bulb. Between the dermal papilla and the epithelial cells inside the hair bulb, all of the BMZ components are evident, with the exception of the BP230.[1,2] The reduced expression of all BMZ components outside the hair bulb and the complete absence of BP230 at the dermal papilla junction seem to be responsible for the incomplete ultrastructure of hemidesmosomes in these regions.

Desmosomes are important in hair structure and function. These components include the desmogleins 1 and 3 (Dsg 1 and Dsg 3), desmoplakins, plakophilin, and plakoglobin. Dsg 3 has been identified as a major component of murine and human hair follicle.[3] In humans Dsg 3 shows the following pattern of expression in the outer root sheath (ORS): in the infundibulum, Dsg 3 immunopositivity is present predominantly in the basal cells, similar to the adjacent epidermis. In the isthmus, Dsg 3 immunopositivity in the suprabasal cells of the ORS is gradually lost toward the infundibulum. Below the isthmus, basal cells of the ORS show weak staining and Dsg 3 is present uniformly in all suprabasal cells of the ORS. This transition in Dsg 3 staining of the ORS correlates with the histologic onset of trichilemmal keratinization, which is characterized by abrupt keratinization lacking a granular layer, and a corrugated luminal surface.[4]

Taken together, these findings show that in normal conditions the BMZ components show normal expression at the upper portions of the hair follicle and a gradual decrease in staining in the transient regions of the hair follicles (ie, at the

Funding Sources: None.
[a] Department of Dermatology and Cutaneous Surgery, University of Miami Miller School of Medicine, 1600 North West 10th Avenue, RSMB – 2023A, Miami, FL 33136, USA
[b] Department of Dermatology, St George Hospital, University of New South Wales, Gray Street, Kogarah, Sydney, NSW 2217, Australia
* Corresponding author.
*E-mail address:* atosti@med.miami.edu

Dermatol Clin 29 (2011) 503–509
doi:10.1016/j.det.2011.03.007

level of the hair bulb).[5] The complete structure of the hemidesmosomes is then responsible for the stabilization of the upper follicle to the surrounding connective tissues, whereas the incomplete hemidesmosome structure may facilitate the movement of the transient region.

Blistering of the scalp, involving lamina lucida and below, usually leads to scarring alopecia secondary to the inflammatory process in the interfollicular epidermis and in the upper portion of the hair follicle. This is the cause of alopecia in the junctional and dystrophic forms of epidermolysis bullosa (EB), as reviewed elsewhere by Tosti and colleagues.[6] Herein, we discuss the presence of alopecia in the most common acquired forms of bullous disorders (**Table 1**).

## PEMPHIGUS GROUP

Hair loss as a feature of pemphigus has been reported in several animal species such as dogs, cats, goats, and horses.[7,8] On the other hand, although scalp involvement is common in pemphigus vulgaris (PV) and pemphigus foliaceus (PF), hair loss is rarely reported. Furthermore, the literature is not precise on the presentation and pathogenesis of hair loss in the reported cases.

### Rodent Models

#### Dsg 3 knockout mouse model

Genetically engineered mice that lack the desmosomal proteins Dsg 3 or desmocollin 3 have been used to study the pathologic mechanisms underlying acantholytic disorders.[9] Koch and colleagues[10] showed that mice without Dsg 3

(Dsg 3−/− knockout mice) not only developed mucous membrane and skin lesions like pemphigus patients but also developed hair loss. Hair was normal through the first growth phase around day 20; however, when the hair follicles entered the telogen phase, mice with a targeted disruption of the Dsg 3 gene lost hair in a wavelike pattern from the head to the tail. Hair then regrew and was lost again in the same pattern with the next synchronous hair cycle. Gentle hair pulls with adhesive tape showed that anagen hairs were firmly anchored but telogen hairs came out in clumps. In normal mice telogen hairs are retained until anagen hairs replace them underneath to prevent bald areas from forming and ascertain the synchronous cycling nature of the hair. Histology of bald skin areas in Dsg 3−/− mice showed cystic telogen hair follicles without hair shafts. Histology of hair follicles in early telogen, just before clinical hair loss occurred, showed acantholysis between the cells surrounding the telogen club and the basal layer of the ORS epithelium. The bald areas were still capable of regrowing hair, indicating that the stem cells in the bulge and the dermal papilla were not affected. The investigators concluded that Dsg 3 is necessary for anchoring the telogen hair club to the ORS and mice devoid of Dsg 3 develop acantholysis in the telogen hair with no defect in the anagen hairs. Telogen hair loss is usually not a feature of pemphigus in humans. However, it is important to consider that the human hair cycle is not synchronous and only 5% to 20% of the follicles in the scalp are in telogen; hair loss can then be subtle if only telogen hairs are affected by the acantholysis.

---

**Table 1**
**Summary of the hair loss patterns in autoimmune bullous diseases**

| Feature | Disease | Significance |
|---|---|---|
| Easily extractable anagen hairs | Pemphigus vulgaris<br>Pemphigus foliaceus | Disease activity |
| Nonscarring alopecia | Pemphigus vulgaris<br>Pemphigus vegetans<br>Pemphigus foliaceus | — |
| Scarring alopecia | Mucous membrane pemphigoid<br>Epidermolysis bullosa acquisita<br>Bullous lupus erythematosus | — |
| Erosive cicatricial alopecia | Brunsting-Perry cicatricial pemphigoid | — |
| Tufted folliculitis | Pemphigus vulgaris | Scarring |
| Scalp scaling and crusting without alopecia | Pemphigus foliaceus | — |
| Scalp scaling and crusting with alopecia | Pemphigus foliaceus | — |
| Pruritic papules | Dermatitis herpetiformis | — |
| Alopecia areata | Pemphigus foliaceus<br>Dermatitis herpetiformis | Coincidental |

### Balding phenotype mouse with bal mutations

Mice with spontaneous mutations of the Dsg 3 gene (balding phenotype mice with homozygous bal[J] and bal[Pas] mutations) develop alopetic lesions accompanied by vesicles on the ventral tongue, mucocutaneous junction of the eyelid, foot pads, and rarely the skin.[11] Dsg 3 is located on mouse chromosome 18 in the region of the balding locus.[12] In the hair follicle separation occurred between the outer layers of the ORS whereas the separation in the epidermis of the skin was clearly formed by cleavage between basal and suprabasal layer (a pattern characteristic for PV). As opposed to the finding that acantholysis developed between telogen club hairs and the ORS in Dsg 3 knockout mice bal[J], in the balding phenotype mice separation of the inner and outer layers of the ORS was most prominent in anagen hair follicles, which resulted in poor anchorage of the hair fiber in the anagen follicle. This finding explains why hairs came out easily in tufts on gentle pulling. The bal mice rarely show cutaneous blisters and do not have circulating pemphigus antibodies against the desmosomes. This characteristic is believed to be because of their thicker hair density and thinner epidermis than humans; blistering was inducible with minor trauma. Murine models have provided compelling evidence that abnormalities in the Dsg 3 gene expression or protein adhesion are followed by defective anchoring of hair shafts within the follicles and alopecia. It is still unexplained why the phase of the hair cycle affected by acantholysis is different in the Dsg 3 knockout mice model (telogen)[10] and the bal mutation model, which is the result of a premature stop codon (insertion of a thymidine in the Dsg 3 gene) (anagen).[11]

### Hair Plucking in the Diagnosis of Pemphigus

Even in patients without alopecia who have pemphigus, plucked hair shafts have been used in lieu of skin biopsies to diagnose pemphigus on direct immunofluorescence, because IgG and C3 are positive in between the ORS cells.[13,14]

### Hair Loss Patterns in Pemphigus

Scalp involvement is common in PV because the hair follicles contain many PV antigens and severe scalp involvement can be a feature of recalcitrant disease. However, hair loss or alopecia is not commonly reported. Different types of hair loss reported in PV include anagen shedding, telogen effluvium (TE), scarring alopecia, and tufted folliculitis.

### Anagen shedding with and without alopecia

Anagen effluvium has been described in 3 patients with PV.[15] In all 3 cases, hair loss was evident as easy shedding within and around erosive lesions on the scalp. All patients regrew hair completely with disease control. The pulled hairs appeared as anagen hairs with normal pigmentation and intact root sheaths. Direct immunofluorescence revealed deposits of IgG and C3 within the ORS where clefts were present. According to the author, the anagen shedding was not related to the erosions and crusts because normal anagen hairs were obtained also from the perilesional area of the scalp. The anagen hairs came out easily with their ORS because of the cleavage within the ORS of the follicles where the pemphigus antibodies bound to the overexpressed desmosomal proteins.[16] The shedding of anagen hair in PV was referred to as Nikolsky sign of the scalp and is considered as a subclinical involvement of the follicle. It heralded pemphigus in one of the reported patients and can possibly be used to verify disease activity. Although this phenomenon has been described as anagen effluvium we believe that anagen shedding is the best term to describe loss of anagen hair in pemphigus. The diagnosis of anagen effluvium generally refers to acute anagen arrest with shedding of dystrophic or broken hair shafts, such as in cases of antimitotic chemotherapy treatment.

### Telogen effluvium

TE is not commonly reported by patients with PV and in our experience is not a feature of the disease. According to Koch and colleagues.[10] this finding may be because human follicles are not synchronized and that telogen loss becomes evident only when severe. Therefore, patients may have mild TE that goes unnoticed. However, these investigators found pathologic evidence of TE in a scalp biopsy of 1 patient.

### Scarring alopecia and tufted folliculitis

One of the authors (DM) has seen a patient who developed scarring alopecia after PV persistently affected an area of his scalp (**Fig. 1**).

There are several case reports on the association between tufted folliculitis, characterized by the emergence of multiple hair shafts from 1 follicular opening, and PV.[17–19] Tufted folliculitis is a long-term complication of PV affecting the scalp and is probably related to infection with subsequent scarring.

Tufted folliculitis was first reported by Saijyo and colleagues,[17] who suggested that the combination of acantholysis and secondary bacterial infection could cause local destruction of the scalp. Jappe and colleagues[18] suggested that in PV anti-Dsg 3 antibodies participate in the pathogenesis of tufted folliculitis by forming the background

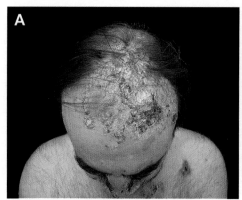
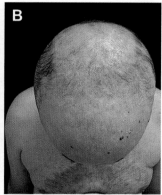

**Fig. 1.** A case of PV affecting the scalp. Note the extensive erosions and hemorrhagic crusts (*A*) healing with scarring alopecia (*B*).

conditions for further inflammatory processes, such as superinfection with bacterial microorganisms. These investigators noticed suprabasal acantholysis in the hair follicles, perifollicular fibrosis around grouped follicles, and normal hair papillae. Petronic-Rosic and colleagues[19] described tufted folliculitis in a patient with PV who developed erosions on the scalp that healed with scars (scarring alopecia). The histopathology revealed several follicles rooted in the subdermis with a common dilated infundibulum in a fibrotic stroma. There were no features of pemphigus in the specimen from the scalp. These investigators explained the development of tufted folliculitis as a host response to the scalp injury in PV: the walls of adjacent follicles are destroyed but the follicular bulbs and papillae remain intact. Because few patients develop tufted folliculitis after scalp involvement of pemphigus this condition cannot be considered characteristic for the disease.

### Pemphigus Vegetans

Pemphigus vegetans rarely affects the scalp. The clinical presentation includes verrucous and vegetating plaques associated with nonscarring alopecia.[20,21]

### Pemphigus Foliaceus

#### Scalp scaling and crusting
PF of the scalp causes erythematous scaly patches that may be misdiagnosed as seborrheic dermatitis (**Fig. 2**).

#### Nonscarring alopecia
Severe alopecia has not been reported in humans, whereas it is common in cats, dogs, and horses.[8,22] Alopecia when present is usually patchy and associated with scalp scaling and crusting (**Fig. 3**).

A case of juvenile PF associated with severe nonscarring alopecia has recently been reported.[22] The scalp was severely involved, with irregularly shaped erythematous and erosive patches of alopecia with strands of residual hair, which was easily extracted. After 5 months of therapy, the erosions healed without scarring and almost complete regrowth of dark and slightly fuzzy scalp hair. At the time of alopecic presentation the patient had extremely high serum levels of circulating anti-Dsg 1 antibodies, which prompted the investigators to consider the possible relationships between this finding and the alopecia. Dsg 1 is mainly present in more differentiated cell populations such as the suprabasal epidermal layer, the inner root sheath of the lower hair follicle, and the innermost layers of the infundibular ORS. Because Dsg 1 is not expressed in the follicular bulge region, this allows the regeneration of the follicular epithelium in PF and prompt hair regrowth.

A case of patchy alopecia areata preceding the onset of a generalized bullous eruption diagnosed as PF has been reported.[23] The patient had complete regrowth of the hair after a course of oral prednisone. However, because the simultaneous

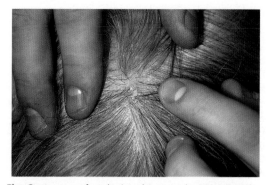

**Fig. 2.** A case of scalp involvement in PF presenting with erythematous scaly lesions without hair loss.

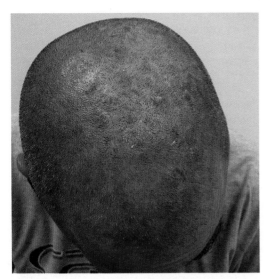

**Fig. 3.** A case of scalp involvement in PF shows diffuse erythematous scaling and crusting covering the entire scalp and resulting in nonscarring patchy alopecia.

occurrence of these 2 disorders has not been subsequently confirmed, it is most probably coincidental.

### Basement Membrane Autoimmune Bullous Disorders Group

To our knowledge there are no reports on hair loss in the different types of bullous pemphigoid. Patients with the corresponding genetic condition affecting the same protein, BP180, who have non-Herlitz junctional EB, have varying degrees of alopecia, depending on whether their *COL17A1* mutations result in no BP180 or reduced BP180.[6] However, there is a form of erosive cicatricial alopecia that some believe to be a form of BP. In 1957 Brunsting and Perry[24] described 7 patients in whom a chronic blistering condition affecting particularly the head and neck resulted in scarring. Six of the 7 patients were balding men and the condition started between the ages of 40 and 70 years. This type of cicatricial pemphigoid has since then been classified by some as a localized form of mucous membrane pemphigoid (MMP) in which mucous membranes are usually spared or as a localized form of bullous pemphigoid.[25] The clinical presentation is that of an extensive erosive scarring alopecia and includes bullous eruptions on the scalp and erosions that heal with scars despite treatment and the main differential diagnosis is erosive and pustular dermatosis of the scalp, infections and EB acquisita (EBA).[26–28] Some investigators believe that Brunsting-Perry cicatricial pemphigoid may represent a clinical variant of EBA.[29,30]

### MMP or cicatricial pemphigoid

MMP can cause cicatricial alopecia when the scalp is affected. One study showed that scalp involvement in MMP is rare, occurring in 4 of 54 patients (7%).[31] A case of MMP with localized scarring, atrophy, and scalp alopecia has been described.[32] It is difficult to explain why targeting of the implicated antigens (BPAG1, BP 230, lam332) in the scalp and development of scarring alopecia occurs only in some patients with MMP. Immune privilege of the hair follicle may be relevant to the sparing of the follicles in most patients with MMP.[33] There may be lack of binding of the autoantibodies to the targeted antigens BP230, BP180, and laminin 332 in the scalp in patients with MMP or there is a universal binding that triggers a scarring response only in some patients.[31]

In dogs affected by MMP, lesions occur on non-hairy regions of the body, and hair loss is not reported.[34]

### Epidermolysis Bullosa Acquisita

EBA can also cause scarring alopecia as a result of antibody formation directed against the noncollagenous domain 1 of collagen VII.[35] Blisters with subsequent scar and milia formation develop in mechanically stressed areas. Direct and indirect immunofluorescence as well as indirect immunofluorescence on salt-split skin is used to exclude the differential diagnosis of bullous pemphigoid.[35] Even severe cases of EBA may have sparing of the scalp, including a case with extensive scarring and contractures with more than 8 esophageal dilatations,[36] suggesting again that immune privilege of the hair follicles may protect them. The corresponding genetic condition, dystrophic EB, usually develops alopecia only in the recessive form in which collagen VII is reduced, and immune privilege is not part of the pathogenesis (**Fig. 4**).[6]

### Bullous Lupus Erythematosus

About 5% of cases of systemic lupus erythematosus (SLE) may be associated with subepidermal blistering and this so-called bullous lupus (BSLE) is caused by autoantibodies directed against the fibronectin III repeat region of collagen VII.[37,38] A significant proportion of SLE cases may have scarring alopecia. The blistering in BSLE is generally on the trunk and limbs, as in inflammatory BP. In view of this, we believe that the alopecia seen in BSLE is a result of their SLE rather than the bullous phenotype and autoantibodies to collagen VII.

### Dermatitis Herpetiformis

The scalp is a common location for lesions of dermatitis herpetiformis, for which the target

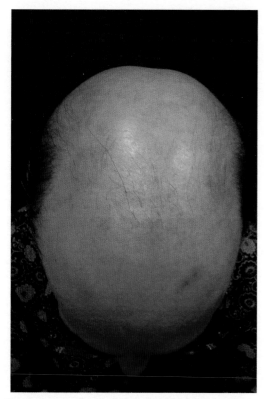

**Fig. 4.** A case of scalp involvement in EBA.

antigen(s) are yet to be precisely defined. In the early stage the scalp, or the scalp and face, may be the only sites affected.[39] The scalp is involved in 30% of patients with dermatitis herpetiformis at some stage of the disease.[40] The presence of intensely irritable papules on the scalp should lead the clinician to search for similar lesions elsewhere. Only in the rare cases when the scalp alone is involved biopsy for light microscopy and direct immunofluorescence can make the diagnosis. Alopecia areata can be associated with celiac disease and occasionally with dermatitis herpetiformis.[41,42]

## REFERENCES

1. Chuang YH, Dean D, Allen J, et al. Comparison between the expression of basement membrane zone antigens of human interfollicular epidermis and anagen hair follicle using indirect immunofluorescence. Br J Dermatol 2003;149(2):274–81.

2. Joubeh S, Mori O, Owaribe K, et al. Immunofluorescence analysis of the basement membrane zone components in human anagen hair follicles. Exp Dermatol 2003;12(4):365–70.

3. Kurzen H, Moll I, Moll R, et al. Compositionally different desmosomes in the various compartments of the human hair follicle. Differentiation 1998; 63(5):295–304.

4. Wu H, Stanley JR, Cotsarelis G. Desmoglein isotype expression in the hair follicle and its cysts correlates with type of keratinization and degree of differentiation. J Invest Dermatol 2003;120(6):1052–7.

5. Al-Refu K, Goodfield M. Basement membrane changes in lichen planopilaris. J Eur Acad Dermatol Venereol 2009;23(11):1289–93.

6. Tosti A, Duque-Estrada B, Murrell DF. Alopecia in epidermolysis bullosa. Dermatol Clin 2010;28(1):165–9.

7. Olivry T, Jackson HA. An alopecic phenotype of canine pemphigus vulgaris? Br J Dermatol 2001; 145(1):176–8.

8. Zabel S, Mueller RS, Fieseler KV, et al. Review of 15 cases of pemphigus foliaceus in horses and a survey of the literature. Vet Rec 2005;157(17):505–9.

9. Ganeshan R, Chen J, Koch PJ. Mouse models for blistering skin disorders. Dermatol Res Pract 2010; 2010:584353.

10. Koch PJ, Mahoney MG, Cotsarelis G, et al. Desmoglein 3 anchors telogen hair in the follicle. J Cell Sci 1998;111(Pt 17):2529–37.

11. Montagutelli X, Lalouette A, Boulouis HJ, et al. Vesicle formation and follicular root sheath separation in mice homozygous for deleterious alleles at the balding (bal) locus. J Invest Dermatol 1997; 109(3):324–8.

12. Ishikawa H, Silos SA, Tamai K, et al. cDNA cloning and chromosomal assignment of the mouse gene for desmoglein 3 (Dsg3), the pemphigus vulgaris antigen. Mamm Genome 1994;5(12):803–4.

13. Schaerer L, Trueb RM. Direct immunofluorescence of plucked hair in pemphigus. Arch Dermatol 2003; 139(2):228–9.

14. Daneshpazhooh M, Asgari M, Naraghi ZS, et al. A study on plucked hair as a substrate for direct immunofluorescence in pemphigus vulgaris. J Eur Acad Dermatol Venereol 2009;23(2):129–31.

15. Delmonte S, Semino MT, Parodi A, et al. Normal anagen effluvium: a sign of pemphigus vulgaris. Br J Dermatol 2000;142(6):1244–5.

16. Wilson CL, Dean D, Wojnarowska F. Pemphigus and the terminal hair follicle. J Cutan Pathol 1991;18(6): 428–31.

17. Saijyo S, Tagami H. Tufted hair folliculitis developing in a recalcitrant lesion of pemphigus vulgaris. J Am Acad Dermatol 1998;38(5 Pt 2):857–9.

18. Jappe U, Schroder K, Zillikens D, et al. Tufted hair folliculitis associated with pemphigus vulgaris. J Eur Acad Dermatol Venereol 2003;17(2):223–6.

19. Petronic-Rosic V, Krunic A, Mijuskovic M, et al. Tufted hair folliculitis: a pattern of scarring alopecia? J Am Acad Dermatol 1999;41(1):112–4.

20. Danopoulou I, Stavropoulos P, Stratigos A, et al. Pemphigus vegetans confined to the scalp. Int J Dermatol 2006;45(8):1008–9.

21. Rackett SC, Rothe MJ, Hoss DM, et al. Treatment-resistant pemphigus vegetans of the scalp. Int J Dermatol 1995;34(12):865–6.

22. Mlynek A, Bar M, Bauer A, et al. Juvenile pemphigus foliaceus associated with severe nonscarring alopecia. Br J Dermatol 2009;161(2):472–4.

23. Rosin MA. Alopecia areata and pemphigus foliaceus. J Am Acad Dermatol 1985;12(5 Pt 1):895–6.

24. Brunsting LA, Perry HO. Benign pemphigold: a report of seven cases with chronic, scarring, herpetiform plaques about the head and neck. AMA Arch Derm 1957;75(4):489–501.

25. Ahmed AR, Kurgis BS, Rogers RS 3rd. Cicatricial pemphigoid. J Am Acad Dermatol 1991;24(6 Pt 1):987–1001.

26. Martin JM, Pinazo I, Molina I, et al. Cicatricial pemphigoid of the Brunsting-Perry type. Int J Dermatol 2009;48(3):293–4.

27. Iwata H, Aoyama Y, Esaki C, et al. Cicatricial pemphigoid with prominent alopecia. Eur J Dermatol 2007;17(4):338–9.

28. Elston GE, Harman KE. Recurrent blistering of the scalp with scarring. Clin Exp Dermatol 2006;31(4):605–6.

29. Kurzhals G, Stolz W, Maciejewski W, et al. Localized cicatricial pemphigoid of the Brunsting-Perry type with transition into disseminated cicatricial pemphigoid. Report of a case proved by preembedding immunogold electron microscopy. Arch Dermatol 1995;131(5):580–5.

30. Baldwin H, Lynfield Y. Brunsting-Perry cicatricial pemphigoid precipitated by trauma. Arch Dermatol 1991;127(6):911–2.

31. Ball S, Walkden V, Wojnarowska F. Cicatricial pemphigoid rarely involves the scalp. Australas J Dermatol 1998;39(4):258–60.

32. Bairstow B. Cicatricial pemphigoid. Arch Dermatol 1971;104(4):454–5.

33. Westgate GE, Craggs RI, Gibson WT. Immune privilege in hair growth. J Invest Dermatol 1991;97(3):417–20.

34. Olivry T, Dunston SM, Schachter M, et al. A spontaneous canine model of mucous membrane (cicatricial) pemphigoid, an autoimmune blistering disease affecting mucosae and mucocutaneous junctions. J Autoimmun 2001;16(4):411–21.

35. Finner A, Shapiro J. Scarring alopecia. In: Blume-Peytavi U, Tosti A, Whiting DA, Trueb R, editors. Hair growths and disorders. Berlin: Springer-Verlag; 2008. p. 227–53.

36. Shipman AR, Agero AL, Cook I, et al. Epidermolysis bullosa acquisita requiring multiple oesophageal dilatations. Clin Exp Dermatol 2008;33(6):787–9.

37. Barton DD, Fine JD, Gammon WR, et al. Bullous systemic lupus erythematosus: an unusual clinical course and detectable circulating autoantibodies to the epidermolysis bullosa acquisita antigen. J Am Acad Dermatol 1986;15(2 Pt 2):369–73.

38. Gammon WR, Murrell DF, Jenison MW, et al. Autoantibodies to type VII collagen recognize epitopes in a fibronectin-like region of the noncollagenous (NC1) domain. J Invest Dermatol 1993;100(5):618–22.

39. Bjornberg A, Hellgren L. Dermatitis herpetiformis. A laboratory and clinical investigation based on a numerical study of 53 patients and matched controls. Dermatologica 1962;125:205–25.

40. Dawber R. Diseases involving the scalp. In: Dwaber R, de Berker D, editors. Diseases of the hair and scalp. Oxford (UK): Blackwell Science; 1997. p. 523.

41. Madan V, Gupta U, Gupta DK. Dermatisis herpetiformis and alopecia areata. A rare association in two sisters. Indian J Dermatol Venereol Leprol 2003;69(1):46–7.

42. Corazza GR, Andreani ML, Venturo N, et al. Celiac disease and alopecia areata: report of a new association. Gastroenterology 1995;109(4):1333–7.

# Nail Involvement in Autoimmune Bullous Disorders

Antonella Tosti, MD[a],*, Marisa André, MD[b],
Dédée F. Murrell, MA, BMBCh, FAAD, MD, FACD[c]

**KEYWORDS**

- Pemphigus vulgaris • Paronychia • Onychomadesis
- Onycholysis • Bullous pemphigoid • Pterygium

## IMMUNOLOGIC CHARACTERISTICS OF THE NAIL APPARATUS

Sinclair and colleagues[1] showed that staining with the epidermal hemidesmosome antigens BP230 kDa, BP180 kDa, and monoclonal antibodies to individual $\alpha6$ and $\beta4$ chains of $\alpha6$ $\beta4$ integrin did not differ in the nail apparatus from normal skin. The lamina lucida and the dermal proteins were also normally expressed in the same distribution as the ubiquitous basal membrane zone (BMZ) antigens, including type IV collagen and laminin 332. All the BMZ antigens and components are also normally expressed in the proximal nail fold, nail matrix, and hyponychium. The desmosomal antigens in this compartment include desmogleins 1 and 3 as in the skin, but the keratin differentiating factors are different.

The normal human nail immune system is very similar to the hair follicle immune system, including a known area of relative "immune privilege" in the proximal nail matrix, which can constitute a safeguard against autoimmunity. Distribution and functional markers of acquired and innate cutaneous immunology differ between the human skin immune system (number and function of antigen-presenting cells are substantially lower in the nail immune system than in the epidermis, with a down-regulation of major histocompatibility complex class II and CD209 expression by Langerhans cells in the proximal nail matrix); natural killer and mast cells are reduced or have diminished function around the human nail apparatus.[2]

## NAIL INVOLVEMENT IN PEMPHIGUS VULGARIS

Patients with pemphigus vulgaris (PV) may present with nail abnormalities, which occasionally can precede skin findings. Nail lesions often relapse just before generalized disease exacerbation or recurrence. Severe nail changes are often associated with extensive and severe disease.[3,4] Nail involvement was previously believed to be rare[3,5–11]; however, the most recent PV prospective study involving 79 patients found that 34.2% had nail changes.[12,13] Patients with a longer duration of disease and accumulated inflammation are more likely to present with nail changes. Fingernails are more commonly affected, especially the first three,[6,9–12,14,15] possibly because of more local trauma associated with greater activity of these fingers (**Fig. 1**). The most common manifestation of PV is paronychia, which can be followed by onychomadesis.[11,14,16] However, severe nail dystrophy, discoloration of the nail plate, and even occasionally destruction of the nail plate

Funding Sources: None.
[a] Department of Dermatology and Cutaneous Surgery, Miller School of Medicine, University of Miami, 1600 NW, 10th Avenue, RMSB, Room 2023-A, Miami, FL 33136, USA
[b] Clínica Universitária de Dermatologia, Hospital de Santa Maria, Centro Hospitalar Lisboa Norte, Avenue, Prof. Egas Moniz, 1649-035 Lisbon, Portugal
[c] Department of Dermatology, St George Hospital, University of New South Wales, Gray Street, Kogarah, Sydney, NSW 2217, Australia
* Corresponding author.
*E-mail address:* atosti@med.miami.edu

Dermatol Clin 29 (2011) 511–513
doi:10.1016/j.det.2011.03.006

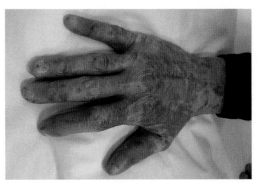

**Fig. 1.** Epidermolysis bullosa acquisita and nail loss and dystrophy.

can occur.[5] A report in the literature associates hemorrhagic nail abnormalities with poor prognosis in patients with PV.[13]

## Paronychia

Depending on the location of acantholysis in the nail folds, different nail changes may result.

When the dorsal nail folds are affected, patients present with acute periungual inflammation and bullous lesions, which may be hemorrhagic. When the ventral nail fold is affected, bullae are not visible and the clinical manifestations are indistinguishable from chronic paronychia. The affected nail shows periungual erythema and swelling, with loss of the cuticle, exudation, and crusting around the nail fold. Secondary colonization with bacteria and yeasts may occur.

## Onychomadesis/Beau lines

The periungual inflammation can affect matrix keratinization and result in Beau's lines or nail shedding (onychomadesis).[10,17,18] Habibi and colleagues[16] reported these signs in one-third of patients with nail changes caused by PV. Nail matrix damage can also cause nail plate surface abnormalities, such as onychoschizia, cross-ridging, pitting, and trachonychia.

## Onycholysis

Subungual bullae cause nail bed detachment with onycholysis, which is often hemorrhagic. Subungual hemorrhages and subungual hyperkeratosis[15,16] have also been described. In one unusual report, a patient with PV had vegetative verrucous lesions on the periphery of fingernails and digits (mimicking warts) and bullous and vegetating lesions on both feet, with nail plate destruction of two toenails.[19]

Onychomycosis is reported in 25% of patients with PV, with increased prevalence among patients undergoing immunosuppressive therapy.[5,11,19]

## Diagnosis

The easiest and most painless method of diagnosing PV of the nail is to obtain a biopsy specimen from perilesional skin of the proximal nail fold and perform direct immunofluorescence testing. A positive result will reveal intercellular fluorescence with IgG immunoglobulins and C3. Tzanck tests are difficult to obtain from the ventral nail fold but are very useful in cases of periungual or subungual bullae.[6] Paronychia from PV exacerbation is important to distinguish from other similar clinical presentations, such as acute paronychia from viral (namely herpes simplex infection), bacterial infection, or chronic paronychia. Paronychia in PV has a specific histopathologic feature: suprabasal acantholysis without spongiosis or exocytosis. Bacterial and fungal cultures to exclude superinfection should be performed.

## Treatment

Nail PV responds to systemic therapy similarly to other dermatologic manifestations, although it may take longer to resolve. Sometimes, when colonization or superinfection occurs, an associated topical treatment might be helpful.

## Nail Disorders and Pemphigoid Group

Nail involvement in bullous pemphigoid is not common and, in most reports, was not confirmed by a nail biopsy.[20–23] The changes in the nails are thought to be from an immunologic reaction with anti–bullous pemphigoid antigen.[20]

Most commonly bullous pemphigoid affects the nail folds, but the nail bed or matrix can also be involved; the location of the blistering in the different constituents of the nail apparatus will determine the different nail signs (see **Fig. 1**). Paronychia and onychomadesis can occur, as in PV.[22] Nail scarring with atrophy or even permanent loss of the nails has been reported in several cases.[20–22]

Pterygium of the fingernails has been described in a few patients with cicatricial pemphigoid.[23,24]

## NAIL INVOLVEMENT IN OTHER BULLOUS AUTOIMMUNE DISEASES

The circulating IgG autoantibodies in epidermolysis bullosa acquisita (EBA) react with a type VII collagen (290-kDa dermal protein), which is the main constituent of anchoring fibrils located at the dermal–epidermal junction, an adhesion molecule of the extracellular matrix in epithelial basement membranes. The literature contains two case reports of EBA with dystrophic fingernails and toenails, and even nail loss (see **Fig. 1**); both patients had extremity involvement.[24] Patients with EBA may have blisters, erosions, milia formation (result from scarring), nail fragility,[20] and dystrophic nail plates. In one report a patient had a severe 9-year evolution EBA with mutilating acral involvement, syndactyly, complete nail loss, and extensive scarring lesions on the scalp. This patient had circulating IgG autoantibodies to type VII collagen at a much higher titer than those typically found in other individuals with EBA.[25,26] The 290-kDa protein ($\alpha$-chain of type VII collagen) can be detected with circulating autoantibodies using an immunoblotting assay.[27]

## REFERENCES

1. Sinclair RD, Wojnarowska F, Leigh IM, et al. The basement membrane zone of the nail. Br J Dermatol 1994;131:499–505.

2. Ito T, Ito N, Saathoff M, et al. Immunology of the human nail apparatus: the nail matrix is a site of relative immune privilege. J Invest Dermatol 2005;125:1139–48.

3. Schlesinger N, Katz M, Ingber A. Nail involvement in pemphigus vulgaris. Br J Dermatol 2002;146:836–9.

4. Diaz RR, Llamazares JA, Rodriguez-Peralto JL, et al. Nail involvement in pemphigus vulgaris. Int J Dermatol 1996;35(8):581–2.

5. Engineer L, Norton LA, Ahmed R. Nail involvement in pemphigus vulgaris. J Am Acad Dermatol 2000;43: 529–35.

6. Ptsatsi A, Sotiriou E, Devliotiou-Panagiotidou D, et al. Pemphigus vulgaris affecting 19 nails. Clin Exp Dermatol 2008;34:204–5.

7. Kim BS, Song KY, Youn JL, et al. Paronychia- a manifestation of pemphigus vulgaris. Clin Exp Dermatol 1996;21:315–7.

8. Baumal A, Robinson MJ. Nail bed involvement in pemphigus vulgaris. Arch Dermatol 1973;107:751.

9. Kolivras A, Gheeraert P, André J. Nail destruction in pemphigus vulgaris. Dermatology 2003;206:351–2.

10. Apalla Z, Chaidemenos G, Karakatsanis G. Nail unit involvement during severe initial pemphigus vulgaris development. Eur J Dermatol 2009;19(3):290–1.

11. Carducci M, Calcaterra R, Franco G, et al. Nail involvement in pemphigus vulgaris. Acta Derm Venereol 2008;88:58–9.

12. Serratus BD, Rashid R. Nail disease in pemphigus vulgaris. Dermatol Online J 2009;15(7):2.

13. Reich A, Wisnicka B, Szepietowski JC. Haemorrhagic nails in pemphigus vulgaris. Acta Derm Venereol 2008;88:542.

14. Cahali JB, Kakuda EY, Santi CG, et al. Nail manifestations in pemphigus vulgaris. Rev Hosp Clin Fac Med Sao Paulo 2002;57(5):229–34.

15. Dhawan S, Zaias N, Pena J. The nail fold in pemphigus vulgaris. Arch Dermatol 1990;126:1374–5.

16. Habibi M, Mortazavi H, Shadianloo S, et al. Nail changes in pemphigus vulgaris. Int J Dermatol 2008;47:1141–4.

17. Berker DD, Dalziel K, Dawber RP, et al. Pemphigus associated with nail dystrophy. Br J Dermatol 1993;129:461–4.

18. James D, Yancey KB. Passive transfer of autoantibodies from a patient with mutilating epidermolysis bullosa acquisita induces specific alterations in the skin of neonatal mice. Arch Dermatol 1995;131: 590–5.

19. Mascarenhas R, Fernandes B, Reis JP, et al. Pemphigus vulgaris with nail involvement presenting with vegetating and verrucous lesions. Dermatol Online J 2003;9(5):14.

20. Namba Y, Koizumi H, Kumakiri M, et al. Bullous pemphigoid with permanent loss of the nails. Acta Derm Venereol 1999;79:480–1.

21. Gualco F, Cozzani E, Parodi A. Bullous pemphigoid with nail loss. Int J Dermatol 2005;44:967–8.

22. Tomita M, Tanei R, Hamada Y, et al. A case of localized pemphigoid with loss of toenails. Dermatology 2002;204:155.

23. Barth JH, Wojnarowska F, Millard PR, et al. Immunofluorescence of the nail bed in pemphigoid. Am J Dermatopathol 1987;9(4):349–50.

24. Burge SM, Powell SM, Ryan TJ. Cicatricial pemphigoid with nail dystrophy. Clin Exp Dermatol 1985; 10:472–5.

25. Borradori L, Caldwell JB, Briggaman RA, et al. Passive transfer of autoantibodies from a patient with mutilating epidermolysis bullosa acquisita induces specific alterations in the skin of neonatal mice. Arch Dermatol 1995;131:590–5.

26. Yeh SW, Ahmed B, Sami N, et al. Blistering disorders: diagnosis and treatment. Dermatol Ther 2003;16:214–23.

27. Baran R, Juhlin L. Photoonycholysis. Photodermatol Photoimmunol Photomed 2002;18:202–7.

# Objective Scoring Systems for Disease Activity in Autoimmune Bullous Disease

Deshan F. Sebaratnam, MBBS (Hons)[a,b],
Dédée F. Murrell, MA, BMBCh, FAAD, MD, FACD[c],*

**KEYWORDS**

- Autoimmune bullous disease • Pemphigus
- Objective scoring systems • PDAI • ABSIS

Autoimmune bullous disease (AIBD) encompasses a range of rare dermatoses such as pemphigus and bullous pemphigoid characterized by the development of autoantibodies directed against keratinocyte epitopes. The clinical presentation of AIBD is heterogeneous, but all manifest by the formation of bullae and erosions. Due the rarity of these diseases, there is a paucity of studies in the literature guiding clinicians in the optimal evidence-based management of AIBD.[1] A recent systematic review of outcome measures in pemphigus over the past 25 years identified 116 different measures across 96 articles.[2] Most studies employ outcome measures based on non-validated subjective or nonspecific ratings of disease activity and, because of the variety of measures employed (including lesion counts, complete healing of lesions, duration of remission, number of recurrences, etc), a significant obstacle in comparing therapeutic modalities is the absence of uniform outcome measures across studies for correlation. This is particularly relevant because of the rarity of AIBD, which means that studies often have lower patient numbers with

meta-analysis combing studies only possible if uniform outcome measures are available. A number of scoring systems have been developed in recent years in an attempt to provide an objective measure to assess disease activity in AIBD. Such measures function alongside the clinical assessment of patients, allowing objective assessment of disease activity in a patient and the monitoring of disease trajectory over time. These measures can also be used as outcome measures in clinical trials to quantify the effectiveness of clinical intervention.

One of the earliest disease activity scores employed was the Pemphigus Area and Activity Score (PAAS).[3] The PAAS divides the body into four divisions (head, trunk, upper limbs, and lower limbs). Each division is assigned a score based on the number of new blisters, extension of existing blisters, and the presence of the Nikolsky sign; then multiplied by the area involved and an index, with the four scores then totaled. Patients with mucosal involvement are also assigned a mucous membrane score by adding the number of mucosal sites involved to a severity score to

Conflict of interest: The senior author is part of the International Pemphigus and Pemphigoid Consensus Group.
<sup>a</sup> Department of Dermatology, St George Hospital, Grey Street, Kogarah, Sydney, NSW 2217, Australia
<sup>b</sup> Faculty of Medicine, University of New South Wales, Kensington, Sydney, NSW 2052, Australia
<sup>c</sup> Department of Dermatology, St George Hospital, University of New South Wales, Gray Street, Kogarah, Sydney, NSW 2217, Australia
* Corresponding author.
*E-mail address:* d.murrell@unsw.edu.au

ascertain a mucous membrane score. As one of the earliest scoring systems, the PAAS was one of the first objective tools to be employed in the setting of AIBD. It has the advantage of scoring cutaneous and mucosal lesions separately. Additionally, it employed the Nikolsky sign, which is a sensitive but not necessarily specific marker of disease activity. However, the system was limited by the fact that scores were weighted heavily by the area of skin involvement and the inability to detect small changes in disease activity. Furthermore, the tool was not truly objective as severity was assessed with variables graded "mild," "moderate," and "severe" dependent on the user's discretion. Last, lesion counting is notoriously inaccurate when there are a high number of lesions assessed by intra-rater and inter-rater validity studies, and such studies were not performed on this system.

Another scoring system employed in a study reviewing the incidence of remission in pemphigus patients graded disease activity on a score from 0 to 10.[4] Extent was scored from 0 to 4 depending on whether predefined areas of the body were affected and therapy was scored from 0 to 6 depending on the dose of oral corticosteroid and the need of adjuvant immunosuppression. Although this system had the advantage of considering therapeutic data, this was also overrepresented in its use as a proxy for disease activity with clinical information only reviewed superficially and the scoring system never validated.

Another study investigating the correlation between antibody titers and clinical severity in pemphigus used a simple arbitrary scale of 0 to 3 to assess cutaneous and oral lesions.[5] Skin lesions were graded as quiescent (no lesions), mild (<5 discrete lesions), moderate (6–19 discrete lesions), or severe (>20 lesions or extensive confluent erosions). Oral lesions were graded as quiescent (no lesions), mild ($\leq$3 erosions), moderate (4–9 erosions or general desquamative gingivitis), or severe ($\geq$10 lesions or extensive, confluent erosions or generalized desquamative gingivitis with discrete erosions at other sites). This simple tool allows an expedient and objective assessment of disease activity but not with the sensitivity required to effectively detect changes in disease status. More importantly, it relies on the number of blisters present, rather than the size of each blister, the area involved, or the severity of the lesions. Again, no independent validity assessments of this score were performed.

A retrospective case series of pemphigus patients stratified disease severity into four categories based on body surface area (BSA) involvement and functional impairment.[6] Patients were classified as having mild disease ($\leq$10% BSA involvement or disease limited to oral mucosa, ability to carry out activities of daily living [ADL] without discomfort), moderate (10%–25% BSA involvement, able to carry out ADL with discomfort), severe (25%–50% BSA involvement and oral involvement, unable to carry out ADL), or extensive (>50% BSA involvement with mucosal involvement, bedridden or has complications). Whereas this was useful for a gross assessment of disease severity, much like earlier scoring systems,[5] the categories are obviously too broad to accurately detect changes to pemphigus activity and were not constructed with this aim. Furthermore, disease extent was combined with a functional scale and the two variables did not necessarily correlate.

A novel approach to assessing disease activity in oral pemphigus was devised by Saraswat and Kumar.[7] The scoring system is divided into two parts: assessing the extent of disease and the consequent functional impairment. Eleven sites in the oral cavity (the upper and lower labial mucosa, upper and lower gingival mucosa, left and right buccal mucosa, dorsal and ventral lingual mucosa, hard and soft palate, and uvula) are assigned a score of 0 or 1 depending on the presence or absence of lesions, regardless of severity. A functional assessment is determined using a modified version of the validated grading system employed in gastroenterology,[8] which utilizes information relating to the frequency of pain and bleeding with nine different food groups to evaluate functional impairment. The investigators put forward that, because oral lesions tend to coalesce, lesion counts are not a valid measure in this setting. Additionally, patients can show an improvement in odynophagia and their ability to eat solids without gross changes to lesion appearance and so a consideration of function is warranted. Obviously, this tool is constrained by the fact that it is limited to oral lesions and of little utility to patients without oral involvement; nevertheless, it paved the way for future validated scoring systems.

Part of the difficulty in devising an objective scoring system for AIBD is the clinical heterogeneity amongst the blistering dermatoses. A tool needs to be general enough to capture the areas predominating in each blistering disease but specific enough to identify changes in a given patient's disease activity. The Autoimmune Bullous Skin Disorder Intensity Score (ABSIS) was devised by Eming and Hertl in Germany, with the aim of developing a scoring system sensitive enough to capture such changes in disease activity in AIBD.[9] Scoring is based on the extent of BSA involved and the quality of the skin lesions. The extent of BSA affected is estimated using the "rule of nines" in which defined areas of the body are equivalent to 9% or multiples of 9%. This value is then multiplied by an index reflecting the most dominant lesion present: 1.5 (erosive, exudative lesions, bullae, or Nikolsky sign positivity), 1.0 (erosive, dry lesions), or 0.5 (reepithelialized lesions) (**Fig. 1**). Oral involvement is evaluated using a modified version of the grading system employed by Saraswat and Kumar.[7] These results are tabulated to give a total score ranging from 0 to 206: 150 for skin involvement, 11 for oral involvement, and 45 for oral functional impairment. The

Date:

Patient's weight (kg):

| Legend for weighting factor (most dominant appearance of skin lesions): | |
|---|---|
| 1.5 | Erosive, exudative lesions |
| 1 | Erosive, dry lesions |
| 0.5 | Reepithelialized lesions |

| Skin Involvement (Max BSA) | Patient's BSA | Weighting factor |
|---|---|---|
| Head & neck (9%): | | |
| L Arm including hand (9%): | | |
| R Arm including hand (9%) | | |
| Trunk (front & back) (36%): | | |
| L Leg (18%): | | |
| R Leg (18%): | | |
| Genitals (1%): | | |

(Skin involvement total score: % BSA x weighting factor = 0-150 points)

Oral Involvement:

   I.    Extent (enter 1 for presence of lesions, 0 absence of any lesion):

| Upper gingival mucosa | | Tongue | |
|---|---|---|---|
| Lower gingival mucosa | | Floor of the mouth | |
| Upper lip mucosa | | Hard palate | |
| Lower lip mucosa | | Soft palate | |
| Left buccal mucosa | | Pharynx | |
| Right buccal mucosa | | | |

(Total score ranges from 0-11)

Severity (discomfort during eating/drinking)

| Food | Level | Factor of Discomfort | Severity score |
|---|---|---|---|
| Water | 1 | | |
| Soup | 2 | | |
| Yogurt | 3 | | |
| Custard | 4 | | |
| Mashed potatoes/ scrambled egg | 5 | | |
| Baked fish | 6 | | |
| White bread | 7 | | |
| Apple/ raw carrot | 8 | | |
| Fried steak/ whole-grain bread | 9 | | |

(Severity score = Level multiplied by the factor of discomfort = 0-45 points)

| Legend for factor of discomfort | |
|---|---|
| 1 | Pain/bleeding occurred always |
| 0.5 | Pain/bleeding occurred sometimes |
| 0 | Never experienced problems |

**Fig. 1.** ABSIS Scoring Sheet. (*Reprinted from* Rosenbach M, Murrell D, Bystryn JC, et al. Reliability and convergent validity of two outcome instruments for pemphigus. J Invest Dermatol 2009;129(10):2404–10; with permission.)

ABSIS score has had two validity studies performed on it.[10,11]

The Pemphigus Disease Area Index (PDAI) was developed by international consensus by the International Pemphigus Definitions Committee, led by Victoria Werth and Dédée Murrell, over a 3-year period as a measure to objectively assess bullous disease activity.[12] The skin and scalp are

### Skin

| Anatomical Location | Activity — Erosion/Blisters or new erythema | Number of lesions if ≤3 | Damage — Post-inflammatory hyperpigmentation or erythema from resolving lesion |
|---|---|---|---|
| | **0** absent<br>**1** 1-3 lesions, up to one >2 cm diameter, none > 6<br>**2** 2-3 lesions, at least two > 2 cm diameter, none > 6cm<br>**3** >3 lesions, none > 6 cm diameter<br>**5** >3 lesions, and/or at least one >6 cm diameter<br>**10** >3 lesions, and/or at least one lesion >16 cm diameter or entire area | | **0** absent<br>**1** present |
| Ears | | | |
| Nose | | | |
| Rest of the face | | | |
| Neck | | | |
| Chest | | | |
| Abdomen | | | |
| Back, buttocks | | | |
| Arms | | | |
| Hands | | | |
| Legs | | | |
| Feet | | | |
| Genitals | | | |
| **Total skin** | /120 | | /12 |

### Scalp

| Scalp | Erosion/Blisters or new erythema | Number of lesions if ≤3 | Post-inflammatory hyperpigmentation or erythema from resolving lesion |
|---|---|---|---|
| | **0** absent<br>**1** in one quadrant<br>**2** two quadrants<br>**3** three quadrants<br>**4** affects whole skull<br>**10** at least one lesion > 6 cm | | **0** absent<br>**1** present |
| **Total Scalp** | /10 | | /1 |

### Mucous Membrane

| Anatomical Location | Erosion/Blisters | Number of lesions if ≤3 |
|---|---|---|
| | **0** absent<br>**1** 1 lesion<br>**2** 2-3 lesions<br>**5** >3 lesions or 2 lesions >2 cm<br>**10** entire area | |
| Eyes | | |
| Nose | | |
| Buccal mucosa | | |
| Hard palate | | |
| Soft palate | | |
| Upper gingiva | | |
| Lower gingiva | | |
| Tongue | | |
| Floor of mouth | | |
| Labial bucosa | | |
| Posterior pharynx | | |
| Anogenital | | |
| **Total Mucosa** | /120 | |

**Total Activity Score:** [　　　]          **Total Damage Score:** [　　　]

**Fig. 2.** Pemphigus Disease Area Index (PDAI). (*Reprinted from* Rosenbach M, Murrell D, Bystryn JC, et al. Reliability and convergent validity of two outcome instruments for pemphigus. J Invest Dermatol 2009;129(10): 2404–10; with permission.)

assessed for disease extent and damage and the oral mucosa is assessed for extent alone (**Fig. 2**). In the skin assessment, 12 anatomic sites (ears, nose, face, neck, chest, abdomen, back and buttocks, arms, hands, legs, feet, genitals) are reviewed and assigned a score according to disease extent: 0 (no lesions), 1 (1–3 lesions, all ≤6 cm, up to 1 >2 cm), 2 (2–3 lesions, all ≤6 cm, at least 2 lesions >2 cm), 3 (>3 lesions, all ≤6 cm), 5 (>3 lesions and/or 1 lesion >6 cm), or 10 (>3 lesions and/or at least one lesion >16 cm). When a score of 1 or 2 is given, a lesion count is also incorporated with a score of 1 given if one lesion is present, 1.3 for two lesions and 1.6 for three lesions. The twelve sites are also reviewed for the presence of post-inflammatory hyperpigmentation or erythema from resolving lesions and assigned a score of 0 (absent) or 1 (present) to assess damage. Damage scores are not included in the overall extent score – they are there to remind graders that not all visible lesions represent activity. The scalp is assigned a score based on the presence of bullae, erosions, or new erythema of 0 (no activity), 1 (one quadrant affected), 2 (two quadrants affected), 3 (three quadrants affected), 4 (whole scalp affected), or 10 (at least one lesion >6 cm). A damage score of 0 or 1 is given to the entire scalp based on the presence of features previously described for the skin damage score. Mucosal activity is assessed by reviewing 12 mucosal sites (eyes, nose, buccal, hard palate, soft palate, upper gingiva, lower gingiva, tongue, floor of mouth, labial mucosa, posterior pharynx, anogenitalia) and assigning a score based on the presence of erosions and blisters: 0 (absent), 1 (1 lesion), 2 (2–3 lesions), 5 (>3 lesions or 2 lesions >2 cm), or 10 (entire area). The total possible score for the PDAI ranges from 0 to 130 for the skin score (120 points for body, 10 points for scalp) and up to 120 points for mucosal activity; with 13 points for damage. These are not combined. Validation studies, both in person and by photovalidation, have been conducted for the PDAI.[10,11]

A recent study compared the ABSIS and PDAI to evaluate the interrater and intrarater reliability of the two instruments.[10] Ten dermatologists travelled to the University of Pennsylvania and evaluated 15 pemphigus patients using the ABSIS, PDAI, and the Physician's Global Assessment (PGA)—a ten point visual analog scale which was used to evaluate convergent validity given no gold standard exists to measure disease activity. Physicians and patients were divided into two groups with half the physicians scoring patients with the ABSIS first, then the PDAI and PGA, with the order reversed in the second group. Each physician returned to the original group 2 hours

later and re-rated two randomly assigned patients. The patients evaluated had mild-moderate disease with the highest patient score less than 25% of the maximum score for both the PDAI and the ABSIS. Both instruments demonstrated validity when compared with the PGA with a correlation of 0.60 (0.49–0.71) for the PDAI and 0.43 (0.30–0.55) for the ABSIS. Interrater reliability had an overall intraclass correlation coefficient (ICC) of 0.76 (0.61–0.91) for the PDAI, 0.77 (0.63–0.91) for the ABSIS, and 0.44 (0.22–0.65) for the PGA. Accordingly, the ABSIS was slightly better in terms of reliability of scores between physicians. However, for skin activity, the PDAI activity score had an ICC of 0.86 and the ABSIS 0.39, suggesting that the PDAI might be better at detecting differences in cutaneous disease. Intrarater reliability was 0.98 (0.96–1.0) for the PDAI, 0.80 (0.65–0.96) for the ABSIS, and 0.75 (0.55–0.94) for the PGA—indicating that PDAI scores were more reproducible. One of the limitations of the study was that the patients evaluated all had mild disease, so these results may not be relevant to patients with a more significant burden of disease. However, the results from the study indicate that the PDAI demonstrates reasonable convergent validity and is a more reliable measure to assess bullous disease activity. Led by Pascal Joly and Michael Hertl, these two scoring systems are currently being prospectively evaluated in relation to acutely presenting pemphigus patients in European centers (predominantly) to observe how they correlate in the more extensive setting.

## SUMMARY

Objectively evaluating disease activity in AIBD is important in terms of the clinical assessment of patients and as an outcome measure for clinical trials. Measures need to be general enough to capture the specific issues for the differing bullous dermatoses but specific enough to capture any changes to disease status for a patient. Different tools have been put forward over the last 15 years, but presently the PDAI and ABSIS seem to be the most promising tools to assess disease activity in AIBD. Further studies need to be performed to validate such measures. Correlations with autoantibody titers and quality of life instruments are possible avenues for the future. Work has already been done to make these tools easier to use clinically, such as the development of a software program by Hertl's group to facilitate electronic completion of the PDAI and ABSIS and software to capture these scores and convert these into decision making tools for clinicians.[13] The assessment of disease activity in AIBD will continue to be an important area of research in the future, as it will function as the cornerstone for future clinical trials to help physicians decide the best evidence-based approach to management in this setting.

## REFERENCES

1. Martin L, Murrell D. Treatment of pemphigus: the need for more evidence. Arch Dermatol 2008;144(1):100–1.
2. Martin L, Murrell D. Measuring the immeasurable: a systematic review of outcome measures in pemphigus. Australas J Dermatol 2006;47(Suppl 1):A32–3.
3. Agarwal M, Walia R, Kochhar AM, et al. Pemphigus Area and Activity Score (PAAS)—a novel clinical scoring method for monitoring of pemphigus vulgaris patient. Int J Dermatol 1998;37(2):158–9.
4. Herbst A, Bystryn JC. Patterns of remission in pemphigus vulgaris. J Am Acad Dermatol 2000; 42(3):422–7.
5. Harman KE, Seed PT, Gratian MJ, et al. The severity of cutaneous and oral pemphigus is related to desmoglein 1 and 3 antibody levels. Br J Dermatol 2001;144(4):775–80.
6. Mahanjan VK, Sharma NL, Sharma RC, et al. Twelve-year clinico-therapeutic experience in pemphigus: a retrospective study of 54 cases. Int J Dermatol 2005;44(10):821–7.
7. Saraswat A, Kumar B. A new grading system for oral pemphigus. Int J Dermatol 2003;42(5):413–4.
8. Dakkak M, Bennet JR. A new dysphagia score with objective validation. J Clin Gastroenterol 1992; 14(2):99–100.
9. Pfutze M, Niedermeier A, Hertl M, et al. Introducing a novel Autoimmune Bullous Skin Disorder Intensity Score (ABSIS) in pemphigus. Eur J Dermatol 2007; 17(1):4–11.
10. Rosenbach M, Murrell D, Bystryn JC, et al. Reliability and convergent validity of two outcome instruments for pemphigus. J Invest Dermatol 2009;129(10): 2404–10.
11. Lin J, Marinovic B, Fiveson D, et al. Photovalidation for two outcome instruments for pemphigus. In: Programs and abstracts of the JC Bystryn Pemphigus and Pemphigoid Meeting: from the bench to the bedside. Maryland; 2010.
12. Murrell D, Dick S, Ahmed A. Consensus statement on definitions of disease, end points, and therapeutic response for pemphigus. J Am Acad Dermatol 2008;58(6):1043–6.
13. Sebaratnam D, Venugopal S, Murrell D. The development of an Excel program to compare disease-specific instruments for assessing activity and the extent of autoimmune bullous disease. Australas J Dermatol 2009;50(Suppl 2):A48.

# Pemphigus and Quality of Life

Shien-Ning Chee, MBBS,
Dédée F. Murrell, MA, BMBCh, FAAD, MD, FACD*

**KEYWORDS**

- Pemphigus • Quality of life • Skin • Autoimmune condition

Skin diseases are rarely life threatening, but their impact on a patient's quality of life (QOL) can be massive. For example, the impact of psoriasis on QOL has been found to be comparable with the impact of heart failure.[1] Contributing factors include physical discomfort, time spent on treatment, staining of sheets and clothes with skin scales or blood, and the visible nature of skin diseases, which often brings negative reactions from the public, thus diminishing self-esteem.[2]

Measurement of the impact of disease on QOL is of utmost importance in dermatology and interest in the area has been recently growing.[1] QOL is increasingly recognized as an important outcome for evaluating effectiveness of care, capturing aspects of patients' health status that are important for the patient, but may not correlate with clinical severity as assessed by physicians.[3]

Pemphigus is a skin disease on which few QOL studies have been conducted, and for which a disease-specific QOL questionnaire has not yet been developed.

## ABOUT PEMPHIGUS

Pemphigus is a group of autoimmune blistering diseases characterized by loss of adhesion between keratinocytes giving rise to blister formation. The intraepithelial blister formation is caused by acantholysis: the loss of adhesion between keratinocytes caused by autoantibodies directed against the intercellular adhesion structures.[4]

The different forms of pemphigus may be distinguished by the specificity of the autoantibodies for different targets or by the location of blister formation. With the most common form, pemphigus vulgaris (PV), blisters are located just above the basal skin layer. With pemphigus foliaceus (PF), blisters occur within the upper layers of the epidermis. Other subtypes of the pemphigus group are paraneoplastic pemphigus (usually occurring in patients with lymphoma) and drug-induced pemphigus. Rare pemphigus variants include pemphigus herpetiformis and pemphigus erythematosus.[4]

## INSTRUMENTS THAT HAVE BEEN USED TO STUDY QOL IN PEMPHIGUS

There are a wide variety of QOL measures. They may categorized as genetic, skin specific, or disease specific.[5]

Generic measures allow for comparisons across all diseases. The Medical Outcome Study 36-item Short-form Survey (SF-36) is a generic instrument that measures health-related QOL and is thus useful in comparing QOL in patients with pemphigus with the general population. It uses a multi-item scale that assesses 8 health concepts[6]: (1) limitations in physical activities because of health problems, (2) limitations in social activities because of physical or emotional problems, (3) limitations in usual role activities because of physical health problems, (4) bodily pain, (5) general mental health, (6) limitations in usual role activities because of emotional problems, (7) vitality, and (8) general health perceptions. A score of 0 to 100 is calculated for each domain, with higher scores correlating with better QOL.[5]

Skin-specific measures used in dermatology allow for comparisons across skin diseases. The Dermatology Life Quality Index (DLQI) was derived

Department of Dermatology, St George Hospital, University of New South Wales, Gray Street, Kogarah, Sydney, NSW 2217, Australia
* Corresponding author.
*E-mail address:* d.murrell@unsw.edu.au

Dermatol Clin 29 (2011) 521–525
doi:10.1016/j.det.2011.03.009

from patients with a variety of skin diseases and provides a simple method of scoring the impact of skin disease on QOL.[7] There are 10 questions covering symptoms and feelings (items 1 and 2), daily activities (items 3 and 4), leisure (items 5 and 6), work and school (item 7), personal relationships (items 8 and 9), and treatment (item 10). Each question has 4 possible responses: "not at all," "a little," "a lot," or "very much," with scores of 0, 1, 2, and 3 respectively. "Not relevant" is also scored as 0. The scores of each question are added to give a DLQI score, with a possible maximum of 30 and minimum of 0. A higher score indicates greater impairment of QOL. Healthy individuals have an average score of 0.5.[8]

The Skindex is another skin-specific measure. It was designed to assess the effect of symptoms and the burden on social function and emotional state.[1] The original Skindex consisted of 61 items but it has now been refined to questionnaires of 29, 17, and 16 items (Skindex-29, Skindex-17, and Skindex-16, respectively) to decrease respondent burden and improve discrimination and evaluation.[9] With dermatologic measures focusing specifically on skin-related issues, they are useful in instances such as comparing patients with different skin diseases, or detecting changes in the effects of skin disease on patients in clinical trials or longitudinal studies.

Psychiatric-related measures are also used in the study of QOL in pemphigus. Psychiatric morbidity is important among patients with skin diseases,[3] and the prevalence of depression among dermatologic patients is high at 25% to 40% compared with only 2% to 5% in the general population.[10] The 12-item General Health Questionnaire (GHQ-12) measures psychological distress and can help detect nonpsychotic disorders such as depression and anxiety. Each item has a 4-point scale with questions such as, "in the last weeks, did you feel under strain?." The higher the score, the greater the likelihood of a minor nonpsychotic psychiatric disorder. GHQ positivity is the cutoff score at which a minor psychiatric disorder such as depression or anxiety is likely.[11]

The Ministry of Health, Labor, and Welfare in Japan has its own burden of disease measure. This questionnaire asks about the ability to independently perform common activities of daily living (ADLs) including bathing, eating, cooking, shaving or applying make-up, using a toilet, traveling by public transportation, and driving.[12]

## PREVIOUS QOL STUDIES ON PEMPHIGUS

There have been only 5 published studies on QOL in pemphigus. One published in Japan by Masahiro and colleagues,[12] 1 in Germany by Mayrshofer and colleagues,[13] another in Morocco by Terrab and colleagues,[14] and 2 published by the same group in Rome by Paradisi and colleagues[11] and Tabolli and colleagues.[15]

Masahiro and colleagues[12] administered the Japanese Ministry of Health, Labor, and Welfare burden of disease measure to 380 patients with pemphigus. Patients with pemphigus retained good ADLs. Of the patients surveyed, 99.7% were able to feed themselves and use the toilet independently, 97% were able to shave or apply make-up by themselves, 96.5% were able to bathe, 90.8% were able to use public transportation, 85.2% could cook, and 82.3% could drive. However, pemphigus was found to have a large impact on finances. Fifty-four percent of patients reported an increased expenditure because of disease, 42% reported decreased income, and 41% described themselves as being in poverty because of factors such as costly medications and expensive transport to and from hospital. These figures were increased by approximately 20% in patients described as having severe pemphigus.

Mayrshofer and colleagues[13] studied 27 patients who attended dermatology clinics at the universities of Dresden, Erlangen, Kiel, Mannheim, Munich, and Wurzburg between January 1996 and October 2001. The patients had a primary diagnosis of PV and received the German DLQI. The average age of the patients was 55.9 years and 40% were men. The average DLQI score was 10 out of 30. Physical symptoms, such as itch, burning pain, and blistering were most responsible for impairment of QOL. Patients with itching had an average DLQI score of 11.5, compared with 7.9 for those without itching. Those with burning had an average score of 10.8, which was twice as high as patients who reported no burning sensations. Patients with blisters involving mucous membranes also had worse QOL, averaging 10.4, whereas those without had a score of 9.3.

Bullous pemphigoid (BP) and PV are similar in that they are both blistering autoimmune diseases. However, the DLQI score of 6.92 for BP is much less than that for PV, perhaps because of the rarity of mucosal membrane involvement in BP,[13] or because it responds to lower doses of drugs, which results in fewer side effects. For example BP typically needs no more than 0.5 mg/kg/day prednisone[16] whereas pemphigus usually needs at least 1 mg/kg/day starting dose and sometimes higher.[17] The study concludes that the DLQI may be useful as an additional measure of response to treatment in patients with pemphigus.[13]

However, QOL is a complex area affected by many factors, and the DLQI has some limitations in assessing pemphigus. The questionnaire was constructed using data from 120 patients and only 1 of these patients had blisters, whereas there were at least 10 cases of eczema, 14 cases of psoriasis, and 15 of acne. Thus, it is likely that the DLQI is more applicable for measuring QOL in patients with eczema, psoriasis, or acne than that of patients with pemphigus. In addition, the scoring reflects the bias of the question selection and it is possible that patients with pemphigus place emphasis on aspects of handicap not covered by the DLQI, or no emphasis on some of the questions mentioned in the DLQI.[8] The DLQI also asks only about the previous week, which may miss flares in chronic disease. The average PV DLQI score of 10 is higher than that for BP and rosacea, but lower than that for atopic eczema, which, with an average DLQI score of 12.5, rates most highly on this scoring system. The common, non–life threatening basal cell carcinoma (BCC) does not have much effect on QOL, with an average score of 2.[13]

Terrab and colleagues[14] conducted another study on patients with pemphigus in Morocco using the SF-36 as well as another questionnaire on the impact of pemphigus on self-perception, social relationships, and behavior. These questionnaires were given to 30 patients with pemphigus and 60 healthy adults between January and August 2002. To be included in the pemphigus group, patients had to have bullous dermatitis with fluid-filled bullae with intraepidermal division on a cutaneous biopsy, the presence of acantholytic cells, and immunoglobulin deposition in the epidermis under direct immunofluorescence. For every person with pemphigus, there were 2 controls of the same age and sex who were seeing a dermatologist for an acute, nonhandicapping problem such as warts or benign cutaneous tumors. Because of the high illiteracy rate in Morocco, the questionnaires were filled out by investigators, not patients (the survey was originally designed for either self-administration or administration by a trained interviewer in person or by telephone). To minimize bias, 1 investigator completed the questionnaires for all participants, whether they were literate or not.[6]

The SF-36 showed decreased mean scores for the pemphigus group compared with controls in all dimensions except for physical pain and alteration in general status of health. Most affected by pemphigus were physical and emotional statuses, particularly if there was facial involvement and large extent of lesions. Results also varied with profession. Seventy percent of affected patients

were ashamed of their appearance, and 60% of those were extremely worried about what others thought of their illness. Sixty percent had lost self-confidence and 82% were very concerned with repercussions on their sex life. Popular beliefs may have been a contributing factor, because skin illnesses in Morocco are believed to be contagious, associated with poor hygiene, or linked to unconventional sexual practices, and, when treatment is unfavorable, the disease is deemed incurable. Other factors found to further decrease QOL were repeated hospitalizations, difficult or costly management, and social concerns such as marriage prospects for young women.[14]

Because the SF-36 is a general health measure, it is likely to be less specific for pemphigus than the DLQI. It has been frequently criticized when used for documenting changes after medical intervention because it is a general health status survey that is not as responsive as a disease-specific survey. However, in the case of pemphigus, there are no disease-specific questionnaires and only generic ones are available. Another problem with the SF-36 is often seen in the subscales of (1) limitations in physical activities because of health problems, and (6) limitations in usual role activities because of emotional problems. Many patients score 0 for these scales before treatment (indicating a worst-case response), and 100 after treatment (indicating a lack of problems), limiting the ability to detect any further improvement because it is impossible to score more than 100.[18]

Tabolli and colleagues[15] also used the SF-36 to investigate 58 patients with either PV or PF. Two questionnaires from The Institute for Personality and Ability Testing were used to measure anxiety and depression. Similar to previous studies, Tabolli and colleagues found that mucocutaneous involvement, severe pemphigus as measured by physicians, and more recent onset correlated with worse health status as measured by the SF-36. Better health status was seen in men and patients with PF. Terrab and colleagues[14] and Tabolli and colleagues[15] concluded that the management of pemphigus must take into account its impact on various aspects of patients' lives.

A fourth study by Paradisi and colleagues[11] used a larger sample of 126 patients with pemphigus. Dermatologists scored patients' disease severity and patients were asked to complete the SF-36, the Skindex-29 and the GHQ-12. Participating in the study were 112 patients with PV (67 women, 45 men, mean age 52.2 years), 10 with PF (8 women, 2 men, mean age 55.1 years), 2 with paraneoplastic pemphigus and 2 with linear immunoglobulin A pemphigus. Both dermatology-specific (using the Skindex-29) and general health (using the SF-36) question-naires found a strong impact of pemphigus on QOL, with women being affected more than men. No difference was seen for age. Worse QOL was also found in those on less than 10 mg/d of steroids (compared with more than 10 mg/d), those with both mucous and cutaneous involve-ment, and those with 2 or more comorbidities (reflecting adverse effects of long-term treatment).

GHQ positivity was detected in 40% of patients with pemphigus, and 70% of patients with PF. These percentages are very high compared with the general population scores of 10%. GHQ posi-tivity correlated with clinical severity. The SF-36 also correlated strongly with clinical severity of PF. However, there was weaker correlation with PV. Paradisi and colleagues[11] suggest that psychological distress and personality disorders may play a role in disease development, mainte-nance, and progression, which in turn would affect QOL. They conclude that, to properly measure patients' health status, a generic and a derma-tology-specific QOL tool should be used, with a psychiatric-oriented questionnaire to help select patients who would benefit from psychological support in addition to their standard treatment.

There were several contrasts to the findings of Tabolli and colleagues. Paradisi and colleagues[11] found that there was poorer QOL for patients with PF than PV, there was no change in role activ-ities because of emotional problems (item 2 on the SF-36), and that QOL was most affected in patients who had had the disease for 3–4 years (not those with recent disease onset). The discrep-ancies between these studies further suggest the need for a disease-specific measure to accurately measure QOL in pemphigus. Although disease-specific measures cannot be used to compare with other groups of disease, they are most sensi-tive to changes in QOL. No disease-specific measures have yet been published for pemphigus.

## APPLICATION OF QOL QUESTIONNAIRES

There are many benefits in using QOL assess-ments. They may inform clinicians about the severity of the patient's illness as well as how treatments are affecting a patient's QOL (for example, adverse side effects). An understanding of QOL may also improve communication and shared decision making between the physician and patient.[19] A more satisfied patient in turn adheres to treatment better, maintains a more stable relationship with the physician, has relief from anxiety, and holds increased sense of personal control of events, all of which contribute to the recovery process.[3]

However, many health care professionals do not implement QOL assessments in their practice. This omission may be because they have limited resources, limited time, or do not have the appro-priate instruments. Many clinicians are less familiar with administering or interpreting QOL assess-ments than with other tests (such as imaging or physiologic tests), and sometimes view QOL as providing soft data as opposed to hard data that may be obtained in a laboratory. Many find that it is more difficult to incorporate QOL assessments with the elderly because of a higher rate of illit-eracy, lower completion rates, cognitive disorders, and comorbidities.[19]

For acceptability of QOL questionnaires, patients prefer questions with fewer answer options, and questions and answers in the form of words rather than numbers. Questionnaires that did not ask overly personal, sensitive, or irrel-evant questions were also favored.[19]

## SUMMARY

QOL assessments are not yet widely used in dermatology, although interest in the area is growing. Pemphigus is a disease that greatly affects QOL, as shown by measures such as the DLQI and SF-36. However, these questionnaires each have limitations. Developing a disease-specific measure for pemphigus would be of great benefit for both patients and their health practi-tioners, and this is something that our group has been working on since 2007.[20–23]

## ACKNOWLEDGMENTS

The authors would like to thank the independent learning program of the University of New South Wales for enabling Shien-Ning Chee to work on QOL in pemphigus with Dedee Murrell, John Frew for translating the German QOL study, James Drummond for translating the French study, and James McMillan, previously of Hokkaido University in Sapporo, for translating the Japanese study.

## REFERENCES

1. Abeni D, Picardi A, Pasquini P, et al. Further evidence of the validity and reliability of the Skindex-29: an Italian study on 2,242 dermatological outpatients. Dermatology 2002;204:43–9.

2. Maroti M, Ulff E, Wijma B. Quality of life before and 6 weeks after treatment in a dermatological outpa-tient treatment unit. J Eur Acad Dermatol Venereol 2006;20(9):1081–5.

3. Renzi C, Tabbolli S, Picardi A, et al. Effects of patient satisfaction with care on health-related quality of

life: a prospective study. J Eur Acad Dermatol Venereol 2005;19:712–8.

4. Hertl M. Autoimmune disease of the skin. 2nd edition. Wien (Austria): Springer-Verlag; 2005.

5. Bhosle M, Kulkarni A, Feldman S, et al. Quality of life in patients with psoriasis. Health Qual Life Outcome 2006;4(35):1–7.

6. Ware J, Sherbourne C. The MOS 36-item short-form health survey. Med Care 1992;30(6):473–83.

7. Finlay A. Quality of life measurement in dermatology: a practical guide. Br J Dermatol 1997;136(3):305–14.

8. Finlay A, Khan G. Dermatology Life Quality Index (DLQI) - a simple practical measure for routine clinical use. Clin Exp Dermatol 1994;19:210–6.

9. Nijsten T, Sampogna F, Chren M, et al. Testing and reducing Skindex-29 using Rasch analysis: Skindex-17. J Invest Dermatol 2006;126:1244–50.

10. Cohen A, Ofek-Schlomai A, Vardy D, et al. Depression in dermatological patients identified by the mini international neuropsychiatric interview questionnaire. J Am Acad Dermatol 2005;54(1):94–9.

11. Paradisi A, Sampogna F, Di Pietro C, et al. Quality-of-life assessment in patients with pemphigus using a minimum set of evaluation tools. J Am Acad Dermatol 2009;60(2):261–9.

12. Masahiro S, Shigaku I, Yutaka I, et al. An investigation of quality of life (QOL) of pemphigus patients in Japan (First report). Jpn J Dermatol 2000;110: 283–8.

13. Mayrshofer F, Hertl M, Sinkgraven R, et al. [Significant decrease in quality of life in patients with pemphigus vulgaris. Results from the German Bullous Skin Disease (BSD) Study Group]. J Dtsch Dermatol Ges 2005;3(6):431–5 [in German].

14. Terrab Z, Benchikhi H, Maaroufi A, et al. Qualite de vie et pemphigus [Quality of life and pemphigus]. Ann Dermatol Venereol 2005;132(4): 321–8 [in French].

15. Tabolli S, Mozzetta A, Antinone V, et al. The health impact of pemphigus vulgaris and pemphigus foliaceus assessed using the medical outcomes study 36-Item Short Form Health Survey Questionnaire. Br J Dermatol 2008;158(5):1029–34.

16. Kirtschig G, Middleton P, Bennett C, et al. Interventions for bullous pemphigoid. Cochrane Database of Systematic Reviews 2010;10:CD002292.

17. Martin LK, Agero AL, Werth V, et al. Interventions for pemphigus vulgaris and pemphigus foliaceus. Cochrane Database of Systematic Reviews 2009;1: CD006263.

18. Kiebzak G, Pierson L, Campbell M, et al. Use of the SF36 general health status survey to document health-related quality of life in patients with coronary artery disease: effect of disease and response to coronary artery bypass graft surgery. Heart Lung 2002;31(3):207–13.

19. Perry S, Kowalski T, Chang C. Quality of life assessment in women with breast cancer: benefits, acceptability and utilization. Health Qual Life Outcome 2007;5:24.

20. Chee S, Martin L, Murrell D. The development of a specific quality of life score for patients with pemphigus. Australas J Dermatol 2008;49(Suppl 1):A42.

21. Chee S, Martin L, Murrell D. The development of a quality of life instrument specific for pemphigus. J Invest Dermatol 2009;129:2908–23.

22. Sebaratnam D, Chee SN, Venugopal S, et al. Advances in the clinical assessment of autoimmune bullous disease: the development of a disease-specific quality of life instrument - the ABQOL. J Invest Dermatol 2009;129:2908–23.

23. Hanna A, Sebaratnam D, Chee S, et al. The development of a disease-specific quality of life instrument for autoimmune bullous diseases - the ABQOL [poster], in Medical Dermatology Society Meeting. Miami, March 5, 2010.

# Index

*Note:* Page numbers of article titles are in **boldface** type.

## A

ABSIS. See *Autoimmune Bullous Skin Disorder Intensity Score.*

Acantholysis
  and fogo selvagem, 416, 417

Acquired autoimmune bullous diseases
  diagnostic immunofluorescence for, 365–371

AIBD. See *Acquired autoimmune bullous diseases.*

Alopecia. See *Hair loss.*

Alternative complement cascade
  and epidermolysis bullosa acquisita, 497

Anagen shedding
  and hair loss patterns, 505

Anchoring fibrils
  and epidermolysis bullosa acquisita, 485, 489, 490

Animal models
  and bullous pemphigoid, 439–444
  of epidermolysis bullosa acquisita, 495, 497, 498
  of hair loss, 504, 505

Autoantibody-induced tissue damage
  and epidermolysis bullosa acquisita, 495–497, 499

Autoantigen
  and fogo selvagem, 416

Autoimmune bullous disorders
  nail involvement in, 511–513

Autoimmune Bullous Skin Disorder Intensity Score, 516–519

Autoimmune diseases
  and comorbidity, 397

Autoimmune response
  and fogo selvagem, 416

Autoimmunity
  and HLA class, 384
  and pemphigus vulgaris, 381–388

## B

Basement membrane autoimmune bullous disorders
  and hair loss, 507

Basement membrane zone
  and hair loss, 503

Basement membrane zone diseases
  patterns of immunofluorescent staining for, 370, 371

Beau lines
  and pemphigus vulgaris of the nail, 512

BMZ. See *Basement membrane zone.*

BP. See *Bullous pemphigoid.*

BP180
  and bullous pemphigoid, 427, 430, 432–434

BP230
  and bullous pemphigoid, 427, 430–433

Brunsting-Perry pemphigoid
  and epidermolysis bullosa acquisita, 487

Bullous autoimmune diseases
  and biopsy and blood sample, 365, 366
  diagnostic immunofluorescence for, 365–371
  and direct immunofluorescence, 366
  and indirect immunofluorescence, 366
  patterns of immunofluorescent staining for, 368–371
  and salt-split skin test, 366–368

Bullous invasion
  and fogo selvagem, 414

Bullous lupus erythematosus
  and hair loss, 507

Bullous pemphigoid
  and associated diseases, 428–430
  and BP180, 427, 430, 432–434
  and BP230, 427, 430–433
  and clinical criteria, 431, 432
  clinical features of, 428
  and collagen XVII, 439–441
  diagnosis of, 431–433
  diagnostic algorithm for, 431
  diagnostic enzyme-linked immunosorbent assay for, 432, 433
  diagnostic immunofluorescence for, 366–368, 370
  differential diagnosis for, 433, 434
  and direct immunofluorescence, 432
  in elderly patients, 428
  epidemiology of, 427, 428
  and hemidesmosomal target proteins, 427, 430–434
  histopathology of, 432
  and IgE antibodies against collagen XVII, 443, 444
  and immunoblot, 433
  and immunohistochemistry, 432
  and immunoprecipitation, 433
  and indirect immunofluorescence, 432
  major pathogenic antigen in, 439–441
  and mortality, 434
  and noncollagenous 16A domain, 439–442
  pathogenesis of, 439–444
  prognosis for, 434
  and target antigens, 430, 431
  and trigger factors, 428–430
  unusual clinical variants of, 428

Dermatol Clin 29 (2011) 527–533
doi:10.1016/S0733-8635(11)00086-6
0733-8635/11/$ – see front matter © 2011 Elsevier Inc. All rights reserved.

# Moving?

## Make sure your subscription moves with you!

To notify us of your new address, find your **Clinics Account Number** (located on your mailing label above your name), and contact customer service at:

**Email: journalscustomerservice-usa@elsevier.com**

**800-654-2452** (subscribers in the U.S. & Canada)
**314-447-8871** (subscribers outside of the U.S. & Canada)

**Fax number: 314-447-8029**

**Elsevier Health Sciences Division**
**Subscription Customer Service**
**3251 Riverport Lane**
**Maryland Heights, MO 63043**

*To ensure uninterrupted delivery of your subscription, please notify us at least 4 weeks in advance of move.

ELSEVIER